P9-CWD-564

RAMAMURTI'S
ORTHOPAEDICS
IN
PRIMARY CARE
Second Edition

RAMAMURTI'S
ORTHOPAEDICS
IN
PRIMARY CARE

Second Edition

EDITED BY

Gerald G. Steinberg, M.D.
Professor of Orthopaedics
Department of Orthopaedics
University of Massachusetts Medical Center
Worcester, Massachusetts

Carlton M. Akins, M.D.
Associate Professor of Orthopaedics
Department of Orthopaedics
University of Massachusetts Medical Center
Worcester, Massachusetts

Daniel T. Baran, M.D.
Professor of Orthopaedics
Department of Orthopaedics
University of Massachusetts Medical Center
Worcester, Massachusetts

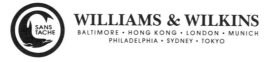

WILLIAMS & WILKINS
BALTIMORE • HONG KONG • LONDON • MUNICH
PHILADELPHIA • SYDNEY • TOKYO

ISBN 0-683-07928-X

90000

9 780683 079289

Editor: Michael Fisher
Associate Editor: Carol Eckhart
Copy Editor: Ann Donaldson
Designer: Norman W. Och
Illustration Planner: Wayne Hubble
Production Coordinator: Adèle Boyd-Lanham
Cover Designer: Norman Och

Copyright © 1992
Williams & Wilkins
428 East Preston Street
Baltimore, Maryland 21202, USA

All rights reserved. This book is protected by copyright. No part of this book may be reproduced in any form or by any means, including photocopying, or utilized by any information storage and retrieval system without written permission from the copyright owner.

Accurate indications, adverse reactions, and dosage schedules for drugs are provided in this book, but it is possible that they may change. The reader is urged to review the package information data of the manufacturers of the medications mentioned.

Printed in the United States of America

First Edition 1979

Library of Congress Cataloging-in-Publication Data

Ramamurti's orthopaedics in primary care / edited by Gerald G. Steinberg. — 2nd ed.
    p.   cm.
  Rev. ed. of: Orthopaedics in primary care / Chinni Pennathur Ramamurti. c1979.
  Includes bibliographical references and index.
  ISBN 0-683-07928-X
  1. Orthopedics. I. Ramamurti, Chinni Pennathur, 1922–   Orthopaedics in primary care. II. Steinberg, Gerald G.   III. Title: Orthopaedics in primary care,
  [DNLM: 1. Orthopedics. 2. Primary Health Care. WE 168 R1652]
RD731.R25 1992
617.3—dc20
DNLM/DLC
for Library of Congress   91-27870
                                        CIP

97 98 99 00
8 9 10

ACKNOWLEDGMENTS

The editors would like to gratefully acknowledge the following individuals for their committed work in the preparation of *Orthopaedics in Primary Care, Second Edition:*

The contributing authors for their expertise and devotion to the field of orthopaedics.

Elizabeth Chickering and Janet Walzer for their editorial assistance and manuscript coordination.

Joy D. Marlowe for her excellent line drawings, interpretation of the authors' descriptions, and finesse in accommodating the contributors' schedules.

Beth Maynard and Charlene Baron for their biomedical artwork, photography, and technical assistance.

Robbie Prendergast for her computer assistance and project management.

Rachel Goldfarb and Caroline Kuzia for their word-processing of the chapters.

CONTRIBUTORS

Carlton M. Akins, M.D.
Associate Professor of Orthopaedics, Department of Orthopaedics, University of Massachusetts Medical Center, Worcester, Massachusetts

Daniel T. Baran, M.D.
Professor of Orthopaedics and Medicine, Department of Orthopaedics and Medicine, University of Massachusetts Medical Center, Worcester, Massachusetts

Thomas F. Breen, M.D.
Assistant Professor of Orthopaedics, Department of Orthopaedics, University of Massachusetts Medical Center, Worcester, Massachusetts

Dudley A. Ferrari, M.D.
Assistant Professor of Orthopaedics, Department of Orthopaedics, University of Massachusetts Medical Center, Worcester, Massachusetts

Nelson M. Gantz, M.D., F.A.C.P.
Chairman of Medicine and Chief of Infectious Disease, Polyclinic Medical Center, Harrisburg, Pennsylvania

David F. Giansiracusa, M.D.
Associate Chairman, Department of Medicine, University of Massachusetts Medical Center, Worcester, Massachusetts

Thomas P. Goss, M.D.
Professor of Orthopaedics, Department of Orthopaedics, University of Massachusetts Medical Center, Worcester, Massachusetts

M. Timothy Hresko, M.D.
Assistant Professor of Orthopaedics, Department of Orthopaedics, University of Massachusetts Medical Center, Worcester, Massachusetts

Anna M. Korkis, M.D., P.A.
150 Franklin Ave., Ridgewood, N.J. 07450, 201-444-0009

Walter J. Leclair, M.D.
Assistant Professor of Orthopaedics, Department of Orthopaedics, University of Massachusetts Medical Center, Worcester, Massachusetts

John J. Monahan, M.D.
Professor of Orthopaedics, Department of Orthopaedics, University of Massachusetts Medical Center, Worcester, Massachusetts

William J. Morgan, M.D.
Assistant Professor of Orthopaedics, Department of Orthopaedics, University of Massachusetts Medical Center, Worcester, Massachusetts

Arthur M. Pappas, M.D.
Professor and Chairman of Orthopaedics, Professor of Pediatrics, Departments of Orthopaedics and Pediatrics, University of Massachusetts Medical Center, Worcester, Massachusetts

Yvonne A. Shelton, M.D.
Assistant Professor of Orthopaedics and Pediatrics, Departments of Orthopaedics and Pediatrics, University of Massachusetts Medical Center, Worcester, Massachusetts

Gerald G. Steinberg, M.D.
Professor of Orthopaedics, Department of Orthopaedics, University of Massachusetts Medical Center, Worcester, Massachusetts

Steven L. Strongwater, M.D.
Associate Professor, Department of Rheumatology, Internal Medicine, University of Massachusetts Medical Center, Worcester, Massachusetts

Thom H. Tarquinio, M.D.
Assistant Director of Orthopaedic Rehabilitation, St. Vincent Hospital, Worcester, Massachusetts

Anthony K. Teebagy, M.D.
Assistant Professor of Orthopaedics, Department of Orthopaedics, University of Massachusetts Medical Center, Worcester, Massachusetts

CONTENTS

PREFACE

Although the evaluation and treatment of musculoskeletal problems typically comprises nearly 25% of primary care practice, there are few texts of adequate scope and depth dedicated to this subject. This text is offered as an easily accessible reference for the primary care or emergency room practice dealing with musculoskeletal problems. This second edition of the original *Orthopaedics in Primary Care* maintains a generally regional chapter organization. Each of the regional chapters contains a review of the essential anatomy, pertinent physical examination, and discussion of the common nontraumatic and traumatic conditions of the region. Chapter 15 specifically deals with principles of pediatric problems, and Chapters 10, 11, and 16 deal with more general topics. Although the chapters have different authors, we have maintained consistent organization and presentation of the material.

Unlike the first edition, each of the chapters in the second edition have been contributed by authors with subspecialty expertise. Care has been taken, however, to keep the scope and depth of discussion appropriate for the primary care setting. The authors have made a special effort to make specific recommendations regarding the need for referral versus definitive treatment by the primary care provider. It is hoped that the information in this text will allow the interested primary care provider to proceed with definitive treatment or appropriate referral. To the extent that we meet that objective, we will meet our overriding goal: the improved care of the patients we all serve.

Gerald G. Steinberg, M.D.

FOREWORD

Approximately 25% of patients seen in the primary care office present with complaints related to the musculoskeletal system.

General knowledge of the musculoskeletal system is important for timely diagnosis and comprehensive treatment of patients, either by the primary care physician or in conjunction with an orthopaedist. This knowledge enhances patient care and keeps the primary care physician informed and involved.

The editors have kept this goal of improved patient care foremost in mind in this second edition of Ramamurti's *Orthopaedics in Primary Care.* Their expertise and commitment to the field of orthopaedics is reflected in the contents of this edition, which is thorough and covers a wide range of issues related to orthopaedics.

This text will benefit the readers of the first edition, as well as the primary care physician, nurse practitioner, physical assistant, and all health care professionals.

Arthur M. Pappas, M.D.

CHAPTER 1

Cervical Spine

John J. Monahan, M.D.

Essential Anatomy

FUNCTIONAL UNITS OF THE CERVICAL SPINE (FIG. 1.1)

A functional unit of the spine consists of any two adjacent vertebrae and their articulations with one another. The cervical spine (C-spine) contains eight functional units, five of which are alike and three of which (the first, second, and last) are unique.

The first functional unit is the articulation between the occiput and the first cervical vertebra (the atlantooccipital joint, Fig. 1.2).

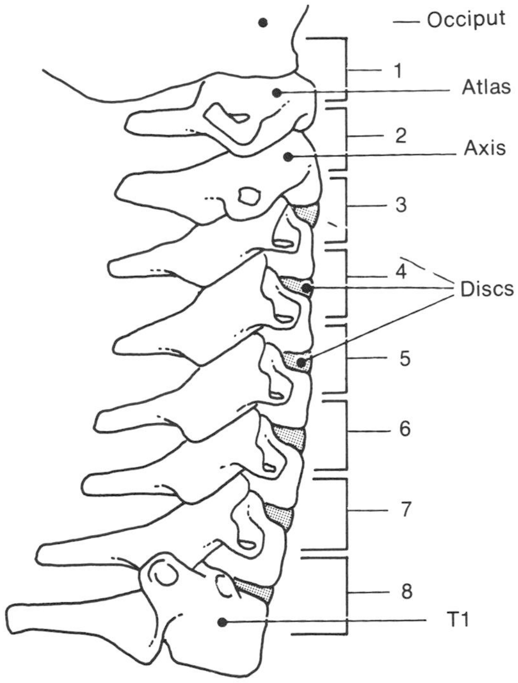
Occiput
1
Atlas
2
Axis
3
4
Discs
5
6
7
8
T1

Figure 1.1. The eight functional units.

This unit is controlled partially by short, deep muscles anteriorly and posteriorly that extend only the width of the segment. Its movement allows for about one-third of full flexion and extension and for about 50% of lateral bending of the head and neck.

The second functional unit is the articulation between the first and second cervical vertebrae (the atlantoaxial joint, Fig. 1.3). It too is controlled partially by short, deep muscles anteriorly and posteriorly that extend across only the second unit and the first two units. The movement of the second unit allows for 50% of the rotational range of motion of the head and neck.

Weight is borne across each of the first two units of the spine on the broad surfaces of the facet joints.

The next five functional units are the articulations between the second through the seventh cervical vertebrae (Fig. 1.4). These units are controlled by long and short deep muscles anteriorly and posteriorly, the scalenus muscles at middle depth, and the sternocleidomastoid and trapezius muscles superficially. Their movement allows for about two-thirds of full flexion and extension, about 50% of rotation, and about 50% of lateral bending. In contrast to the first two units, these five units bear weight on three broad surfaces, the two facets and the vertebral bodies. The facet articulations are synovial joints, and the body articulations are fibrocartilaginous joints (the intervertebral discs). The facet articulations are in the same plane as the intervertebral disc. The postero-

(AP)   (LAT)

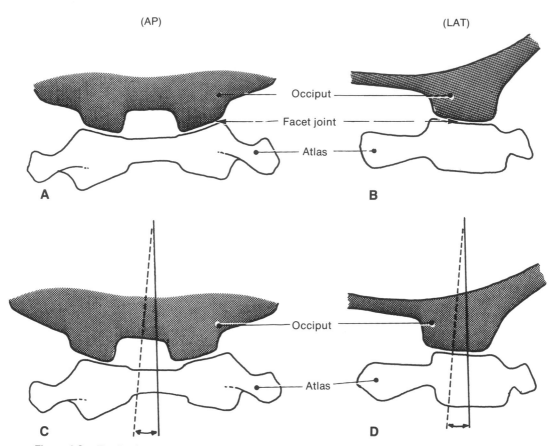

Figure 1.2.   The first functional unit: the atlantooccipital joint. *A* and *B*, neutral. *C*, lateral bending. *D*, nodding.

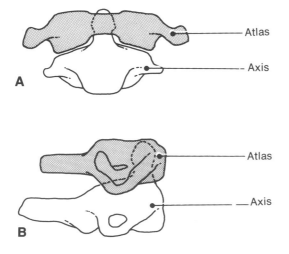

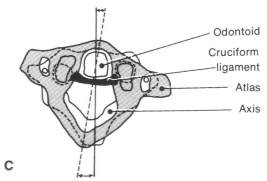

Figure 1.3.   The second functional unit: the atlantoaxial joint. *A*, anteroposterior, neutral. *B*, lateral. *C*, superior, rotated.

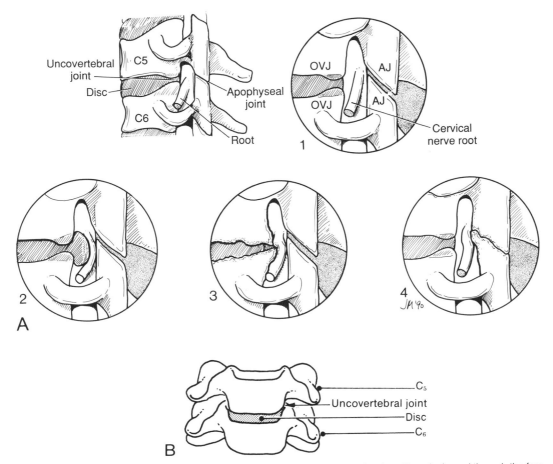

Figure 1.4. *A*, normal and abnormal relationships of a cervical nerve root passing from the spinal canal through the foramen. *1*, normal. *2*, disc protrusion. *3*, oncovertebral osteophyte. *4*, apophyseal osteophyte. *B*, the five similar functional units: articulations between the second and seventh cervical vertebrae.

lateral margins of the bodies project slightly beyond the disc to form a synovial joint, the uncovertebral joints, across each functional unit. The uncovertebral joints are vulnerable to wear and tear and frequently develop degenerative osteophytes.

The cervical nerve roots exit through the foramen formed by the uncovertebral joint anteriorly and the facet joint posteriorly. Thus, the roots are vulnerable to acute impingement during subluxation of any of the units, and to compression caused by posterolateral herniation of disc material or protrusion of bony spurs from the uncovertebral and facet joints (Fig. 1.2). The movements of the cervical spine allow for the most severe injuries and greatest wear and tear across the units between C-4 and C-7. The nerve roots passing through the intervertebral foramina of these units are, respectively, the fifth, sixth, and seventh.

The last functional unit is the articulation between C-7 and T-1 (Fig. 1.5). The C-7 vertebra is unique in two respects: its upward-directed facets are cervical-like and its downward-directed facets thoracic-like, and its body is nearly of thoracic dimension. (The body of each lower cervical vertebra from C-3 to C-7 is slightly larger than its superior neighbor.) These unique characteristics

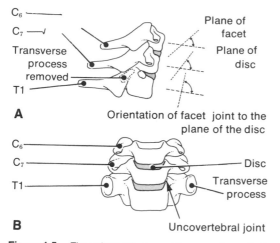

Figure 1.5.   The unique structure of the seventh cervical vertebra.

make the last functional unit of the cervical spine like a thoracic unit, in that the larger vertebral bodies of C-7 and T-1 bear the bulk of the weight across the unit and the facet articulations are nearly at right angles to the intervertebral disc. These near-perpendicular articular surfaces allow the unit limited movement in flexion, extension, and rotation. Severe injury or wear and tear across this unit is unusual.

SOFT TISSUES OF THE CERVICAL SPINE

The soft tissues of the cervical spine include the deep fascia, many layers of muscle, the thick ligaments, the synovia of the facet joints, and the intervertebral disc.

Deep Fascia (Fig. 1.6)

The deep fascia consists of three layers of dense connective tissue that separate the neck into compartments. The superficial layer lies beneath the platysma and surrounds all of the deeper structures of the neck. It splits to invest the sternocleidomastoid and strap muscles anteriorly, and the trapezius posteriorly. The prevertebral layer surrounds the cervical spine and the deep muscles that cling to the spine anteriorly and posteriorly. The pretracheal layer surrounds

the trachea, esophagus, thyroid, and parathyroid. All three layers fuse to form the carotid sheath which surrounds the carotid artery, the internal jugular vein, and the vagus nerve.

Muscles (Fig. 1.7)

The muscles of the neck accessible to physical examination anteriorly are the accessory muscles of the pharynx and larynx, which in aggregate are often called the strap muscles, and the sternocleidomastoid muscle. The muscles accessible posteriorly and laterally are the trapezius and parts of the splenius capitis and cervicis, the levator scapulae, and the scalene muscles. The diagnosis of muscular injury depends on the discovery of tenderness in these muscles. While deeper muscles that surround and lie on the cervical spine are affected in painful processes, the effect cannot be isolated by physical examination.

Ligaments (Fig. 1.8)

The ligamentum nuchae is the most superficial of ligaments. It represents a thin extension of the supraspinous and interspinous ligaments outward between the trapezius muscles. While the supraspinous and interspinous ligaments are distinct entities in the dorsal and lumbar spine, in the neck they merge and lose their identities in the ligamentum nuchae. With the neck in full flexion, the ligamentum nuchae can be palpated distinctly as it extends from the spine of the seventh cervical vertebra to the prominence of the occiput. This is the only ligament that can be distinguished as such by palpation. The capsular ligaments of the facet joints surround each facet joint, extending between the margins of the two articular surfaces. Palpation through the scalene and splenius muscles allows the examiner to detect the facet column. The joints as such cannot be distinguished by palpation, and tenderness of the ligaments cannot be distinguished from tenderness of

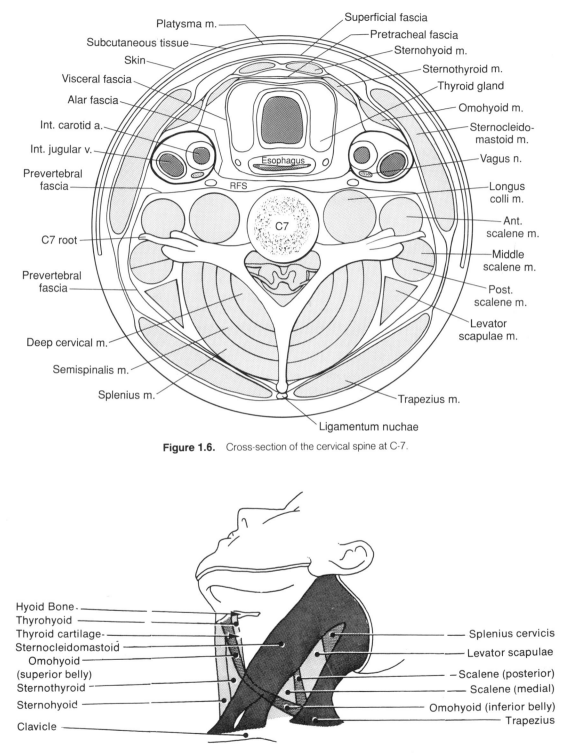

Figure 1.6. Cross-section of the cervical spine at C-7.

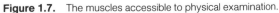

Figure 1.7. The muscles accessible to physical examination.

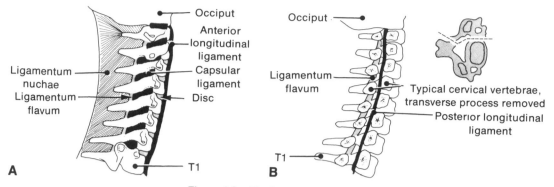

Figure 1.8.   The ligaments of the neck.

the overlying muscles. Localized tenderness does, however, indicate potential pathology, superficial or deep.

The posterior longitudinal ligament passes the length of the spinal column, lying against the posterior walls of the vertebral bodies and discs. The anterior longitudinal ligament passes the length of the spinal column, lying against the anterior walls of the vertebral bodies and discs. The ligamenta flava are a series of short ligaments that pass between the lamina of the posterior arches of each functional unit along the length of the spine.

All of these ligaments are pain-sensitive.

Synovia of the Facet Joints (Fig. 1.8)

A synovial membrane lies beneath the capsular ligaments and invests and lubricates the articulations of the facets. It may be stretched along with the capsule when the facet joints are subluxated, and it has been postulated that it may be pinched between facet surfaces when they move on one another in slight malalignment. As may be true of all synovial joints, local degenerative and various "systemic" events may provoke an inflammation within the synovium. All of these processes result in a painful synovitis.

Intervertebral Disc (Fig. 1.8)

The disc consists of two parts, a springy outer ring of interwoven fibrocartilaginous bands called the anulus, and a "hydroelas-

tic," gelatinous inner core called the nucleus pulposus. Young discs are thick, malleable, and elastic, while old discs are thin, rigid, and brittle. Thus, greater forces are required to injure young discs than old ones. The forces that injure discs may injure the anterior and/or posterior longitudinal ligaments as well. Disc material displaced against the posterior longitudinal ligament may also protrude far enough to compress the adjacent nerve root, producing radicular pain and dysfunction. The disc anulus also contains pain-sensitive nerve endings. Therefore, the pain directly attributable to a disc injury is the pain from the disc, injured nerve root (radiculopathy), injured spinal cord (myelopathy), and/or injured anterior or posterior longitudinal ligament.

Evaluation of the Patient with Neck Symptoms
HISTORY

Since the neck is a complex structure made up of multiple organ systems, a meticulous history is necessary to define the specific system or systems involved. The pathologic process may be local or referred from the upper abdomen, thorax, upper extremities, scalp, temporomandibular joint, or teeth. The clinical characteristics include pain, abnormal posture or range of motion, and neurologic or vascular dysfunction. The history of the present illness should include the how, what, when, and where of onset of symptoms; details of possible congenital, infectious, inflammatory, traumatic, endocrine, metabolic, or tumor processes; description of pain pattern; description of any deformity; and description of muscle weakness and/or associated disturbance of sensory function or bowel and bladder sphincter control.

PHYSICAL EXAMINATION

The techniques and emphasis of the physical examination of the neck vary with the etiology of neck symptoms: nontraumatic or traumatic.

Inspection

The patient with a traumatic C-spine injury should have been immobilized in a neck brace at the scene of the injury. In addition, the patient should be attached to a spine board. The neck should be in the neutral or the least deformed position possible without using undue force or causing pain. Inspection of the patient with a suspected spinal injury must be carried out in the brace with the patient's neck in a neutral or near-neutral position. The primary care physician should look for obvious swelling, asymmetry, discoloration, tracheal deviation, respiratory distress, or malalignment of the cervical spine. The patient's neck should not be moved until fracture, dislocation, or unstable ligament injury have been ruled out. The patient with complete cord injury is usually able to identify pain at the site of injury, but the observer notes anesthesia below this level. The sensory loss may mask visceral injuries involving the chest or the abdominal cavity. Suspicion of injury above C-5 should trigger concern for possible respiratory compromise (the diaphragm is innervated by C-3 through C-5).

In the nontraumatic case, the patient is inspected as he or she walks into the examining room and undresses to the waist. The examiner notes abnormal posture or motion

(splinting or guarding) and diminished range of motion. Local or diffuse swelling, rashes, discoloration, or scars of the neck and upper extremities are observed. The chest, upper abdomen, scalp, temporomandibular joint, and teeth may need to be inspected.

Palpation

In both traumatic and nontraumatic cases, palpation may reveal areas of tenderness, swelling, induration, asymmetry, or malalignment in the bony and soft tissues of the neck. Anterior bony landmarks include the hyoid bone at the C-3 level, thyroid cartilage at the C-4/C-5 level, and first cricoid ring at the C-6 level. Posteriorly, the occiput, inion, superior nuchal line, mastoid process, spinous processes, and apophyseal joints are examined. The examination of the anterior soft tissues includes the sternocleidomastoid muscles, strap muscles, scalenus muscles, lymph nodes, thyroid gland, carotid pulses, and supraclavicular fossa (e.g., clavicle fractures, cervical ribs, or superior sulcus tumors). Posteriorly, the trapezius and paraspinous muscles, lymph nodes, greater occipital nerve, and superior nuchal ligament (which extends from the occiput to the C-7 spinous process) are examined.

In traumatic cases, active or passive range of motion should not be tested until appropriate radiographic studies rule out fracture or dislocation.

Range of Motion

The range of motion of the C-spine is age-dependent, i.e., tends to diminish with aging. The normal painless range of motion of the C-spine in a young adult is approximately 45° of flexion (the patient is able to touch chin to chest), approximately 45° to 60° of extension, and approximately 80° of rotation (the patient is able to rotate the head from side to side so that the chin is almost in line with the shoulder). Lateral bending, in which the patient tries to touch the ear to the shoulder, should be approximately 45° toward each shoulder.

NEUROLOGIC EXAMINATION
Neurologic Anatomy

There are eight cervical nerves. The individual spinal cord segments correspond to the vertebral segments. One through seven exit on top of their respective vertebrae; the eighth exits between C-7 and T-1. T-1 exits below the T-1 vertebra. The brachial plexus is composed of nerves emanating from C-5 to T-1. As the individual roots travel from the spine to the upper extremity, they form specific trunks, divisions, cords, and peripheral nerves at specific anatomic levels. Impingement of these specific structures produces characteristic signs and symptoms.

Sensory Distribution

From C-2 to T-1, each root supplies sensation to a portion of the extremity in a succession of dermatomes around the extremity. These dermatomal distributions are variable, but the following autonomous zones for each root are useful, though approximate, clinical indices. C-2 supplies the area 2 inches below the tip of the ear, C-3 the base of the neck, C-4 the top of the shoulder, C-5 the lateral arm at the shoulder, C-6 the lateral aspect of the forearm and tip of the thumb, C-7 the tip of the middle finger, C-8 the medial border of the hand, and T-1 the medial aspect of the lower arm.

Motor Distribution and Deep Tendon Reflexes

Roots C-3/C-5 via the phrenic nerve innervate the diaphragm; respiratory paralysis may be present and assisted ventilation necessary with injuries proximal to C-4. C-5 innervates the deltoid and biceps muscles, and is responsible for the biceps deep tendon reflex. C-6 supplies the wrist extensors (extensor carpi radialis longus and brevis) and abductor and extensors of the thumb, and is responsible for the brachioradialis reflex. C-7 innervates the triceps, wrist flexors, and finger extensors, and controls the triceps reflex. C-8 supplies innervation to the finger flexors, and has no deep tendon reflex. T-1 innervates the intrinsic muscles of the hand, which include the dorsal interossei and the abductor digiti quinti. There is no definable reflex.

The examiner should also test the function of the intrinsic neck muscles in flexion, extension, lateral rotation, and lateral bending. The primary flexor is the sternocleidomastoid, innervated by the spinal accessory or 11th cranial nerve. Secondary flexors are the scalenus and paravertebral muscles. Primary extensors are the splenius, semispinalis, capitis (paravertebral extensor mass), and trapezius, innervated by the spinal accessory or 11th cranial nerve. The sternocleidomastoid muscle is responsible for lateral rotation. Primary muscles acting in lateral bending are the scalenus anticus, medius, and posticus, innervated by the anterior primary divisions of the lower cervical nerves.

Special Tests

Distraction Test.   The distraction test is performed by cupping the patient's chin and occiput and gently lifting the head. Distraction opens up the foramen, intervertebral space, and apophyseal and uncovertebral joints. This relieves pressure on the nerve root exiting through the foramen and sensitive para-articular tissues, protruding discs, inflamed synovia, or degenerative osteophytes of the adjacent synovial joints. A positive test (i.e., pain relief) indicates a potential source of pathology within the vertebral complex.

Compression Test.   The compression test is the opposite of the distraction test. It is performed by gently pushing directly down on the patient's head. The axial loading precipitates or aggravates the pain when the foramen and its contained nerve root, intervertebral space, and degenerated synovial joints are compressed.

Valsalva Test. The patient bears down as if moving the bowels. The examiner notes aggravation of pain as the intrathecal pressure increases. Space-occupying lesions in the cervical canal, such as herniated discs or tumors, cause local and/or radicular pain corresponding to the level of C-spine pathology.

Swallowing Test. Dysphagia or pain on swallowing may be caused by cervical spine pathology, such as bony protuberances, osteophytes, or soft tissue swelling.

Adson's Test. (See section on "Thoracic Outlet Syndrome.") The test is used to determine compression of the brachial plexus and/or subclavian artery.

RADIOLOGIC EXAMINATION
Diagnostic Studies

In trauma cases, a lateral cervical spine x-ray should be taken early in the course of the examination, usually during the primary survey immediately after the life-threatening problems are identified and controlled. The lateral x-ray should be taken with the neck in neutral in a nonradiopaque cervical brace. All seven cervical vertebrae must be identified. If C-7 and T-1 cannot be seen, the attending physician should pull the patient's shoulders down gently while the x-ray is being taken. If C-7 and T-1 cannot be seen in the routine lateral view, a lateral swimmer's view, which is a slightly oblique lateral view of the cervical spine, is obtained. This allows the physician to assess spinal injuries and determine the need for further spine x-rays. Once the patient is stable, the full C-spine x-ray series is completed, including anteroposterior (AP), oblique cervical, and open-mouth odontoid views. Tomography and/or computed tomography (CT) may be necessary to make a radiologic diagnosis. After studies have ruled out fracture or dislocation, stress films should be taken if stability of the C-spine is in question. The study should be performed with caution and supervised by the physician. It includes two lateral x-rays of the cervical spine with the neck moved actively with guidance into the maximum flexed and maximum extended positions within the limits of pain.

X-ray Review

In trauma cases, x-rays should be examined for the alignment of the vertebral bodies and any displacement of bone fragments into the spinal canal. The segments of the vertebral complex involved in the fractures (Fig. 1.9) should be identified. For the evaluation of stability, the spine may be divided into three segments. The first segment in-

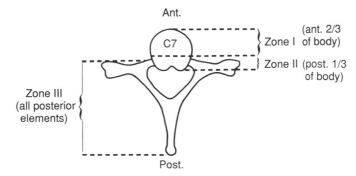

Figure 1.9.   Structural segments of a cervical vertebra. Fractures involving more than one segment are usually unstable.

cludes the anterior longitudinal ligament and anterior two-thirds of the vertebral body; the second segment is composed of the posterior third of the vertebral body including the posterior longitudinal ligament; and the third segment is composed of the posterior elements (facet joints, neural arch and processes) of the vertebral complex (Fig. 1.9). If a fracture or ligamentous disruption involves two or more of the three segments of the vertebral complex, the injury is considered unstable. When assessing the lateral spine, the distance between the pharynx and the anterior-inferior border of C-3 is measured. The prevertebral soft tissue thickness at this level should be less than or equal to 5 mm. Increase in this area of density suggests a vertebral fracture because it could represent a hematoma secondary to the fracture. Any angulation of two adjacent vertebrae greater than 11° more than the angulation between each of those vertebrae and their adjacent vertebrae indicates instability of the cervical spine. Any translation of one vertebra upon another, either anterior, posterior, lateral, or combinations thereof, greater than 3.5 mm also indicates instability. Any evidence of instability requires orthopaedic and/or neurosurgical referral. While waiting for the consultant, the cervical spine should continue to be immobilized.

In nontraumatic cases of neck pain, routine C-spine x-rays are also taken, i.e., AP, lateral, both obliques, and odontoid views. In addition to the interpretive criteria described for traumatic cases, evidence of destruction (lytic lesion) or increased bone production (blastic lesion) are sought, as well as narrowing or hypertrophic changes of the disc or apophyseal joints, calcific deposition within the disc space, and associated soft tissue changes. Additional studies such as tomography, CT scan, magnetic resonance imaging (MRI), and bone scan are often indicated for further evaluation, but this is usually a decision made after orthopaedic referral.

Nontraumatic Conditions of Childhood

CONGENITAL MUSCULAR TORTICOLLIS

Congenital muscular torticollis is a contracture of one of the sternocleidomastoid muscles, more commonly seen on the right side. The cause of this deformity is unknown, but a traumatic etiology has been postulated. The deformity is characterized by a "cock robin" position of the head in which the head is tilted toward the side of the shortened muscle and the chin rotated to the contralateral side. On a pathologic section of excised specimens, the muscle appears to be replaced by fibrous tissue.

Clinical Characteristics

At birth, the child may be normal or present with the characteristic torticollis. In children who are normal at birth, the deformity and mass in the sternocleidomastoid usually becomes obvious at 2 to 3 weeks. As the child grows, the abnormal posture progresses and there are secondary structural changes in the face and skull resulting in asymmetric molding of these structures. Palpation reveals a firm, nontender, fusiform mass within the substance of or replacing the sternocleidomastoid muscle. When present at birth, it commonly enlarges over the subsequent several weeks. Regression of the "tumor" usually occurs over a period of 2 to 6 months.

Without treatment, facial asymmetry, including changes in the levels of the ears and eyes, may develop. The superficial and deep muscular tissue of the neck may become shortened.

Because there is an increased incidence of clubfeet, congenital hip dysplasia, and other congenital abnormalities in patients with torticollis, these infants should be carefully examined. There is a significant history of difficult delivery in patients with torticollis, and infants with such a history should be carefully checked for this deformity. Infants with congenital torticollis do not have any neurologic abnormality. While there may be pain with passive stretching, there is no pain at rest.

X-ray studies are usually unremarkable in the muscular type of torticollis. They should be carried out since there are congenital bony deformities of the C-spine (Klippel-Feil syndrome and primary cervical synostosis) that should be ruled out. Differential diagnosis should also include traumatic conditions, such as fracture or rotatory subluxation, inflammation of the cervical lymph nodes, and tumors of the spinal cord or brain.

Treatment

Early recognition and treatment are indicated. Stretching of the involved sternocleidomastoid muscle should be performed several times a day. A good stretching program is usually successful. The physician or an experienced physical therapist should instruct the parents in the technique of stretching. One hand is utilized to stabilize the chest and shoulders while the other hand tilts the head away from the contracted muscle and rotates the chin toward the contracted side. Each stretching maneuver is best held to a count of 10 with 15 repetitions. The initial tenderness of the muscle mass with stretching subsides gradually and a great majority of infants respond to these conservative measures.

If the deformity does not respond to passive stretching in 1 to 2 months, orthopaedic referral is indicated. If a child is over 1 year of age at initial presentation, the contracture and progressive deformity are probably best treated by surgical release of the sternocleidomastoid muscle.

KLIPPEL-FEIL SYNDROME

Klippel-Feil syndrome is a congenital fusion of two or more cervical vertebrae. Clinically, the neck is short, stiff, and webbed. The hairline is horizontal. This syndrome is often associated with torticollis. These patients should be referred for orthopaedic evaluation.

Nontraumatic Conditions in Adulthood
DEGENERATIVE DISEASE

As in the thoracic and lumbosacral spine, a theoretical scheme of spinal degeneration provides a good perspective for the primary care physician in evaluating patients with degenerative conditions of the cervical spine. This theory proposes that facet joint synovitis, hypermobility, and progressive degeneration are "natural" consequences of aging and the repetitive trauma of "normal" activity. The facet joint changes occur along with degenerative changes in the intervertebral disc, which begin with marginal tears of the anulus and progress to radial tears and disc herniation. Subluxation of the facet joints with enlargement of the articular processes occur in parallel with disc resorption and spinal osteophyte formation. In the cervical spine, the uncovertebral joints may be severely involved in this process. In the early phases of this degenerative process, patients may be identified as having "facet joint syndrome" or after relatively minor trauma, the patient may develop an "acute disc herniation." It is important to recognize that the facet joint and the discs are each one part of the motion segment and it is unlikely that there is isolated trauma or inflammation in one part of the spinal unit without associated abnormalities in the complementary parts.

Acute Disc Herniation

Acute disc herniation in the cervical spine is less common than in the lumbar region. The syndrome may be triggered by an acute injury to the disc with or without underlying degenerative changes. It may also present with little or no remembered trauma and is frequently associated with degenerative changes of the intervertebral disc. With herniation of the disc, there may be irritation of an associated nerve root or other nerve endings in the disc complex, i.e., anulus fibrosus or posterior longitudinal ligament. A disc herniation, consequently, may cause true radicular pain or nonradicular referred pain felt in the upper extremity. In true radicular pain, the signs and symptoms vary with the level of nerve root irritation.

Clinical Characteristics. C-4/C-5 (fifth root) causes neck, shoulder, and lateral arm pain and motor weakness of the deltoid and biceps. Sensation is diminished over the lateral upper arm with an autonomous zone over the lateral deltoid. The biceps reflex may be diminished.

C-5/C-6 (sixth root) causes pain in the neck with variable radiation into the occiput and/or interscapular area, posterolateral aspect of the shoulder, lateral aspect of the upper arm and forearm, and the thumb and index finger. Sensory dysfunction in the lateral forearm, thumb, and index finger may be noted. There may be weakness of the biceps, long abductor and extensor of the thumb, and wrist extensors. The brachioradialis reflex is usually diminished.

C-6/C-7 (seventh root) causes neck pain with variable radiation into the occiput and shoulder or interscapular region, lateral aspect of the upper arm and forearm, and occasionally the volar aspect of forearm, ulnar aspect of the hand, and fourth and fifth fingers. Sensory loss involves the fourth and fifth fingers. Muscle weakness is evident in the triceps, wrist flexors, and finger extensors. The triceps reflex is usually diminished.

C-7/T-1 (eighth root) causes neck pain with variable radiation into the occiput, interscapular region, medial aspect of the upper arm, and forearm. Motor weakness involves the deep and superficial finger flexors. Sensory dysfunction occurs along the C-8 dermatome on the ulnar aspect of the distal forearm and hand.

T-1/T-2 (T-1 root) pain involves the neck, with variable referral to the occiput and interscapular region. Usually, pain is felt in the medial aspect of the arm. Sensory deficits are noted in the medial side of the proximal half of the forearm and distal half of the upper arm. Motor weakness involves the finger abductors. No deep tendon reflex is associated with the T-1 root.

Pain from an acute disc herniation is usually aggravated by coughing, sneezing, straining, and activities involving prolonged abnormal positioning, especially fixed flexion or extension with rotation. Lifting, pushing, and pulling may trigger pain. There is tenderness to palpation over the posterior elements of the spinous process of the involved root or over the facet joints. Gentle manual traction tends to relieve pain, while compression of the spine increases pain. Further physical findings include pain on active or passive motion of the C-spine with an overall diminished range of motion. There may be abnormal posture of the C-spine with flattening of lordosis or development of torticollis. The pain is relieved somewhat by bringing the patient's ipsilateral hand up behind the neck. Pain is aggravated by hyperextension and rotation of the neck to the involved side. There is usually associated muscle spasm of the paravertebral muscles, and occasionally the more anterior muscle groups. There may be trigger points in the interscapular region.

X-ray studies may be normal, or may reveal degenerative changes or disc space narrowing. If there is no response to initial conservative treatment, orthopaedic referral is indicated. CT scan, MRI studies, myelogram, or bone scan may be indicated to further evaluate the patient. Electromyography (EMG) and nerve conduction studies are useful in delineating a specific radiculopathy.

Treatment. Conservative treatment is recommended for acute disc herniation. The keystone is rest. Rest may be defined as limiting the patient's activities of daily living to a point where he or she is comfortable. If the patient is having severe pain, especially when associated with neurologic dysfunction, strict bed rest is indicated (bathroom privileges are allowed). A position of comfort, utilizing soft (not foam rubber) pillows, elevation of the head of the bed, and a soft cervical collar (Fig. 1.10) when necessary, is recommended. Bed rest is continued with the neck protected in a cervical collar until the patient can sit, stand, and walk comfortably in the collar. At this point, ambulatory activity is allowed as tolerated. The period of bed rest is usually 2 to 10 days. While on bed rest, the patient may maintain muscle tone in the trunk and lower extremities by an isometric exercise regimen.

If the signs and symptoms are moderate, relative rest is indicated utilizing a firm or soft cervical collar to provide comfort and support to the cervical spine. Limited activities are permitted as tolerated, using pain as the limiting factor.

The rest regimen may be supplemented by intermittent cervical traction, unless this makes the patient more uncomfortable. Careful positioning for traction is essential (Fig. 1.11). Traction should begin with the neck in a comfortable position, usually slight flexion. The neck should be well supported, with the halter applying a distractive force

posteriorly below the occiput. Traction for 20 minutes 4 times a day should begin with light weight, i.e., 5 to 7 pounds with the patient supine in bed, or 10 to 12 pounds with the patient sitting. Weight should be increased gradually as tolerated for as long as the traction affords relief, up to a maximum of 10 to 15 pounds with the patient supine in bed, or 20 to 25 pounds with the patient sitting. Before traction, moist heat should be applied to the neck for 15 to 20 minutes, with gentle massage of the area as tolerated.

Medications may include nonsteroidal anti-inflammatory drugs, muscle relaxants, and analgesics.

If the patient does not respond to these conservative measures within 2 to 3 weeks, additional studies as well as orthopaedic or neurosurgical consultation are indicated. If the patient demonstrates progressive weakness, sensory loss, or loss of bowel or bladder control at any point in the program, immediate consultations should be obtained.

If the patient has improved on the conservative program (i.e., the patient is comfortable under rest conditions and range of motion and motor strength of the neck are improving without precipitating pain), rehabilitative measures are indicated. These measures involve a physical therapy pro-

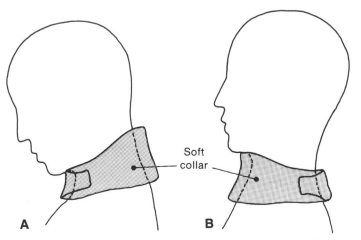

Figure 1.10. Applications of the soft collar. *A,* flexion. *B,* extension.

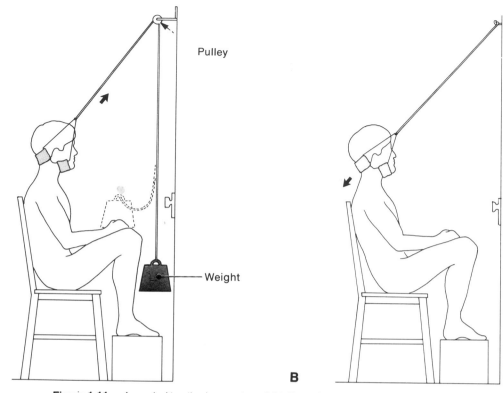

Figure 1.11. *A*, cervical traction by counterweight. *B*, cervical traction by body weight.

gram to gain full functional range of motion and strength of the C-spine and the affected extremity. The program begins with active range of motion exercises and isometric exercises and progresses to isotonic exercises of the neck and involved upper extremity, while maintaining a mobilizing and strengthening program for the trunk and lower extremities. During the rehabilitation period, patients should be encouraged to perform activities of daily living as tolerated to lessen the overall period of disability and hasten full recovery.

Rehabilitation also involves weaning the patient from the restrictions imposed during the acute phase. The patient should be weaned from bed rest by initiating progressive periods of ambulation over the day. Initially, the neck is protected by a cervical collar. The three or four periods out of bed each day are gradually lengthened. The patient is taught to avoid pain, or better, to recognize the warnings that precede pain (e.g., fatigue, dull burning ache) and indicate that the patient is proceeding too quickly.

The cervical collar is gradually discontinued. The progressive isometric and isotonic exercises are continued 3 to 5 times a day for 5 to 7 minutes each session, while the periods out of the collar are gradually extended in 20- to 30-minute increments, beginning with 15 to 20 minutes every 2 to 3 hours. Pain should be avoided while reducing time in the collar.

The author suggests that the weaning process be carefully monitored over 2 to 3 weeks to avoid prolonged immobilization and its attendant chronic pain syndrome with persistent pain, muscle atrophy, stiffness, depression, and disability.

The patient should be guided back to full activity when he or she is out of the collar and comfortable with the physical therapy program. A general aerobic exercise program should be prescribed. Walking is excellent. Swimming is equally beneficial, but occasionally causes recurrent pain and spasm with specific strokes that stress the neck improperly.

The patient should avoid lifting, pushing, pulling, or using the hands above shoulder level. Malpositioning should be discouraged, i.e., prolonged neck flexion while typing or the extension/rotation that occurs when falling asleep while sitting with the head unsupported. An early return to rigorous sports is discouraged, and contact sports are contraindicated. Most patients can return to sedentary occupations in 2 to 4 weeks, while manual laborers may require a waiting period of 6 to 8 weeks or longer.

Chronic Degenerative Disease of the Cervical Spine, Cervical Spondylosis, Osteoarthritis

The constellation of symptoms grouped under these diagnostic categories occur in an older population, usually over age 45. The underlying pathology of the intervertebral disc, facet and uncovertebral joints, and ligaments has been described. While these conditions are often more benign in their clinical presentation than an acute cervical disc syndrome, they are frequently associated with true radiculopathy because of the relationship of the nerve root to the surrounding structures, as demonstrated in Figure 1.4*A*.

Clinical Characteristics. Pain may be limited to the involved facet joints, but is more often a generalized ache in the cervical spine without a radicular component. There may be referred, nonradicular shoulder and arm pain. If there is nerve root involvement, true radiculitis or radiculopathy may be noted with sensory and motor dysfunction. The pattern of symptoms is dependent on the nerve root involved, as discussed above.

Treatment. Symptoms usually respond to the traction program as described above. Further treatment is the same as that described under "Acute Disc Herniation."

Acute Cervical Myalgia (Muscular Wryneck)

Wryneck is a symptom complex; its etiology is unclear. It appears to be some type of soft tissue inflammation or irritation, either in the muscles, ligaments, or facet joints (synovia).

Clinical Characteristics. Onset is gradual, usually without history of significant trauma. Onset may be associated with exposure to cold, with tension or anxiety, or with repetitive motion or prolonged positioning of the C-spine. Pain is felt in one of the posterior cervical triangles. Occasionally, pain may be referred into the ipsilateral shoulder, interscapular region, and occiput. Range of motion is usually diminished. The greatest restriction is in those directions that stretch the affected muscle groups. A tender focus is often discovered by careful palpation of the trapezius, splenius capitis, and levator scapulae on the painful side (Fig. 1.6). This area is often indurated and exhibits crepitus on deep palpation. Palpation over the spinous processes has no effect on pain. X-rays are within normal limits.

Treatment. Acute cervical myalgia is treated as a mild cervical sprain (see section on "Cervical Sprains and Strains"), except that the exercise regimen is initiated as early as possible and emphasizes movements that stretch the tender muscle. The condition tends to clear spontaneously in 7 to 10 days, with no significant sequelae.

Rheumatoid Arthritis

Rheumatoid arthritis may involve the cervical spine, as it does other parts of the axial and appendicular synovial joints. The reader is referred to Chapter 12 for a discussion of the underlying pathology. Cervical instability is the most serious and potentially life-threatening sequela of rheumatoid arthritis of the cervical spine.

Clinical Characteristics. The history and physical findings include neck pain with occipital and lower cervical radiculopathy, neck crepitus, variable signs of cervical myelopathy, and generalized signs and symptoms of the disease process. Significant laboratory abnormalities include elevated erythrocyte sedimentation rate and the presence of rheumatoid factors. X-rays reveal osteopenia, joint space narrowing, soft tissue swelling about involved joints, bone erosions near the capsular attachments of involved joints, and joint malalignment and subluxation.

Treatment. General treatment of C-spine rheumatoid arthritis consists of rest, gentle massage, soft cervical collar, isometric neck exercises within pain tolerance, and intermittent heat, i.e., 15 minutes 3 times a day (a hot shower in the morning to "loosen up" is an excellent technique). Medications begin with salicylates. If these do not provide adequate pain control, nonsteroidal anti-inflammatory drugs are utilized. Rheumatologic consultation determines the role of further pharmacologic therapy.

Surgical treatment must be considered in those instances where the disease has progressed to produce joint instability. There are three basic types of instability: atlantoaxial impaction (platybasia), C-1/C-2 subluxation, and subluxations of the lower cervical vertebrae, most common at the C-3/C-4 level. The reported incidence of instability in rheumatoid arthritis ranges from 43 to 86%. These lesions are expected to progress. Lateral cervical spine films in neutral, flexion, and extension are useful for evaluating the degree of instability and platybasia. Initially, cervical bracing is a reasonable treatment. If neurologic signs of cord or root entrapment are present or if there is evidence of instability on x-ray, orthopaedic referral is indicated for possible decompression and/or stabilization. An incidence of

neurologic deficits of 7 to 34% and sudden death of 10% have been reported.

FIBROMYALGIA

Fibromyalgia includes myofascial pain syndrome, extraarticular rheumatism, and fibrositis. It affects musculoskeletal tissues other than joints, including muscle, tendon, fascia, bursa, ligament, and synovial sheath. There may be a psychologic overlay.

Clinical Characteristics

These entities present a spectrum of signs and symptoms. A common form is characterized by multiple localized sites of deep tenderness in the trapezius, rhomboids, and levator scapulae. These are considered trigger points. Diffuse aching of more than 3 months' duration and sleep disturbances in a patient under age 50 are characteristic of this disorder. Physical findings include normal C-spine range of motion, normal motor strength, and exquisitely tender "trigger points" in the above-mentioned muscle groups. The EEG is usually abnormal and indicative of sleep disturbance. X-rays are within normal limits.

Treatment

Treatment should include reassurance, psychotherapy, and physical therapy, i.e., intermittent heat, massage, gentle active range of motion exercises, and isometric programs. Vacation or rest is recommended to relieve stress. Medications include amitriptyline, salicylates, nonsteroidal anti-inflammatory drugs, and occasional local injection of trigger points with lidocaine with or without corticosteroids. Addictive drugs should be avoided. Prognosis is poor with chronic relapses.

OSTEOPOROSIS

This generalized disease of bone affects the cervical spine as it does other parts of the axial and appendicular skeleton. It is discussed fully in Chapter 14.

THORACIC OUTLET SYNDROME

The thoracic outlet syndrome presents as neck and shoulder pain with radicular or nonradicular referred pain into the upper extremity with variable neurovascular signs and symptoms. It results from compression of the brachial plexus and the subclavian vessels, usually at one of three sites as they pass through the neck and superior thoracic outlet toward the axilla: (*a*) supraclavicular, (*b*) costoclavicular, and (*c*) infraclavicular (Fig. 1.12). These anatomic zones define the three subgroups that comprise the thoracic outlet syndrome.

Essential Anatomy and Pathomechanics

As the plexus descends toward the first rib (Fig. 1.12) it passes through the first zone of potential entrapment (supraclavicular), which is a triangular area bounded by the anterior scalene muscle, the middle scalene muscle, and the first rib. Distally in this zone, the plexus is joined by the subclavian artery and vein from below. This segment of the neurovascular bundle may be compressed by (*a*) an enlargement of the transverse process of C-7 (cervical rib), (*b*) a fibrous band that extends from the C-7 transverse process of C-7 to the first rib (pseudocervical rib), (*c*) degenerative arthritis of the first costovertebral joint, (*d*) hypertrophy or spasm of the anterior and/or medial scalene muscles, or (*e*) any process that causes traction on the neurovascular bundle as it crosses the first rib, such as poor posture, kyphosis, muscle weakness, heavy breasts, or obesity.

The second point of potential compression is the costoclavicular area (Fig. 1.12), which involves impingement of the neurovascular bundle as it enters a rigid narrow space formed by the clavicle superiorly and the first rib inferiorly. This space may be further narrowed by abnormal configuration of the first rib or clavicle caused by trauma, tumor, or inflammation; elevation of the first rib; or drooping of the shoulder girdle from backpacking or weight lifting.

The third point of compression is at the coracoid process (infraclavicular zone) (Fig. 1.12). The neurovascular bundle is trapped between the pectoralis minor and the rib cage, where the bundle is sharply angulated during hyperabduction and extension of the shoulders. Symptoms develop when pa-

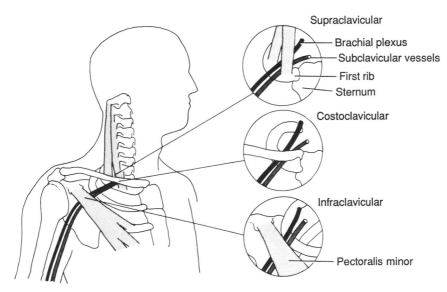

Figure 1.12.   Point of neurovascular compression in the thoracic outlet.

tients work for prolonged periods with the arms stretched overhead or sleep with the shoulders hyperabducted.

Clinical Characteristics

The essential picture of the thoracic outlet syndrome, whether supraclavicular, costo-clavicular, or infraclavicular, is similar since it usually involves compression of the inferior trunk of the brachial plexus, which makes up the ulnar nerve. The pain pattern usually extends from the neck or shoulders into the ulnar aspect of the arm, forearm, and ring and little fingers. Occasionally it involves the entire hand. Depending on the relative involvement of the neurovascular elements, there is a spectrum of either non-radicular referred pain associated with deep, diffuse, ill-defined aching, heaviness, weakness, burning, edema, discoloration, temperature changes, and painful throbbing of the fingers; or a more defined radicular referred pain pattern with associated specific motor, sensory, and deep tendon reflex aberrations. A positive Adson's test (Fig. 1.13) (producing a diminished radial pulse and/or precipitation or aggravation of the patient's symptoms in the involved extremity) is often a useful confirmatory test for the syndrome. X-rays of the neck, chest, and shoulder should be obtained. Other studies may be deferred to the time of referral if symptoms do not respond to treatment.

Differential Diagnosis

The thoracic outlet syndrome must be differentiated from the subclavian steal syndrome, in which blood is diverted from the cerebral circulation, causing CNS neurologic symptoms and signs with the upper extremity symptoms of the thoracic outlet syndrome. It is not usually precipitated by Adson's test and it is differentiated by a subclavian arteriogram, which shows blockage of the subclavian artery proximal to the origin of the vertebral artery.

Other entities to be included in differential diagnosis are cervical disc syndrome, cervical spondylosis, Pancoast tumor, carpal tunnel syndrome, or entrapment of the ulnar nerve at the elbow or wrist. Conditions to be excluded are reflex sympathetic dystrophy, occlusions of the axillary and brachial artery or vein, and brachial neuritis.

Treatment

The first choice in management is a conservative program. Treatment goals for the three types of thoracic outlet syndrome are the same, i.e., increase the space of the thoracic outlet and lessen pressure on the neurovascular elements. The program includes correction of faulty posture and body mechanics; manual stretching to increase mobility of the neck, shoulder girdle, and first and second ribs; and a specific home program. At home, the patient performs deep diaphragmatic breathing for relaxation, cervical-dorsal glide to stretch the neck, and strengthening exercises for the neck and shoulder girdle. The patient must also work to correct faulty sleeping or occupational habits. Patients must avoid slumped positions, round shoulders, and carrying heavy objects in the hands or over the shoulders. They minimize overhead activity and support their arms when sitting. They are instructed to avoid overexertion. Patients must avoid prone sleeping with the head rotated and extended and shoulders hyperextended or hyperabducted. It may be beneficial if a physical therapist manages the exercise and postural program.

It is reasonable to continue conservative treatment as long as the patient responds. If the signs and symptoms do not improve or if they increase, the patient should be referred to a surgeon for further evaluation and possible surgical intervention. This may involve resecting the constricting structure, e.g., the cervical rib and its fibrous attachments, or a portion of the scalenus anterior and medius muscles, or the first rib.

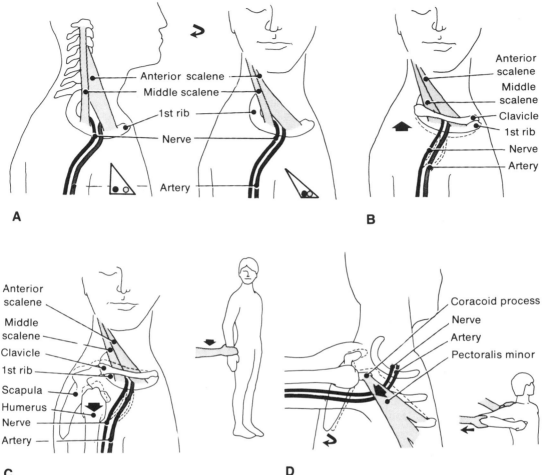

Figure 1.13. Mechanisms of the Adson's test. *A,* rotation of the head and neck toward the affected side compresses the neurovascular structures between the anterior and middle scalene muscles. *B,* a full inspiration elevates the first rib which thus stretches out the neurovascular structures and also further narrows their passage between the first rib and the middle and anterior scalene muscles. *C,* downward traction on the arm stretches out the neurovascular structures and also narrows their passage between the first rib and the clavicle. *D,* abduction and extension of the shoulder stretches out the neurovascular structures and retracts the scapula, thereby stretching the pectoralis minor tightly over the ribs, narrowing the neurovascular passage between the pectoralis minor and the ribs.

Traumatic Conditions of Childhood

ROTATORY SUBLUXATION OF C-1 ON C-2

Rotatory subluxation of the atlantoaxial joint is a relatively common problem in children. It may be the result of an injury, or may present without a history of significant trauma. In these circumstances, it often occurs in association with pharyngitis. It is thought that the inflammation, edema, and hyperemia lead to weakening of the supportive ligaments at C-1/C-2, allowing the facet joints to subluxate spontaneously or as a consequence of an otherwise minor injury.

Clinical Characteristics

The diagnosis is based on a fixed, painful torticollis with muscle spasm. Cervical spine x-ray, particularly open-mouth odontoid view, reveals the pathognomonic asymmetry of the C-1/C-2 joint with the odontoid deviated to one side.

Treatment

Treatment consists of bed rest, analgesics, and constant head-halter traction until painful spasm subsides and the subluxation reduces. After reduction, the child's neck should be protected in a soft cervical collar (Fig. 1.10) until the neck is completely comfortable and stable with a full, painless cervical range of motion. If the subluxation does not respond to traction within 5 to 7 days, an orthopaedic surgeon should be consulted.

BIRTH INJURIES OF THE BRACHIAL PLEXUS

The two common types of brachial plexus injury, Erb's palsy and Klumpke's palsy, are caused by strong lateral flexion of the infant's head and neck, producing traction on the brachial plexus. These injuries occur during a difficult delivery in which there is cephalopelvic disproportion, when the infant must be extracted quickly to ensure viability.

Clinical Characteristics

Erb's palsy is the more common of the two conditions. The infant presents with mixed sensory and motor defects of the upper trunks (C-5/C-6). While occasionally transient and reversible, it usually results in residual paralysis and sensory deficits of the shoulder and upper arm. Typically, the arm is motionless and lies adducted and extended in internal rotation at the infant's side. The hand and wrist are usually functional.

Klumpke's palsy is a rare condition. It involves the lower trunks (C-8/T-1), resulting in a flail hand and wrist with atrophy of the forearm. The upper arm is functional. Spontaneous recovery is not likely.

Treatment

The treatment for both types of palsy is gentle passive range of motion exercises of the paralyzed muscle groups to prevent contractures. These exercises should be taught to the family so that the routine can be carried out several times each day. Reconstructive surgery is sometimes useful to improve function of the impaired extremity. Orthopaedic consultation is necessary.

Traumatic Conditions in Adulthood
CERVICAL SPRAINS AND STRAINS

The exact nature of injury to the cervical spine depends on many variables. The intensity of the injuring force, the degree of protective muscle tone at the time of impact, the underlying strength of the bone and soft tissue, the position of the head and neck at the time of impact, and the presence of a protective support are all significant. Injury may involve the muscular tissue, the anterior and posterior longitudinal ligaments, the capsular ligaments of the facet joints, the intervertebral disc, the bony elements, the cervical nerve roots, and the spinal cord. There may also be injury to the temporomandibular joint, cervical sympathetic chain, and brainstem. Because of the numerous structures potentially involved, the symptoms following cervical injury may be numerous and complex, with an often confusing pattern of localized, referred, and radicular pain.

Most cervical injuries represent a combination of sprain and strain. They are usually the result of hyperflexion and/or hyperextension injuries with or without a rotational component. The injuries are most often sustained in motor vehicle accidents or in sporting activities. The severity of the sprain is determined by a knowledge of the injuring force applied, the severity of symptoms, the physical findings, and careful analysis of x-rays.

Clinical Characteristics

Most patients recall the mechanism of injury, describing it variably as hyperextension, hyperflexion, rotation, or a combination. There may be a history of transient confusion or unconsciousness. Many patients do not note immediate pain, but after several minutes or hours begin to develop pain and a sense of tightness in the neck. Some complain of nausea.

With mild injuries, initial physical examination usually reveals little in the way of abnormal findings. There may be some tenderness or mild restriction of motion, but often there is no tenderness or significant limitation of motion. After several hours or days, however, findings are usually more significant. There may be muscle tenderness, swelling, and spasm. The symptom complex may include pain referred to the interscapular area, shoulders, or upper extremities. There may be a sense of vague numbness, tingling, or heaviness in a nonradicular pattern, or there may be true radicular numbness and muscle weakness. Headaches, dizziness, and visual disturbances may be noted.

With moderate injuries, there may be radicular pain into one or both extremities. Spinal cord injury produces a myelopathy, and the patient may complain of a deep, aching, ill-defined pain about the shoulder girdle and/or pelvis associated with a feeling of weakness and instability in the lower extremities. Nerve root injury causes a radicular pattern of motor, sensory, and reflex signs and symptoms. Injury to the disc complex may cause local and radicular signs and symptoms.

Diagnostic workup should include routine x-rays of the cervical spine. Normal static x-rays support the diagnosis of a mild to moderate soft tissue injury without insta-bility. Plain x-rays also rule out fracture or dislocation. It is important to evaluate the plain films carefully. X-ray demonstration of prevertebral soft tissue widening, particularly in the upper cervical spine, suggests significant injury with hemorrhage and edema. The prevertebral space anterior to C-1 in the normal adult should not exceed 10 mm; at the C-2/C-3 level it should not exceed 5 to 7 mm. The relationship between vertebral bodies must also be assessed. Any anterior or posterior translation greater than 3.5 mm indicates potentially significant soft tissue injury and instability. Any angulation between two vertebrae that is 11° greater than the angulation between adjacent vertebrae also indicates possible instability. It is also important to be aware of any sharp reversal in the normal cervical curve. In the patient who has had a significant injury, stress views (flexion, extension, and possibly traction) should be obtained if there is any question regarding stability.

Treatment of the Stable Cervical Sprain-Strain

The patient who has a neurologic deficit or evidence of an unstable cervical spine injury should be referred promptly for orthopaedic evaluation and treatment. Fortunately, most patients do not have an unstable injury. These patients are treated with rest in a position of comfort, maintained by a soft cervical collar, for 1 to 2 days. For patients with moderate or severe symptoms, bed rest may be necessary. After 3 to 5 days pain usually is less, and by 2 weeks most patients have improved significantly. The soft cervical collar should be used symptomatically in the initial days following the injury. Subsequently, as symptoms resolve and healing occurs, the patient should be encouraged to wean out of the collar to avoid its habitual use. Application of cold packs is usually more effective initially than heat. Cold packs are applied for 15 minutes, 4 to 6 times daily, for the first 2 days. After this, moist heat may be used if symptomatically helpful. Analgesics and muscle relaxants may be used on a symptomatic basis and are helpful, particularly for nighttime pain and spasms that interfere with sleep.

As symptoms subside and healing occurs, exercises to gently stretch muscles and increase motion are encouraged within the limits of comfort. Early motion of a stable C-spine injury (proved by negative stress films) brings about a better result than prolonged immobilization. Gentle active range of motion and isometric exercises are recommended (Fig. 1.14). Isometric neck exercises are simple to perform and can be done independently. Exercises are first performed in the collar, which limits the range of motion. As long as the patient is pain-free, the exercises should be performed for 5 minutes, 3 times a day. Should pain occur, the duration but not frequency of the exercises should be decreased. A physical therapist may be helpful in guiding the patient.

After 2 to 3 weeks of gradual mobilization of the neck, the patient is weaned from the collar and the exercise program expanded appropriately to include isotonic exercises. Once again, care is taken to avoid pain by not overtaxing the healing tissues.

Manipulative treatment is contraindicated in the acute phase of moderate sprain-strains since it may cause additional injury. Cervical halter traction (Fig. 1.11) (steady or intermittent), as described under "Acute Disc Herniation," may assist in mobilizing the spine in those patients with stable injuries in the subacute or chronic phase who

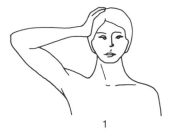

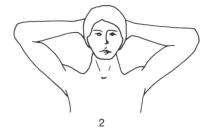

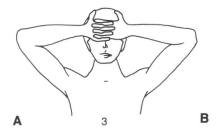

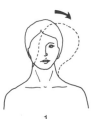

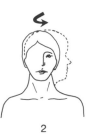

Figure 1.14. Exercises for cervical pain syndromes. *A*, isometric exercises. *1*, press head sideways against the heel of the hand (place the heel of the hand just above the ear), tense, relax, repeat. *2*, clasp hands behind head (over large bony prominence), tense head backward with chin tucked in, relax, repeat. *3*, press forehead against clasped hands, tense muscles without moving head, relax, repeat. *B*, range of motion exercises. Sit in a comfortable chair and take a moment to relax. Shrug shoulders in all directions, both together and alternately, until you relax. Shrug between exercises if you need to relax more. *1*, tip ear toward shoulder, turn to midposition, relax, tip to opposite side, relax, repeat. *2*, turn head and chin toward shoulder, return to midposition, relax, turn toward opposite shoulder, return to midposition, relax, repeat. *3*, tip head forward, return to erect position, relax, repeat.

A 1 2 3 **B** 1 2 3

present with persistent cervical pain, stiffness, tenderness, and muscle atrophy. If traction produces more discomfort, it should be discontinued immediately.

If severe pain persists or symptoms progress after 1 week, the patient should be re-evaluated and it is appropriate to consider repeat x-ray. If the patient does not improve, orthopaedic referral should be made.

While many patients with stable soft tissue neck injuries recover satisfactorily over a 4- to 6-week period, a significant percentage continue to have varying degrees of symptoms several months or years following injury. As would be expected, patients with more severe symptoms initially, x-ray abnormalities (including degenerative disease and sharp cervical curve reversal), and neurologic involvement have a poorer prognosis.

Treatment of the Unstable Cervical Sprain-Strain

These patients should be promptly placed under the care of an orthopaedic surgeon and/or neurosurgeon. These injuries frequently require surgical stabilization or prolonged bracing with a halo brace or halo cast apparatus. In the acute phase, the patient's cervical spine must be immobilized as described earlier in this chapter.

Burner's Syndrome

Burner's syndrome is a variant of the sprain-strain syndrome that occurs in athletes. A ballplayer complains of a transient burning pain in the neck, arm, and possibly hand following an injury that occurs while tackling or blocking an opponent, i.e., when the involved shoulder is depressed and the neck is bent to the opposite side on contact. This may produce injuries to the spinal cord, cervical roots, and supporting tissues of the neck and shoulder, and traction on elements of the brachial plexus. Variable degrees of pain, weakness, paresthesia, and sensory and reflex changes are noted on physical ex-

amination. Pain, tenderness, and limitation of motion of the cervical spine and occasionally the shoulder are present. This is treated as a moderate or severe cervical sprain-strain. Further evaluation is necessary to rule out fracture, dislocation, subluxation, and associated injuries to the cervical disc and root complex at the level of injury, and injury to the brachial plexus. The symptoms usually resolve within a few minutes, but the player should not resume play and should be evaluated by an orthopaedic surgeon.

CERVICAL FRACTURE, DISLOCATION, SUBLUXATION

As with soft tissue injury, the mechanisms of injury causing fracture and/or dislocation of the cervical spine include excessive flexion, extension, bending, rotation, compression, and distraction, alone or more commonly in some combination. A compressive force may produce a burst or explosion-type fracture of the vertebral body with ruptures of the anterior and/or posterior longitudinal ligaments. Extension forces produce fractures of the posterior bony elements with disruption of the anterior longitudinal ligament. Flexion injuries disrupt the posterior longitudinal ligament and compress the vertebral bodies; there may be injury to the facet joint capsule and intervertebral disc. Rotational injuries cause disruption of the ligaments with fracture or dislocation of the facet joints. The vertebral body may also be injured. The injuries that are the result of a combination of forces tend to be more severe and more unstable.

The classification of a fracture-dislocation as stable or unstable is not always a simple judgment. The three-segment concept is helpful in this regard. As described previously (Fig. 1.9), if two of the three segments of the spine are disrupted, the fracture-dislocation is considered unstable. An unstable injury is one that cannot withstand normal physiologic forces without abnormal deformity, and that jeopardizes the underlying spinal cord and/or nerve roots. Such instability may be acute or chronic as a result of late bony deformity. It must also be noted that in the cervical spine, cord injury has been documented in the presence of what appears to be a stable fracture.

Whenever a fracture-dislocation of the cervical spine is noted, the primary care physician's role is to stabilize the spine until orthopaedic and/or neurosurgical care can be instituted. In addition, initial treatment of a patient with a documented spinal cord injury should include the administration of high-dose methylprednisolone. Recent studies indicate that a dose of methylprednisolone 30 mg/kg of body weight administered within 8 hours of injury has a positive effect on neurologic recovery. After this initial bolus, a dose of methylprednisolone 5.4 mg/kg of body weight per hour should be administered for 23 hours.

Below is a brief description of the common fractures and dislocations of the cervical spine:

Fractures of C-1 (the atlas) are caused by axial loading that compresses and explodes the atlas. They are usually not associated with cord injuries. They are, however, unstable and should be treated initially with a rigid neck brace. A neurosurgeon or orthopaedic surgeon should be consulted. Definitive treatment is usually with halo jacket or halo vest for at least 8 weeks, followed by a cervical orthosis.

C-2 fractures usually involve fracture of the odontoid. The success rate for healing depends on the degree of displacement, the age of the patient, and the location of the fracture. Most of these injuries are treated with a halo body jacket, although some injuries with a poor prognosis should be stabilized immediately. Fractures associated with spinal cord injury at this level are often fatal.

In addition to fractures through the odontoid, C-2 fractures may also be through the pedicles. This is the so-called hangman's fracture. These injuries usually unite well when treated with a halo brace.

Fractures of C-3 through C-7 may involve all possible combinations of forces. One of the most severe is the injury caused by combined axial compression force with flexion. This is the common diving accident where the head strikes a solid object. This produces a comminuted fracture of the vertebral body with retropulsion into the spinal canal and injury to the cord. Many of these patients need surgical stabilization.

The common dislocations of the cervical spine usually occur between C-3 and C-7. These involve unilateral or bilateral facet dislocations. The injury is indicated on the lateral cervical spine x-ray by varying degrees of displacement of the superior vertebra anteriorly on the adjoining inferior vertebra. In unilateral facet dislocation, there is approximately a 25% anterior listhesis of the superior on inferior vertebra. In bilateral dislocation, this is usually in the 50% range. In addition to the listhesis, careful review of the x-ray shows the abnormal relationship of the facet joints.

Occipital/C-1 dislocations are rare and almost always fatal. If the patient does not die as a result of this injury, halo immobilization is indicated followed by surgical stabilization.

C-1/C-2 dislocations or subluxations may occur with or without odontoid fracture. One type of C-1/C-2 dislocation is the "adult rotatory subluxation of the atlantoaxial joint," which presents with the same characteristics as the childhood variant but is related to significant injury. This injury occurs when there is a rotational force applied to the head, causing the inferior facet of C-1 to slip forward on the superior facet of C-2. If the articulation becomes fixed in this position, there is marked limitation of motion and a painful posttraumatic torticollis develops. Neurologic deficits often occur. X-rays demonstrate an asymmetry in the position of the odontoid. It is deviated to one side and remains deviated (i.e., fixed subluxation) even with rotation of the head and repeat x-ray. CT scan is helpful in evaluating this.

Injury to the Cervical Disc

Acute cervical disc injuries occur in decreasing frequency between units C-5/C-6, C-6/C-7, and C-7/T-1 (Fig. 1.1). Injury to the disc–annular ligament–posterior ligament complex may result in protrusion or herniation of the nucleus pulposus with subsequent radicular pain patterns, depending on the level of injury. Mechanisms of injury are similar to those producing fracture, dislocation, or subluxation. Clinical features and treatment are described in the section on "Acute Disc Herniation."

SUGGESTED READINGS

Anderson JE. Grant's atlas of anatomy. 8th ed. Baltimore: Williams & Wilkins, 1983.

Bracken MB, Shepard MJ, Collins WF, et al. A randomized, controlled trial of methylprednisolone or naloxone in the treatment of acute spinal-cord injury. N Engl J Med 1990;322(20):1405–1411.

Cervical Spine Research Society Editorial Committee. The cervical spine. 2nd ed. Philadelphia: JB Lippincott Co, 1989.

Committee on Trauma. Advanced trauma life support course instructor manual. Chicago: American College of Surgeons, 1990.

Edmonson AS. Spinal anatomy and surgical approaches. In: Crenshaw AH, ed. Campbell's operative orthopaedics. 7th ed. St. Louis: The CV Mosby Co, 1987:3091–3107.

Evarts C McC, Mayer PJ. Complications. In: Rockwood CA Jr, Green DP, eds. Fractures in adults. 2nd ed. Philadelphia: JB Lippincott Co, 1984:219–294.

Freeman BL III. Fractures, dislocations, and fracture-dislocations of spine. In: Crenshaw AH, ed. Campbell's operative orthopaedics. 7th ed. St. Louis: The CV Mosby Co, 1987:3109–3142.

Grant JCB, Basmajian JV. Grant's method of anatomy by regions, descriptive and deductive. 8th ed. Baltimore: Williams & Wilkins, 1971.

Hollinshead WH. Anatomy for surgeons, vol 3, The back and limbs. 2nd ed. New York: Harper and Row, 1969.

Hoppenfeld S. Physical examination of the spine and extremities. Norwalk, CT: Appleton-Century-Crofts, 1976:105–132.

Iverson LD, Clawson DK. Manual of acute orthopaedic therapeutics. 3rd ed. Boston: Little, Brown and Co, 1987.

Lovell WW, Winter RB, eds. Pediatric orthopaedics. 2nd ed. Philadelphia: JB Lippincott Co, 1986.

Ogden JA. The uniqueness of growing bones. In: Rockwood CA Jr, Wilkins KE, King RE, eds. Fractures in children. Philadelphia: JB Lippincott Co, 1984:1–86.

Pappas AM. Muscles, joints, and ligaments. In: Southmayd W, Hoffman M, eds. Sports health: the complete book of athletic injuries. New York: Quick Fox, 1981:70–85.

Rodnan GP, Schumacher R, Zvaifler NJ, eds. Rheumatoid arthritis. In: Primer on the rheumatic diseases. 8th ed. Atlanta, GA: Arthritis Foundation, 1983:38–48.

Salter RB. Textbook of disorders and injuries of the musculoskeletal system: an introduction to orthopaedics, fractures and joint injuries, rheumatology, metabolic bone disease and rehabilitation. 2nd ed. Baltimore: Williams & Wilkins, 1983.

Sculco TP. Neck pain. In: Beary JF III, Christian CL, Johanson NA, eds. Manual of rheumatology and outpatient orthopedic disorders: diagnosis and therapy. 2nd ed. Boston: Little, Brown and Co, 1987:77–80.

Simeone FA, Rothman RH. Cervical disc disease. In: Rothman RH, Simeone FA, eds. The spine. 2nd ed. Philadelphia: WB Saunders Co, 1982:440–499.

Stauffer ES. Fractures and dislocations of the spine. Part I: the cervical spine. In: Rockwood CA Jr, Green DP, eds. Fractures in adults. 2nd ed. Philadelphia: JB Lippincott Co, 1984:987–1035.

Wood GW. Infections of spine. In: Crenshaw AH, ed. Campbell's operative orthopaedics. 7th ed. St. Louis: The CV Mosby Co, 1987:3323–3345.

Wood GW. Other disorders of spine. In: Crenshaw AH, ed. Campbell's operative orthopaedics. 7th ed. St. Louis: The CV Mosby Co, 1987:3347–3374.

CHAPTER 2

Shoulder and Upper Arm

Thomas P. Goss, M.D.

Essential Anatomy

The shoulder is comprised of four articulations: the glenohumeral joint, the scapulothoracic joint, the acromioclavicular joint, and the sternoclavicular joint. This complex is designed for maximal mobility, allowing the hand to be placed in the near infinite number of positions necessary for upper extremity function.

GLENOHUMERAL JOINT

The glenohumeral joint can be thought of as a "soft tissue articulation" since bony restraint is minimal. The surrounding soft tissues provide both stability and motor function. The glenohumeral joint is therefore the most mobile articulation in the body, but also the most prone to instability when the periarticular soft tissues are damaged. The glenohumeral joint is also a "distractive articulation" as opposed to the "compressive joints" of the lower extremities. This makes it much less prone to degenerative joint disease.

The glenohumeral joint is a ball-and-socket articulation consisting of the small, shallow glenoid portion of the scapula (the socket) and the articular segment of the proximal humerus (the ball). Only one-quarter of the articular surface of the proximal humerus is in contact with the glenoid at any one time. The joint space is surrounded by the synovial membrane and the fibrous capsule, which are attached to the bony glenoid via the glenoid labrum, a fibrocartilaginous structure that surrounds the periphery of the glenoid. There are no ligaments posteriorly, but the glenohumeral joint is stabilized by the superior, middle, and inferior glenohumeral ligaments anteriorly.

One layer more superficial is the musculotendinous (rotator) cuff, which is the confluence of the tendons of four muscles: the subscapularis (upper and lower subscapular nerves), the supraspinatus (suprascapular nerve), the infraspinatus (suprascapular nerve), and the teres minor (axillary nerve). The supraspinatus, infraspinatus, and teres minor muscles arise over the dorsal aspect of the scapula and insert on the greater tuberosity of the proximal humerus. The subscapularis muscle arises over the ventral aspect of the scapula, and inserts on the lesser tuberosity of the proximal humerus (Fig. 2.1). The rotator cuff has four functions: (*a*) it is a soft tissue shock absorber between the proximal humerus and the undersurface of the acromion; (*b*) it lends passive stability to the glenohumeral joint; (*c*) it acts in a dynamic fashion to provide motion at the glenohumeral joint; and (*d*) it actively seats the humeral head firmly into the glenoid fossa so that stronger, more superficial muscles such as the deltoid can optimally move the arm. The blood supply for the articular segment of the proximal humerus enters via the greater and lesser tuberosities.

Between the greater and lesser tuberosities is the biceps groove, which contains the long head of the biceps tendon as it passes

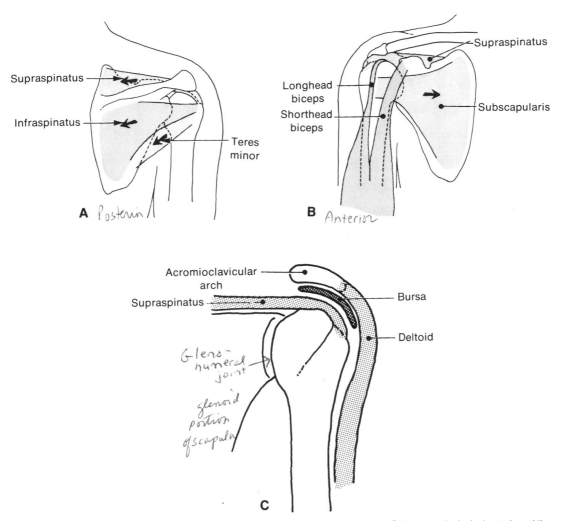

Figure 2.1. *A* and *B,* the musculotendinous cuff. *A,* posterior view; *B,* anterior view. *C,* the acromioclavicular arch and the subacromial bursa.

from its origin at the superior margin of the glenoid to its junction with the short head of the biceps to form the belly of the biceps muscle (musculocutaneous nerve). The short head of the biceps tendon originates at the tip of the coracoid process (Fig. 2.1). The coracoid process is also the origin of the coracobrachialis muscle (musculocutaneous nerve), which lies over the anteromedial aspect of the upper arm deep to the biceps. Posterior to the glenohumeral joint is the teres major muscle (lower subscapular

nerve), which originates from the inferior angle of the scapula and inserts on the anterior aspect of the proximal humerus. The long head of the triceps muscle originates from the inferior aspect of the glenoid and joins the lateral and medial heads distally to form the belly of the triceps muscle (radial nerve).

The acromion process of the scapula is a bony arch that overhangs the proximal humerus. The subacromial bursa lies between the bony acromion and the rotator cuff (Fig.

2.1). The coracoacromial ligament runs from the coracoid process to the anterior margin of the acromion.

The deltoid muscle (axillary nerve) lies just beneath the skin and subcutaneous tissue. It arises from the distal third of the clavicle (anterior deltoid), the acromion (middle deltoid), and the spine of the scapula (posterior deltoid) and inserts over the lateral aspect of the proximal humeral shaft. Finally, within the axilla medial to the glenohumeral joint, lie the brachial plexus and axillary vessels.

The arcs of motion and positions of the arm at the glenohumeral joint are shown in Figure 2.2. The prime controllers of these movements are the following: flexion—anterior deltoid, pectoralis major; extension—latissimus dorsi, posterior deltoid; abduction—middle deltoid, supraspinatus; adduction—pectoralis major, latissimus dorsi, teres major; internal rotation—subscapularis; external rotation—infraspinatus, teres minor.

SCAPULOTHORACIC JOINT

The scapulothoracic articulation is not a true joint. Considerable movement, however, is provided to the shoulder complex as the scapula glides over the posterior thoracic rib cage.

The scapula is a thin, triangular bone with three processes: the spine of the scapula arises over its dorsal aspect and runs laterally to become the acromion process; the glenoid process serves as the socket for the glenohumeral joint; the coracoid process protrudes anteriorly and provides attachment for several tendons and ligaments. The scapula is fixed to the posterior thoracic cage by musculotendinous attachments and a bony strut, the clavicle. The clavicle (via the acromioclavicular and sternoclavicular joints) is, therefore, the only bony connecting link

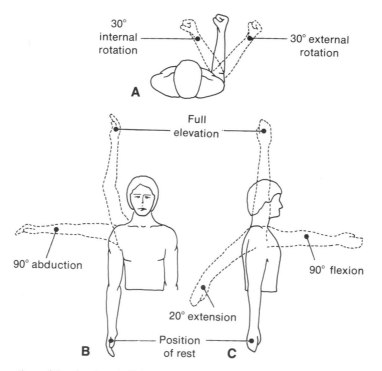

Figure 2.2. The motions of the glenohumeral joint and the positions of the arm at the glenohumeral joint. *A,* internal and external rotation. *B,* abduction-adduction. *C,* flexion-extension.

between the shoulder complex/upper extremity and the rest of the skeleton. Posteriorly, the levator scapulae (deep branches of the cervical plexus), the rhomboideus minor (dorsal scapular nerve), and the rhomboideus major (dorsal scapular nerve) muscles originate from the cervical and thoracic vertebrae and insert onto the upper, middle, and inferior thirds, respectively, of the medial margin of the scapula. The serratus anterior (long thoracic nerve) originates over the anterior aspect of the upper eight to nine ribs and inserts on the inferior angle of the scapula. Superficial to these muscles, the trapezius (spinal accessory nerve and several cervical nerves) arises from the spinous processes of the cervical and thoracic vertebrae, and inserts on the spine and acromion of the scapula. The latissimus dorsi (thoracodorsal nerve) arises from the lower half of the vertebral spine and iliac crest and inserts on the anterior aspect of the upper third of the humerus. Anteriorly, the scapula is controlled by the pectoralis major (medial and lateral pectoral nerves) and pectoralis minor (medial pectoral nerve) muscles, which originate from the anterior thoracic cage and insert on the proximal aspect of the humerus and coracoid process, respectively. These muscles control the stability and provide the six movements of the scapula. These movements and their prime controllers are noted in Figure 2.3.

The bony anchor of the scapula to the thoracic cage is the clavicle, which articulates laterally with the acromion to form the acromioclavicular joint and medially with the sternum to form the sternoclavicular joint.

ACROMIOCLAVICULAR JOINT (FIG. 2.4)

The lateral end of the clavicle articulates with the acromion to form the acromioclavicular (AC) joint. The capsule of the AC joint is reinforced by the superior and inferior acromioclavicular ligaments. A fibrocartilaginous disc is contained within the artic-

ulation. Additional stability is provided by the coracoclavicular ligaments, which run from the coracoid process of the scapula to the undersurface of the clavicle.

STERNOCLAVICULAR JOINT (FIG. 2.5)

The medial end of the clavicle articulates with the sternum to form the sternoclavicular (SC) joint. The capsule of the SC joint is reinforced by the anterior and posterior sternoclavicular ligaments. An intraarticular fibrocartilaginous disc lies within the joint. Additional stability is provided by the costoclavicular ligament, which runs from the medial end of the clavicle to the first rib.

Scapular movement is accompanied by corresponding motion at the AC and SC joints.

UPPER ARM

The structural scaffolding of the upper arm is the humerus. The biceps, coracobrachialis, and brachialis (musculocutaneous nerve) muscles reside within the anterior portion of the upper arm, while the triceps muscle lies posteriorly. The coracobrachialis muscle inserts over the anterior shaft of the humerus, while the brachialis muscle originates over the anterior portion of the humerus. The medial and lateral heads of the triceps muscle originate from the posterior aspect of the humeral shaft (Fig. 2.6). The deltoid muscle inserts over the lateral aspect of the upper third of the humerus (Fig. 2.7).

The radial nerve enters the upper arm via the axilla, posterior to the humerus. It then spirals distally from medial to lateral adjacent to the shaft of the humerus and deep to the medial and lateral heads of the triceps muscle, which it innervates. The nerve is especially vulnerable to injury at two points: (*a*) as it spirals around the midshaft of the humerus posterolaterally, and (*b*) as it enters the forearm between the brachioradialis and biceps muscles. The ulnar nerve courses posterior to the brachial artery along the medial aspect of the upper arm. Proximally, it lies

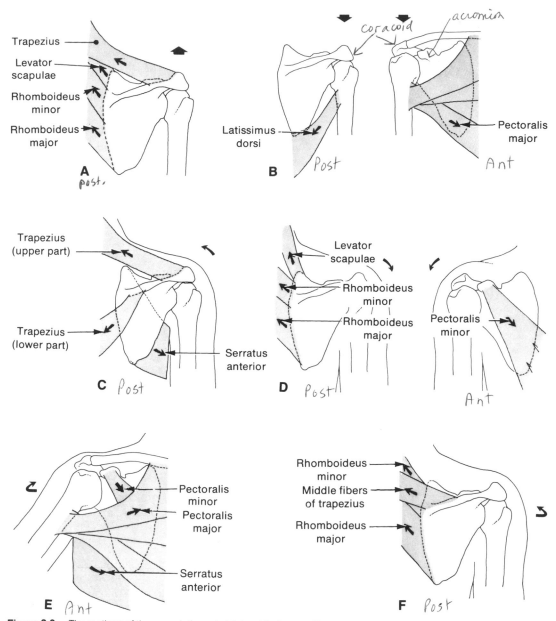

Figure 2.3. The motions of the scapulothoracic joint and their controlling muscles. *A*, elevation, posterior view. *B*, depression; *left*, posterior view; *right*, anterior view. *C*, upward rotation, posterior view. *D*, downward rotation; *left*, posterior view; *right*, anterior view. *E*, protraction, anterior view. *F*, retraction, posterior view.

within the anterior compartment. At the middle third of the arm, it pierces the medial intermuscular septum to enter the posterior compartment. The median nerve runs anterior to the brachial artery along the medial aspect of the upper arm. The musculocuta-

neous nerve lies between the biceps and brachialis muscles and innervates the biceps, brachialis, and coracobrachialis muscles. The axillary nerve curves around the lateral aspect of the upper arm from posterior to anterior and lies deep to the deltoid muscle,

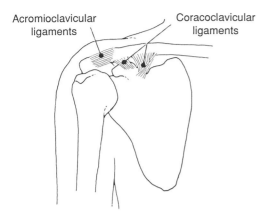

Acromioclavicular ligaments

Coracoclavicular ligaments

Figure 2.4.   The acromioclavicular joint and its ligaments.

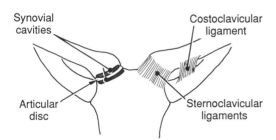

Synovial cavities

Costoclavicular ligament

Articular disc

Sternoclavicular ligaments

Figure 2.5.   The sternoclavicular joint: its synovial cavities, disc, and ligaments.

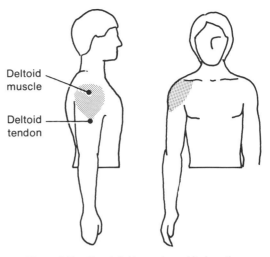

Deltoid muscle

Deltoid tendon

Figure 2.7.   The deltoid muscle and its insertion.

which it innervates. The brachial artery courses with the median and ulnar nerves along the medial aspect of the upper arm, separated from the humerus by the brachialis muscle and the medial head of the triceps muscle.

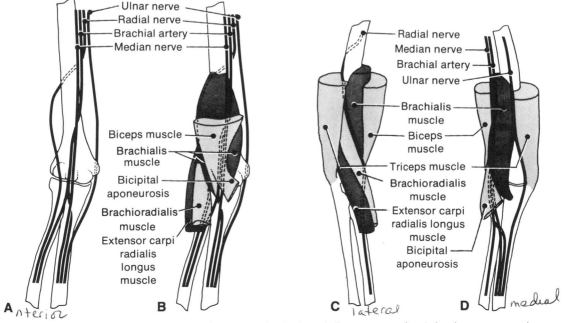

Ulnar nerve
Radial nerve
Brachial artery
Median nerve

Biceps muscle
Brachialis muscle
Bicipital aponeurosis
Brachioradialis muscle
Extensor carpi radialis longus muscle

A *anterior*   B

Radial nerve
Median nerve
Brachial artery
Ulnar nerve

Brachialis muscle
Biceps muscle
Triceps muscle
Brachioradialis muscle
Extensor carpi radialis longus muscle
Bicipital aponeurosis

C *lateral*   D *medial*

Figure 2.6.   Relationships of the muscles and neurovascular structures in the upper arm. *A*, anterior view, neurovascular structures alone. *B*, anterior view with muscles added. *C*, lateral view. *D*, medial view.

Evaluation of the Patient with Shoulder Symptoms

The shoulder region and upper arm are susceptible to a wide variety of disorders, both traumatic and nontraumatic. The initial step in evaluating the individual with symptoms in these areas is to obtain a good history. Questions should first be general. The second group of questions is directed toward specific clinical entities suggested by the patient's responses to the general questions.

The second step is the physical examination. This should begin with a gross visual inspection of the shoulder from all aspects (anterior, posterior, superior, and lateral), looking for deformities, asymmetry, discoloration, muscle atrophy, etc. The region is then palpated for masses, defects, deformities, and areas of tenderness. One should be familiar with the surface anatomy of the area as well as palpable anatomic landmarks: the coracoid process, the biceps tendon, the impingement interval, the SC joint, the AC joint, the trapezius and deltoid muscles, the supraspinatus and infraspinatus fossae, the clavicle, the spine of the scapula, the scapula, the greater tuberosity, and the acromion. The examiner should then put the shoulder through a very gentle passive circular range of motion, followed by having the patient perform the same maneuver actively. The patient is asked to localize any pain that is elicited. The examiner watches for any restriction of motion and keeps a hand on the shoulder, feeling for associated crepitus. The shoulder is then put through a full passive and active range of motion (forward flexion, abduction, adduction, extension, internal rotation behind the back, and external rotation). The examiner notes any associated crepitus and its general location; any associated pain, its location, and the position of the shoulder when it occurs; any asymmetry of glenohumeral-scapulothoracic motion; and any loss/restriction of motion or motor weakness.

A good basic neurovascular evaluation should be undertaken to demonstrate active function of the musculature about the shoulder, including the trapezius, rhomboids, serratus anterior, deltoid, biceps, triceps, and rotator cuff. Median, ulnar, and radial nerve function should be tested and distal pulses palpated. If shoulder instability is suggested by the patient's history, apprehension and stress testing should be performed (Fig. 2.8). If degenerative disease of the AC joint is sus-

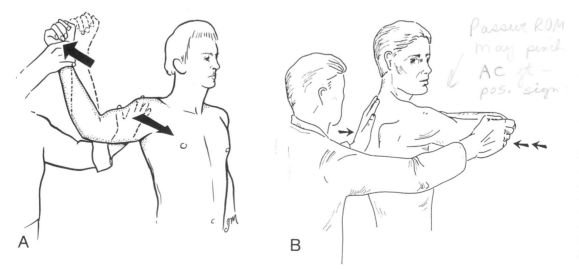

Figure 2.8.   Stress testing of the glenohumeral joint to detect instability. *A*, anterior stress testing. *B*, posterior stress testing. (From Goss TP. Recurrent symptomatic posterior glenohumeral subluxation. Orthop Rev 1988;XVII(10):1024–1032.)

pected, the arm is brought across the chest and the AC joint manually compressed to see whether pain is elicited (Fig. 2.9).

D   A brief examination of the cervical spine and the ipsilateral elbow, forearm, wrist, and hand should also be performed to make sure that "shoulder-upper arm symptoms" are not originating from these areas. Finally, one should remember that shoulder-upper arm symptoms can be referred from the respiratory, cardiovascular, and gastrointestinal systems.

The third step in evaluating the patient is the radiologic examination. The basic shoulder study includes true anteroposterior (AP) (neutral rotation) and axillary views of the glenohumeral joint. Figure 2.10 demonstrates these projections with accompanying line drawings showing the major bony landmarks. One must remember when interpreting an x-ray that this is a two-dimensional representation of a three-dimensional structure. Supplementary views include AP projections of the shoulder with the proximal humerus internally and externally rotated, the transthoracic lateral view, and the tangential or lateral scapula view (Fig. 2.10) as well as AP views of the AC joint with the patient holding weights (Fig. 2.11). Radiologic evaluation of the upper arm consists simply of AP and lateral projections.

More sophisticated diagnostic studies are available if warranted by the specific clinical situation.

Shoulder Physiotherapy and Rehabilitation

For any shoulder disorder, whether traumatic or nontraumatic, maintaining and regaining range of motion, flexibility, and strength are critical to achieving a successful functional result. Consequently, physiotherapy and rehabilitation are extremely important. The specifics of the program vary with the nature of the disorder. There are, however, a few basic principles that should be observed and a general program can be outlined.

BASIC PRINCIPLES

One works for range of motion, flexibility, and strength in six directions: forward flexion, abduction, adduction, extension, internal rotation behind the back, and external rotation. Multiple short exercise sessions are better than a few lengthy sessions to avoid irritating, damaging, or overtaxing the periarticular soft tissues. The general progression is from passive or active-assistive range of motion exercises to isometrics to active strengthening exercises to late stretching and strengthening techniques. Each exercise session should be preceded by local application of moist heat and followed by local application of ice. Range of motion and strengthening exercises are performed with the patient lying supine (gravity assisted) at first. The patient is gradually advanced to stand-

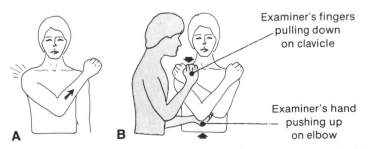

Figure 2.9.   Tests for acromioclavicular pain. *A*, cross-chest maneuver designed to compress the AC joint. *B*, technique used to stress the AC joint in the vertical plane.

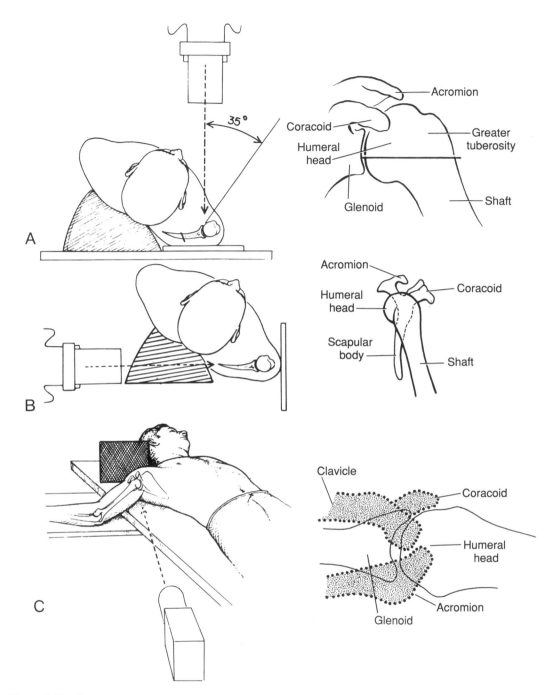

Figure 2.10. Standard radiologic views of the glenohumeral joint. *A,* true AP view of the glenohumeral joint with the arm in neutral rotation. (From Rockwood CA, Green DP, eds. Fractures in adults, vol 1. 2nd ed. Philadelphia: JB Lippincott Co, 1984:679 and 821.) *B,* true lateral projection of the glenohumeral joint. (From Rockwood CA, Green DP, eds. Fractures in adults, vol 1. 2nd ed. Philadelphia: JB Lippincott Co, 1984:679.) *C,* true axillary view of the glenohumeral joint. (From Rockwood CA, Green DP, eds. Fractures in adults, vol 1. 2nd ed. Philadelphia: JB Lippincott Co, 1984:680 and from Neer CS II. Displaced proximal humeral fractures: I. Classification and evaluation. J Bone Joint Surg 1970;52A:1077–1089.)

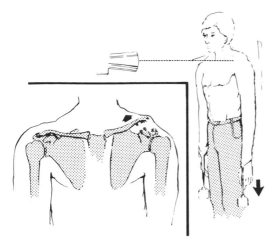

Figure 2.11. Technique for obtaining stress films of the acromioclavicular joint (used to detect injury to the acromioclavicular and coracoclavicular ligaments). (From Rockwood CA, Green DP, eds. Fractures in adults, vol 1. 2nd ed. Philadelphia: JB Lippincott Co, 1984:877.)

ing exercises (against gravity) as symptoms and strength allow. The patient should strive for gentle, relaxed motion without excessive pain, and should not overdo. Any exercise causing lingering pain is temporarily omitted.

GENERAL PROGRAM (FIG. 2.12)

The shoulder should be immobilized until judged to be sufficiently stable or healed to begin physiotherapy. The simplest exercise consists of dependent circular and pendulum range of motion exercises. When healing is sufficient, passive or active-assistive exercises to maintain or regain range of motion and flexibility are begun. When healing, range of motion, and flexibility are satisfactory, active exercises to maintain or regain strength are begun. When healing, range of motion, flexibility, and strength are satisfactory, late stretching and strengthening exercises are prescribed if deficiencies exist. As range of motion, flexibility, and strength improve, the functional capabilities of the shoulder increase accordingly.

Nontraumatic Disorders
GLENOHUMERAL DEGENERATIVE JOINT DISEASE

Degenerative disease of the glenohumeral joint can occur as the result of a number of different processes, including primary

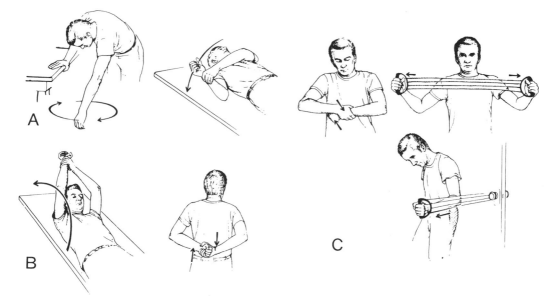

Figure 2.12. Shoulder physiotherapy and rehabilitation. *A*, dependent circular range of motion exercises. *B*, active-assistive range of motion exercises for forward flexion, internal rotation behind the back, and external rotation. *C*, active strengthening exercises. (From Rockwood CA, Green DP, eds. Fractures, vol 1. 1st ed. Philadelphia: JB Lippincott Co, 1975:595.)

osteoarthritis, traumatic articular disruption, posttraumatic and nontraumatic avascular necrosis, as well as a variety of inflammatory arthritides including rheumatoid arthritis and others (Chapter 12). The humeral articular surface, the glenoid articular surface, or both may be involved. Clinical characteristics include the following: shoulder pain that is worse with motion; palpable crepitus on gentle range of motion; restriction of glenohumeral range of motion secondary to pain or mechanical block; and radiologic evidence of degenerative disease, including subchondral cysts, sclerosis, joint space narrowing, marginal osteophytes, and irregularity of the articular surfaces.

Treatment

If disruption of the humeral articular surface is present but the glenohumeral joint space and glenoid appear reasonably normal, referral to an orthopaedist is indicated for consideration of prosthetic replacement of the humeral articular segment. In addition to alleviating the patient's symptoms, this protects the glenoid articular surface from secondary damage and avoids a later total shoulder replacement. If both sides of the articulation are involved, a trial of nonoperative treatment is worthwhile. This consists of avoidance of aggravating positions and activities, rest, application of moist heat, and nonsteroidal anti-inflammatory or analgesic medications. Intraarticular steroid injections may be helpful. Should pain and/or disability become unacceptable, referral to an orthopaedist is indicated for consideration of a total shoulder replacement.

DEGENERATIVE DISEASE OF THE AC AND SC JOINTS

Degenerative disease of the AC and SC articulations can be caused by a variety of processes, including primary osteoarthritis, rheumatoid disease, traumatic articular disruption, etc. Clinical characteristics include the following. Discomfort is localized to the AC or SC articulations and is worse with shoulder motion. There is palpable crepitus over the affected articulation on range of motion. Swelling may be evident and marginal irregularity may be palpable. Pain over the articulation is increased by palpation and during the cross-chest maneuver (Fig. 2.9). Radiologic examination shows evidence of degenerative disease, including subchondral sclerosis, cyst formation, narrowing of the joint space, marginal osteophytes, and irregularity of the articular surfaces.

Initial treatment is nonoperative and includes avoidance of aggravating positions and activities, rest, moist heat, and analgesic medications for discomfort. Anti-inflammatory medications and intraarticular steroid injections may be helpful. If nonoperative treatment is ineffective, referral to an orthopaedist is indicated for consideration of surgical resection of the clavicular portion of the affected articulation.

CHRONIC INSTABILITY OF THE GLENOHUMERAL JOINT

Chronic instability of the glenohumeral joint presents the greatest diagnostic and therapeutic challenge of any of the disorders that affect the shoulder region. There are three types of chronic instability (Fig. 2.13): dislocation, subluxation, and functional instability. Dislocation is an instability in which an applied force causes the apex of the humeral head circumference to move beyond the rim of the glenoid fossa. Subluxation is an instability in which an applied force causes the humeral head to move excessively relative to the glenoid, but short of an actual dislocation. Functional instability means that a piece of tissue, be it a partially attached labral fragment, a loose osseous body, a loose cartilaginous body, etc., becomes intermittently interposed between the glenohumeral articular surfaces, causing the shoulder to catch, slip, or lock (symptoms similar to that of a torn knee meniscus). In addition, one must determine whether the

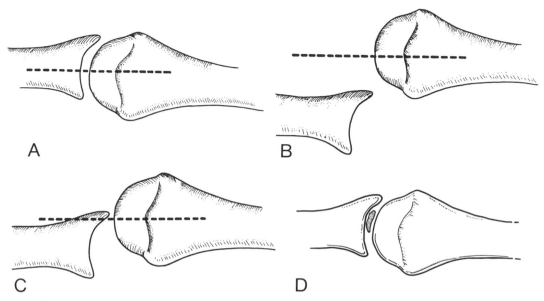

Figure 2.13. Types of chronic glenohumeral instability. *A*, normal relationship. *B*, dislocation (note the apex of the humeral head circumference moves beyond the rim of the glenoid fossa). *C*, subluxation (note the apex of the humeral head circumference moves out to, but not beyond, the rim of the glenoid fossa). (*B* and *C* from Goss TP. Factors to consider in chronic symptomatic shoulder instability. Orthop Rev 1985; XIV(10):27–32.) *D*, functional instability (note the fragment of tissue interposed between the glenohumeral articulating surfaces).

articulation is unstable anteriorly, posteriorly, inferiorly, or in multiple directions (Fig. 2.14).

Chronic (Recurrent) Dislocation

Characteristic clinical features include the following. The patient usually remembers a clear initiating event followed by multiple episodes. Each time the shoulder dislocates, the patient feels the humeral head become caught out of place for a variable period of time, and the patient or someone else must manipulate the shoulder back into place. Each recurrence requires less trauma and each relocation becomes easier. The patient can often relate the dislocation to a specific position of the arm: extension-abduction-external rotation for anterior instability and adduction-forward flexion-internal rotation for posterior instability. Apprehension and stress testing in the direction of instability are generally positive. X-rays of the glenohumeral joint often show an impression de-

fect over the humeral head, and/or a fracture, erosion, or ectopic calcification along the glenoid rim. Prior x-rays showing the articulation actually dislocated confirm the diagnosis. Once the diagnosis is made or suspected, referral to an orthopaedist is in order since surgical repair of the damaged retaining structures is generally indicated.

Chronic (Recurrent) Subluxation

This clinical entity is much more difficult to diagnose than chronic (recurrent) dislocation. This is a milder form of glenohumeral dissociation. Signs and symptoms are similar to those of chronic dislocation, but more subtle. By definition, there is no actual dislocation of the shoulder requiring manipulation by the patient or a companion, but the individual may describe the shoulder as catching, slipping, or going out of place. Patients may describe their arm as transiently "going dead" or may only state that their shoulder is bothering them.

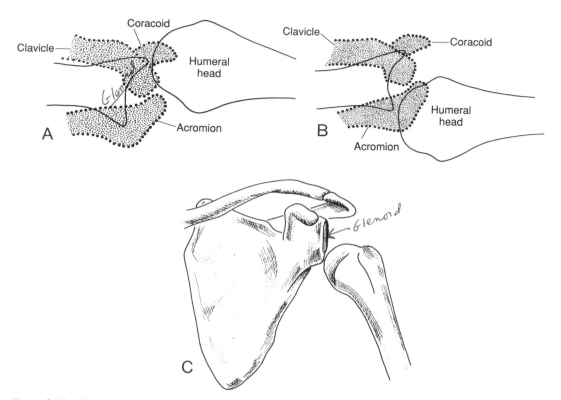

Figure 2.14. Directions of chronic glenohumeral instability. *A*, anterior instability (note the humeral head moves excessively relative to the glenoid toward the coracoid process). *B*, posterior instability (note the humeral head moves excessively relative to the glenoid toward the acromion process). *C*, inferior instability (note the humeral head moves excessively inferiorly relative to the glenoid). (From Goss TP. Factors to consider in chronic symptomatic shoulder instability. Orthop Rev 1985;XIV(10):27–32.)

Treatment. Approximately 50% of individuals with chronic glenohumeral subluxation will respond to a nonoperative therapeutic program consisting of avoidance of aggravating positions and activities, and exercises designed to strengthen stabilizing muscle groups (the forward flexors and internal rotators for anterior instability and the extensors and external rotators for posterior instability). Referral to an orthopaedist is indicated if one suspects the diagnosis but is uncertain, or if the diagnosis is made and nonoperative therapeutic modalities are ineffective. For those individuals who are unresponsive to nonoperative therapy, surgery designed to repair the damaged retaining structures is indicated.

Functional Instability

This clinical entity is particularly difficult to diagnose since signs and symptoms are even more subtle than those of recurrent subluxation. The patient may or may not be able to remember a primary initiating event. Patients may describe the shoulder as catching, slipping, clicking, locking, or may simply say that the shoulder is bothering them. The patient may or may not be able to relate symptoms to certain shoulder positions. Apprehension and stress testing are negative. Routine radiographs are unremarkable unless the cause of the patient's symptomatology is an intermittently interposed intraarticular loose osseous body. Radiographic contrast studies such as glenohumeral CT arthrography and glenohumeral arthrotomography are necessary to reveal the intermittently interposed intraarticular soft tissue responsible for the patient's symptomatology.

Treatment. Once the diagnosis is confirmed or suspected, referral to an orthopaedist is indicated. Definitive treatment involves arthroscopic removal of the intermittently interposed intra-articular tissue responsible for the patient's symptomatology.

IMPINGEMENT SYNDROME

Impingement syndrome is an extremely common shoulder disorder. The space between the undersurface of the anterior acromion and the superior aspect of the proximal humerus is called the impingement interval. This space is normally quite narrow and is maximally narrow when the arm is raised from 60° to 120° of elevation. Several soft tissue structures reside within this interval:

the subacromial bursa, the long head of the biceps tendon, and the rotator cuff (Fig. 2.15). Any condition that further narrows this interval (for example, a calcium deposit, swelling of the soft tissues, excessive overhang of the anterior acromion, etc.) can cause these soft tissues to be "impinged upon." If impingement involves the subacromial bursa, a bursitis occurs; if the long head of the biceps is involved, a bicipital tendinitis results; if the rotator cuff is involved, a rotator cuff tendinitis occurs. These familiar clinical entities are all included under the designation "impingement syndrome."

There are three stages of impingement. Stage I impingement is essentially an inflammation of the soft tissues within the impingement space. This usually occurs in individuals 25 years of age or younger. Stage II impingement usually occurs in individuals between 25 to 40 years of age. The soft tissues within the impingement interval are inflamed, but because these individuals have had multiple episodes in the past, some per-

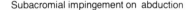

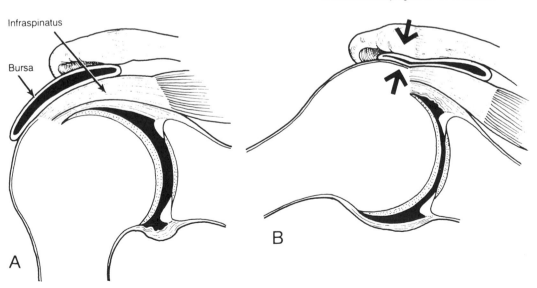

Figure 2.15. Subacromial impingement on glenohumeral abduction. *A*, the impingement interval and associated structures with the arm in neutral position. *B*, subacromial impingement on abduction. (By permission from Rowe CR, Leffert RD. Subacromial syndromes. In: Rowe CR, ed. The shoulder. New York: Churchill Livingstone, 1988:106.)

manent scarring, thickening, or fibrosis is also present. Stage III impingement usually occurs in individuals over 40 years of age who have had multiple episodes of impingement in the past. There is inflammation of the soft tissues in the impingement interval and permanent fibrosis, scarring, or thickening. In addition, either a complete thickness tear of the rotator cuff or a ruptured long head of the biceps tendon as well as associated bone alterations are present.

Clinical Characteristics

Pain is noted over the anterior aspect of the shoulder and may radiate down the front of the arm to, but not below, the elbow. Pain is elicited by palpation over the impingement interval. Pain over the anterior aspect of the shoulder is maximal when the arm is raised from 60° to 120° of elevation (the so-called "painful arc"), and especially with the arm internally rotated. If one injects the impingement interval with lidocaine without epinephrine, the patient's symptoms are transiently relieved (Fig. 2.16). X-rays of the shoulder may show bone spurs over the inferior aspect of the anterior acromion or the distal clavicle; cysts, irregularity, or sclerosis

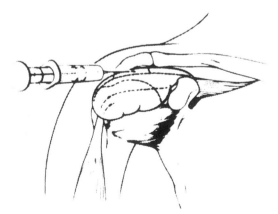

Figure 2.16.   The impingement injection test. (Lidocaine, 5 ml, is injected into the subacromial space. If the patient's symptoms on glenohumeral abduction are relieved, the diagnosis of impingement is highly likely.) (From Neer CS II. Impingement lesions. Clin Orthop 1983;173:70–77.)

over the greater tuberosity; or calcific deposits within the impingement interval.

When bicipital tendinitis is present, maximal discomfort is elicited when one palpates over the biceps groove and rolls the biceps tendon under the examining finger. Elevation of the arm is more painful when the elbow is extended and the forearm supinated, and less painful when the elbow is flexed and the forearm pronated. With the forearm in supination, flexion of the elbow against resistance will often cause pain over the anterior aspect of the shoulder.

In the case of acute subacromial bursitis, onset is abrupt and pain severe. There is tenderness and increased discomfort with shoulder motion. Erythema, edema, and visible swelling over the anterior aspect of the shoulder may be present. Body temperature and erythrocyte sedimentation rate may be elevated.

Characteristic clinical features associated with complete tears of the rotator cuff and ruptures of the long head of the biceps tendon will be discussed later in this chapter ("Stage III Rotator Cuff Syndrome" and "Acute Rupture of the Long Head of the Biceps Tendon").

Treatment

Stage I Impingement. When symptoms are acute, management includes avoidance of aggravating positions and activities (particularly raising the arm from 60° to 120° of elevation), ice packs applied to the anterior aspect of the shoulder, and analgesics. Anti-inflammatory medications are also helpful. Patients should gently put their arm through a full range of motion at least 2 or 3 times a day to prevent adhesive capsulitis. Sling immobilization is helpful. As the patient's symptoms improve, the sling can be discontinued gradually and increased functional use of the shoulder allowed. When the patient is pain-free, physiotherapy is instituted to help the individual regain normal shoulder range of motion, flexibility, and strength. Patients usually improve rapidly.

Stage II Impingement. These individuals tend to be more refractory to treatment. Initial management, however, is exactly the same as for those with Stage I impingement. If unsuccessful, the subacromial bursa can be injected with corticosteroids (Fig. 2.16). The author's preference is to inject 2 mg of methylprednisolone plus 2 ml of 1% lidocaine without epinephrine. Care should be taken to avoid injecting directly into the biceps tendon or the rotator cuff. The injection serves as a diagnostic as well as a therapeutic test. If the lidocaine alleviates discomfort during the 1st hour after the injection, the diagnosis of impingement is confirmed. If the corticosteroid gives lasting relief, so much the better. Corticosteroids cause degenerative changes within the local soft tissues, however, so no one area should be injected more than twice in a year.

Once symptoms have subsided, physiotherapy is prescribed to help the individual regain normal shoulder range of motion, flexibility, and strength. These individuals are told that theirs is a chronic condition and recurrences are common. Activities that require forceful and/or repetitive elevation of the arm through the painful arc are particularly likely to cause a recurrence. They are also encouraged to perform musclestrengthening exercises on a regular basis to help prevent upriding of the proximal humerus and open up the impingement space.

If impingement symptoms persist, referral to an orthopaedist is indicated for consideration of operative intervention. Surgical treatment consists of either an open or arthroscopic procedure designed to decompress/enlarge the impingement interval.

Stage III Impingement. These individuals have sustained either a rupture of the long head of the biceps tendon, or a full thickness tear of the rotator cuff. These clinical entities will be discussed later in this chapter ("Acute Rupture of the Long Head of the Biceps Tendon" and "Stage III Rotator Cuff Syndrome").

MUSCULOTENDINOUS (ROTATOR) CUFF SYNDROME

Lying within the impingement interval, the rotator cuff and particularly the supraspinatus tendon are prone to attritional disease. The same three stages occur as described in the section on "Impingement Syndrome."

Stage I Rotator Cuff Syndrome

This generally occurs in individuals 25 years of age or younger, and is simply a rotator cuff tendinitis secondary to forceful and/or repetitive elevation of the arm. Signs and symptoms are the same as those described for impingement syndrome. Treatment is the same as that described for Stage I impingement syndrome and usually results in rapid improvement.

Stage II Rotator Cuff Syndrome

This is a Stage II impingement lesion, which usually occurs in patients 25 to 40 years of age who have had multiple previous episodes. In addition to inflammation of the rotator cuff, some permanent fibrosis, thickening, or scarring is present and impingement symptoms are evident. Calcific deposits may be noted within the rotator cuff on x-ray. Treatment is the same as that described for Stage II impingement syndrome. If simple nonoperative modalities such as rest, ice followed by heat, analgesics, and oral anti-inflammatory medications are ineffective, the impingement interval may be injected with a corticosteroid plus lidocaine. If symptoms persist or return quickly, referral to an orthopaedist is indicated for consideration of a surgical shoulder decompression.

Stage III Rotator Cuff Syndrome (Fig. 2.17)

This is a Stage III impingement lesion—a complete thickness tear of the rotator cuff.

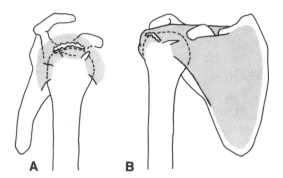

Figure 2.17. A musculotendinous cuff tear. *A,* lateral view. *B,* anterior view.

These individuals are usually 40 years of age or older, and have had multiple episodes of impingement in the past. The rotator cuff gradually degenerates until it finally tears through. Consequently, the process is rather insidious and frequently no significant precipitating traumatic event is noted. Once a complete thickness tear develops, the involved tendons begin to retract, causing the defect to become increasingly large. In addition to the usual impingement symptoms, patients note increasing shoulder pain and crepitus as the proximal humerus begins to rub against the undersurface of the acromion. These individuals also note increasing weakness when trying to elevate and externally rotate their arm. On physical examination, subacromial crepitus is usually palpable during passive and active range of motion of the shoulder. Once the diagnosis is suspected, a shoulder arthrogram should be ordered. If a full-thickness rotator cuff tear is present, dye injected into the glenohumeral joint space escapes through the defect into the more superficial soft tissues.

Treatment of Full-Thickness Rotator Cuff Tears. These individuals should be referred to an orthopaedist for subsequent care. Assuming the patient is amenable and medically fit, the author believes that full-thickness rotator cuff tears should be surgically repaired and the impingement interval decompressed as soon as possible after the

diagnosis is made. As time passes, the tear becomes larger, the patient's signs and symptoms worse, the surgical repair more difficult, and the postoperative result less satisfactory.

ACUTE RUPTURE OF THE LONG HEAD OF THE BICEPS TENDON

The tendon of the long head of the biceps muscle passes through the impingement interval of the shoulder and as a result is subject to degenerative or attritional disease. In individuals under the age of 40, this results in episodes of bicipital tendinitis (Stage I and Stage II impingement; see section on "Impingement Syndrome"), and in individuals usually over the age of 40, a complete rupture of the tendon may occur (Stage III impingement) (Fig. 2.18).

Clinical Characteristics

The individual is usually 40 years of age or older and has had episodes of impingement in the past. The patient reports a sudden and usually painful popping sensation over the anterior upper arm or shoulder during a lifting effort. The retracted belly of the biceps muscle bulges over the anterior aspect of the distal arm and a concavity is visible over the anterior aspect of the proximal arm. The distal bulge is particularly prominent when the elbow is flexed against resistance. The upper arm is painful and tender to palpation for several days following the rupture. Active use of the shoulder and elbow often increases the discomfort. Ecchymosis generally appears over the distal arm and elbow several days after the rupture. As the acute tissue irritation subsides, elbow flexion-forearm supination strength gradually returns, and with exercise can return to near normal. Usually, however, a 5 to 10% deficit persists.

Treatment

Referral to an orthopaedist is indicated. If diagnosed within 5 to 7 days, surgical repair

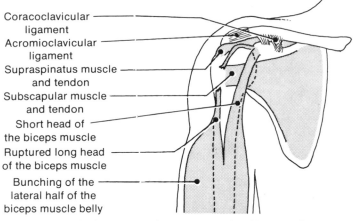

Coracoclavicular ligament
Acromioclavicular ligament
Supraspinatus muscle and tendon
Subscapular muscle and tendon
Short head of the biceps muscle
Ruptured long head of the biceps muscle
Bunching of the lateral half of the biceps muscle belly

Figure 2.18. Rupture of the long head of the biceps tendon.

of the biceps tendon is considered as well as a shoulder decompression to prevent continued impingement. After 7 days, the ruptured tendon is generally too contracted or fibrosed to allow repair. Fortunately, these individuals generally do quite well with conservative nonoperative care, despite the altered cosmetic appearance of their arm and approximately 5 to 10% loss of elbow flexion-forearm supination strength.

ADHESIVE CAPSULITIS (FROZEN SHOULDER)

The shoulder complex is particularly prone to symptomatic stiffness. This is formally known as adhesive capsulitis, but commonly referred to as a frozen shoulder. Anything that causes shoulder discomfort (intrinsic disorders, e.g., fractures, impingement syndrome, etc., or pain referred from another area, e.g., left shoulder pain secondary to angina pectoris or myocardial infarction) can be the initiating event. The patient consciously or subconsciously limits the use of the shoulder because of pain, and soft tissue tightness/stiffness in one or more directions develops. Discomfort then occurs when the patient moves the arm and the contracted soft tissues are stretched. The individual limits motion even more, further stiffness occurs, and a vicious cycle ensues.

The patient eventually seeks medical care because of shoulder pain and limited movement.

Clinical Characteristics

The shoulder is comfortable when at rest. Shoulder motion is limited in one or more directions with pain occurring at the limits of motion. The physical examination is otherwise relatively unremarkable. Usually no local pain to palpation is found. Routine x-rays are generally unremarkable.

Treatment

Treatment consists of breaking up the adhesions and stretching out the contracted soft tissues responsible for the condition. Daily intensive sessions with a physiotherapist for 3 weeks are prescribed and the focus is on manually stretching the shoulder in the direction(s) of limited mobility. The patient is instructed to perform the same exercises 4 times a day at home at evenly spaced intervals. Judicious use of analgesics is often helpful in allowing the individual to perform the stretching exercises optimally. As motion improves, the overall function of the shoulder gradually returns to normal and discomfort subsides. The patient's progress is noted by the physician at 3-week intervals. Physiotherapy should continue until either full range of motion is achieved, or until the patient's improvement plateaus. If the individual's motion plateaus short of normal, the patient and the physician must decide whether the residual symptoms and the shoulder mobility are acceptable. If not, referral to an orthopaedist is indicated for consideration of a manipulation of the shoulder under anesthesia.

MINOR SPRAINS, MINOR STRAINS, CONTUSIONS, AND OVERUSE SYNDROME

The most common injuries to the shoulder and upper arm regions are minor sprains, minor strains, contusions, and overuse syndrome.

Minor sprain: This is a lesser injury to a ligamentous structure produced by an indirect force. The tissues are merely stretched—not ruptured or partially torn.

Minor strain: This is a minor injury to a musculotendinous structure caused by an indirect force. The tissues are merely stretched—not ruptured or partially torn.

Contusion: This is a minor injury to bone and/or soft tissue caused by a directly applied force.

Overuse syndrome: This is a minor injury to bone and/or soft tissue caused by the application of stresses to which the tissues are not accustomed. In general, symptoms do not occur during the activity, but up to 48 hours later.

These injuries share similar clinical features. The patient may or may not be able to remember a specific initiating event, and may or may not be able to localize the symptoms. Swelling, discoloration, or both may be present over the involved area. Pain to palpation is generally present over the involved tissues and shoulder motions that stress or require use of the involved tissues elicit pain. X-rays of the shoulder are unremarkable. The diagnosis is often one of exclusion: one rules out more serious clinical entities.

Treatment

Treatment is similar for each of these clinical entities. The patient is advised to rest the shoulder (avoid aggravating positions and activities) to allow the involved tissues to heal. Local application of ice during the first 48 hours after injury is helpful, followed by local moist heat thereafter. Over-the-counter analgesics are usually sufficient and anti-inflammatory medications may be useful. Sling immobilization may be necessary initially for comfort, but the individual should at least be encouraged to put the shoulder through a full passive/active-assistive range of motion 1 to 2 times a day to prevent adhesive capsulitis. Occasionally, an injection of cortisone into an area of very localized pain will be helpful. The patient should be encouraged to gradually increase the functional use of the shoulder as symptoms resolve. Progressive exercises to regain shoulder range of motion, flexibility, and strength are worthwhile. These patients generally improve fairly rapidly, although symptoms may persist for 4 to 6 weeks. A full functional recovery is the rule.

RADIAL NERVE PALSY

The radial nerve is vulnerable to a compression neuropathy commonly referred to as the "Saturday night palsy." This syndrome of radial nerve dysfunction is caused by prolonged pressure on the nerve for whatever reason at any point along its course down the upper arm. (Individuals acutely intoxicated by a Saturday night binge may fall deeply asleep and remain motionless for a significant period of time with their arm resting against an object, causing compression of the radial nerve. The individual later awakens with a radial nerve palsy, hence the origin of the name). These patients either have difficulty actively extending their wrist and digit metacarpophalangeal joints, or are unable to do so. They also note diminished or absent sensation over the first dorsal web space. These patients should be referred to an orthopaedist for subsequent care; however, treatment consists primarily of reassurance that nerve function will return. The individual is told to avoid positions that apply pressure on the nerve. A removable volar splint is made to hold the wrist and metacarpophalangeal joints in an extended position. Radial nerve function gradually returns over time.

DELTOID TENDINITIS

Forceful, prolonged, and/or repetitive use of the deltoid muscle may result in inflammation of its origin or tendinous insertion. Such involvement of its insertion is fairly common.

Clinical Characteristics

Adults in their middle years or older seem to be most commonly affected. The individual often relates the onset of symptoms to a direct blow to the area, a sudden abduction strain, or an activity involving prolonged or repetitive abduction of the arm. Pain is felt over the deltoid muscle and down the lateral aspect of the arm. The individual may note paresthesias and aching over the entire extremity. Passive range of motion of the shoulder is usually full, though uncomfortable. Pain is especially acute when the arm is actively abducted against resistance. The patient is tender to palpation directly over the deltoid insertion on the lateral aspect of the humerus. X-rays are usually unremarkable.

Treatment

The patient should avoid aggravating positions and activities, particularly forceful and/or repetitive abduction of the shoulder. Use of an arm sling is helpful. The individual is instructed, however, to remove the sling and put the shoulder through a full passive range of motion once or twice a day to prevent adhesive capsulitis. The patient is en-couraged to gradually increase active shoulder motion and use as symptoms subside. Nonprescription analgesics are generally sufficient. Anti-inflammatory medications may be helpful. Local application of ice during the first 48 hours after the onset of symptoms is recommended. Thereafter, application of moist heat to the symptomatic area is helpful. In particularly severe or persistent cases, an injection of corticosteroid plus 1% lidocaine without epinephrine adjacent to, but not within, the affected tendon can result in rapid and complete alleviation of symptoms.

Traumatic Disorders of the Shoulder and Upper Arm

SPRAINS OF THE AC JOINT

A sprain is an injury to the ligamentous structures that stabilize an articulation. Three types of AC joint sprains may occur (Fig. 2.19): Grade I, Grade II (subluxation of the AC joint), and Grade III (dislocation of the AC joint). The mechanism of injury is usually a fall on the acromion process which forces the scapula down and applies stress to the acromioclavicular and coracoclavicular ligaments.

Grade I Sprains of the Acromioclavicular Joint

In this injury, the acromioclavicular ligaments are significantly stressed but not torn. Characteristic clinical features include the following. The patient usually describes an injury in which a significant force was applied to the superolateral aspect of the shoulder, followed by pain over the AC joint. The AC joint is tender to local palpation and painful on attempted shoulder motion. The area may also be slightly swollen. X-rays of the AC joint obtained with the patient standing and holding 10-pound weights in both hands will show a normal relationship between the affected acromion and clavicle.

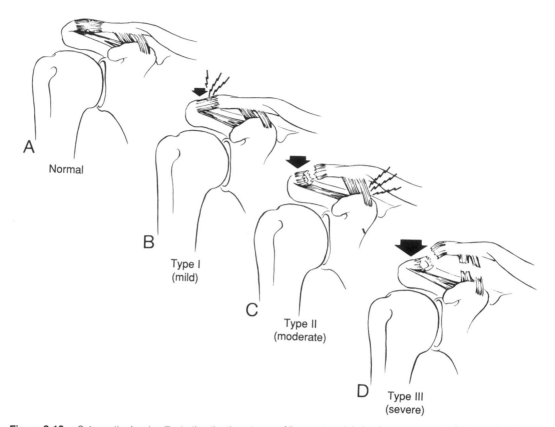

A
Normal

B
Type I
(mild)

C
Type II
(moderate)

D   Type III
(severe)

Figure 2.19.   Schematic drawing illustrating the three types of ligamentous injuries that can occur at the acromioclavicular joint. *A*, normal. *B*, type I: stretched acromioclavicular ligaments. *C*, type II: torn acromioclavicular ligaments and stretched coracoclavicular ligaments allowing partial displacement of the acromioclavicular joint. *D*, type III: torn acromioclavicular and coracoclavicular ligaments allowing complete displacement of the acromioclavicular joint. (From Rockwood CA, Green DP, eds. Fractures, vol 1. 1st ed. Philadelphia: JB Lippincott Co, 1975:729 and from Allman FL Jr. Fractures and ligamentous injuries of the clavicle and its articulation. J Bone Joint Surg 1967;49A:774–784.)

Treatment. The affected extremity is initially immobilized in a sling and swathe dressing for comfort. Functional use of the shoulder is permitted and gradually increased to normal as symptoms allow. Local application of ice is helpful during the first 48 hours, followed by moist heat thereafter as symptoms require. Over-the-counter pain medications should be sufficient.

Grade II Sprains of the AC Joint (Subluxation)

This injury represents a complete tear of the acromioclavicular ligaments. Character-

istic clinical features include the following. The patient usually describes an injury in which a significant force was applied to the superolateral aspect of the shoulder, followed by pain over the AC joint. The AC joint is locally tender to palpation and painful on range of motion of the shoulder. Swelling may be noted over the AC joint. The outer end of the clavicle may be noted to protrude slightly upward. X-rays of the affected AC joint obtained with the patient standing and holding 10-pound weights in both hands reveal that the inferior margin of the distal clavicle lies above the inferior margin but below the superior margin of the acromion.

Treatment. This is a controversial area. Many believe that an acute traumatic subluxation of the AC joint should be treated surgically with an open reduction and internal fixation to restore normal anatomy. Others, including the author, usually prefer to treat this injury in the same manner as the Grade I acromioclavicular sprain. With nonoperative treatment, the end result is usually quite satisfactory, although a prominence of the outer end of the clavicle may remain, a 5 to 10% loss of shoulder strength may occur, and symptomatic degenerative disease of the AC joint may develop at a later date. Referral to an orthopaedist is therefore indicated so that the nonoperative versus operative treatment can be fully discussed. Should symptomatic degenerative disease of the AC joint develop, the therapeutic modalities described in the section on degenerative joint disease of the AC joint are employed.

Grade III Sprains of the AC Joint (Dislocation)

Grade III sprains of the AC joint represent a complete disruption of the acromioclavicular and coracoclavicular ligaments. This injury permits the sternocleidomastoid muscle to pull the clavicle upward, while the weight of the extremity pulls the shoulder downward. Characteristic clinical features include the following. The patient usually describes an injury in which a significant force is applied to the superolateral aspect of the shoulder, followed by pain over the AC joint. The AC joint is markedly tender to local palpation and painful on shoulder range of motion. Swelling and ecchymosis are often present over the AC joint. The outer end of the clavicle is generally noted to be quite prominent superiorly. X-rays obtained with the patient standing and holding 10-pound weights in both hands show superior displacement of the clavicle, such that the in-

ferior margin of the distal clavicle lies at or above the superior margin of the adjacent acromion.

Treatment. Again, controversy exists regarding treatment of these injuries. Some believe that the dislocation should be surgically reduced and internally fixed to restore normal anatomy and, hopefully, normal shoulder function. Others prefer the application of external braces designed to restore the normal relationship between the affected clavicle and the acromion, also in hopes of restoring normal shoulder appearance and function. These braces must be worn continually for 6 weeks, and frequently checked and readjusted. Unfortunately, they often cause skin breakdown, and some displacement frequently occurs as soon as the brace is discontinued. Many, including the author, believe that Grade III sprains can be managed in the same manner as Grade I sprains with very satisfactory functional results. The patient should be aware, however, that there will be a permanent prominence of the distal clavicle and approximately 5 to 10% loss of shoulder strength. As with Grade II sprains of the AC joint, referral to an orthopaedist is indicated so that nonoperative versus operative treatment can be fully discussed.

SPRAINS OF THE SC JOINT

Sprains of the SC joint are uncommon injuries resulting from strong and unusually directed forces applied to the stabilizing ligaments. Three grades of sprains can occur, depending on the severity of the force applied (Fig. 2.20).

Grade I and Grade II (Subluxation) Sprains of the SC Joint

A Grade I sprain represents a stretching or partial tear of the sternoclavicular ligaments, while a Grade II sprain (subluxation) represents a complete tear of the sternoclavicular ligaments. Both injuries cause the individual to present with pain (especially with shoul-

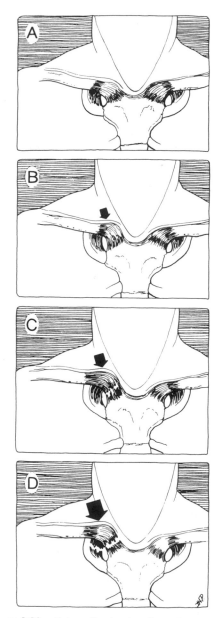

Figure 2.20. Schematic drawing illustrating the three types of ligamentous injuries that can occur at the sternoclavicular joint. *A*, normal. *B*, type I: stretched sternoclavicular ligaments. *C*, type II: torn sternoclavicular ligaments and stretched costoclavicular ligament allowing partial displacement of the sternoclavicular joint. *D*, type III: torn sternoclavicular and costoclavicular ligaments allowing complete displacement of the sternoclavicular joint. (From Post M. The shoulder: surgical and non-surgical management. 2nd ed. Philadelphia: Lea & Febiger, 1988:598.)

der motion), tenderness, and swelling over the involved articulation. Treatment is essentially symptomatic. Sling and/or figure-of-eight splintage is prescribed as necessary for comfort, followed by increase in functional use of the extremity as symptoms allow. Ice is applied to the involved area during the first 48 hours, followed by local moist heat thereafter. Analgesic medications may be needed.

Grade III Sprains (Dislocation) of the SC Joint

In this injury, the costoclavicular ligament as well as the sternoclavicular ligaments are completely torn, allowing the articulation to dislocate either anteriorly or posteriorly.

Clinical Characteristics. Anterior Dislocation: Severe pain and tenderness are present over the SC joint. Any movement of the shoulder causes increased pain. Pain is increased when the patient is supine, and the individual prefers to be in the sitting position, supporting the arm on the injured side. The anteriorly displaced medial end of the clavicle is generally quite visible.

Posterior Dislocation: Severe pain and tenderness are present over the SC joint. Any movement of the shoulder causes increased pain. Pain is increased when the patient is supine and the patient prefers to be in the sitting position, supporting the arm on the injured side. The usually prominent medial end of the clavicle is not visible or palpable because of its posterior displacement. Posterior dislocation of the SC joint may cause pressure on the great vessels, the trachea, or the esophagus. Either the dislocation itself or associated injuries to the chest wall may result in a pneumothorax. These complications are manifested by venous congestion in the neck, partial or complete airway obstruction, and difficulty in swallowing. If the pneumothorax is extensive, the patient may complain of air hunger and breathing may be rapid. Breath sounds are diminished over the area of the pneumothorax. A tension pneumothorax is suggested by the usual signs of vascular collapse.

An x-ray is generally necessary to confirm the diagnosis of a sternoclavicular dislocation (Fig. 2.21). Oblique roentgenograms are often quite helpful since standard AP projections are frequently difficult to interpret. Even more definitive is a CT scan of the articulation.

Treatment (Fig. 2.22). Anterior Dislocation: At least one attempt at a closed reduction is reasonable. Intravenous sedation is usually adequate, but occasionally general anesthesia is necessary. The patient is positioned supine at the edge of a table with a sandbag beneath the scapula. The injured arm is abducted 90° and extended to the point of resistance (about 15°). While traction is being applied to the injured extremity, the medial end of the clavicle is pushed posteriorly. Reduction is usually easy, but generally unstable. A figure-of-eight bandage holding the shoulder back and a sling supporting the arm are then worn for 6 weeks. Strenuous activities are prohibited for an additional 2 weeks. If the dislocation cannot be reduced or the reduction cannot be maintained, an orthopaedist should be consulted. Whether anatomic healing is achieved or not, however, satisfactory painless function usually results.

Posterior Dislocation: An immediate orthopaedic consultation should be requested. When pressure on the great vessels or the trachea is posing a threat to life, reduction of the dislocation becomes an emergency. Unless the patient is in extremis, general anesthesia or intravenous sedation should be used. The patient is positioned supine at the edge of a table with a sandbag beneath the scapula. The arm is abducted 90° and extended to the point of resistance (about 15°). As traction is applied to the extremity, reduction of the dislocation may occur. How-

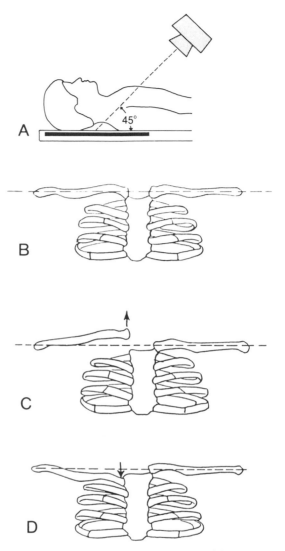

Figure 2.21. Cephalic tilt roentgenogram of the sternoclavicular joint. *A,* positioning of the patient. *B,* normal appearance at the sternoclavicular joint. *C,* when the clavicle is dislocated anteriorly, it is projected above the horizontal plane. *D,* when the clavicle is dislocated posteriorly, it is projected below the horizontal plane. (*B–D* from DePalma AF. Surgery of the shoulder. 3rd ed. Philadelphia: JB Lippincott Co, 1983:452.)

ever, it may be necessary to pull the medial end of the clavicle outward either manually or with a towel clip. In most cases, the clav-

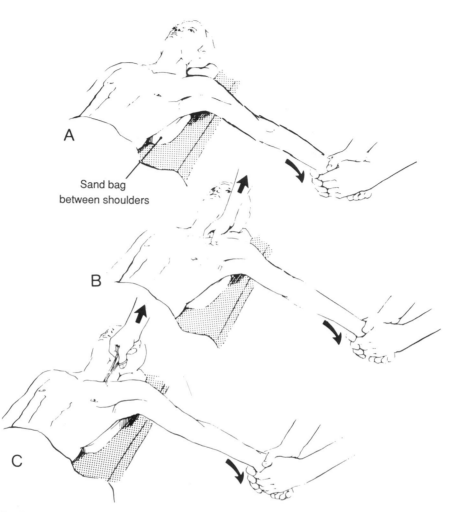

Figure 2.22. Technique for closed reduction of the sternoclavicular joint. *A*, positioning the patient and application of longitudinal traction with the arm in abduction and slight extension. In anterior dislocations, direct anterior pressure may be required to replace the medial end of the clavicle. *B*, in posterior dislocations of the sternoclavicular joint, in addition to traction, it may be necessary to lift the clavicle from behind the manubrium with the fingers. *C*, in difficult cases of posterior dislocation of the sternoclavicular joint, a sterile towel clip may be used to grasp the medial end of the clavicle to lift it laterally and anteriorly. (From Rockwood CA, Green DP, eds. Fractures in adults, vol 1. 2nd ed. Philadelphia: JB Lippincott Co, 1984:929.)

icle will reduce with an notable "pop." Reduction must be achieved and operative intervention may be necessary. Once obtained, the reduction is generally quite stable. A figure-of-eight bandage is then applied and maintained for 6 weeks. Strenuous activities are prohibited for an additional 2 weeks.

ACUTE DISLOCATIONS OF THE GLENOHUMERAL JOINT

The shoulder is the most mobile joint in the body, but also the most prone to instability. Acute dislocations are usually the result of indirect forces applied to the glenohumeral joint, and are most commonly seen in vigorous young and middle-aged adults.

The shoulder can dislocate either anteriorly or posteriorly. Anterior dislocations comprise approximately 95% of such injuries, while posterior dislocations make up the remaining 5%.

Acute Anterior Dislocation of the Glenohumeral Joint (Fig. 2.23)

This injury occurs when the shoulder is forcefully abducted-extended-externally rotated. The humeral head is forced out of the glenoid anteriorly and comes to rest beneath the coracoid process, the clavicle, or the glenoid.

Clinical Characteristics. The arm is held close to the body, slightly abducted and internally rotated. The patient is usually in considerable distress and any attempt to move the shoulder accentuates the pain. The normal contour of the shoulder (convex to the lateral side) is lost. The shoulder appears flattened laterally and unusually prominent anteriorly. X-rays taken in two planes (AP and lateral scapula or axillary views) will confirm the dislocation.

The physician should always look for associated injuries, including proximal humeral fractures (see section on "Fractures of the Proximal Humerus"), avulsion of the rotator cuff (see section on "Musculotendinous (Rotator) Cuff Syndrome"), and injuries to the adjacent neurovascular structures. The axillary nerve is the most likely to be involved. Patients with injuries to this structure are unable to actively contract the deltoid muscle, and note a small area of decreased sensation over the midlateral aspect of the shoulder. The injury is usually a neurapraxia and function gradually returns to normal once the shoulder is reduced. The other nerves in the area are rarely injured, but a thorough neurologic examination should be performed after reduction. Injury to the axillary vessels is also rare, but when it occurs the consequences can be catastrophic. Again, once the shoulder has been reduced, assessment of the vascular integrity of the extremity should be performed.

Treatment. The dislocation should be reduced as soon as possible. Many maneuvers have been described, but two basic principles should be observed: the patient should be completely relaxed, and the maneuver should be done gently to avoid fur-

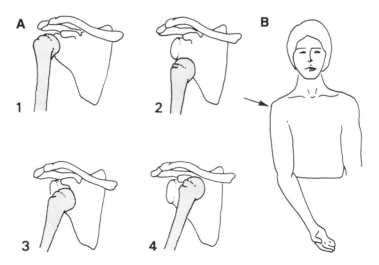

Figure 2.23. Acute anterior dislocation of the glenohumeral joint. *A*, the positions: *1*, normal; *2*, subglenoid; *3*, subcoracoid; *4*, subclavicular. *B*, anterior view of the patient's appearance. The round prominence of the shoulder has shifted anteriorly, leaving the lateral salient flat (*arrow*).

ther damage to the articulation. The author presently sedates patients with intravenous diazepam. The patient is positioned supine on the examining table with the injured arm abducted as far as possible and the elbow flexed to 90°. An assistant stands at the opposite side of the table, passes a sheet around the patient's torso, and holds the sheet to stabilize the patient's upper body. The physician ties another sheet in a loop, stands inside the loop, and also places the loop over the patient's injured arm (Fig. 2.24). The physician then gradually leans back against the looped sheet. This progressive pull down the long axis of the humerus combined with gentle anterior pressure over the shoulder and slight internal rotation usually effects the reduction quickly and easily. After the reduction, x-rays should be obtained in two planes (AP and lateral scapula or axillary views) to be certain that the reduction has been effected and no associated fracture(s) missed. If the shoulder is irreducible, referral to an orthopaedist is indicated.

Following the reduction, the patient's arm is immobilized in a sling and swathe dressing (Fig. 2.25). Individuals over the age of 40 are immobilized for 7 to 10 days for comfort and then encouraged to gradually increase the functional use of their shoulder as symptoms allow. Individuals under the age of 40 are at significant risk for redislocation (the younger they are at the time of the initial dislocation, the higher the risk). Consequently, the author recommends a full 6 weeks of sling and swathe immobilization for these individuals to promote healing of the damaged retaining structures. This is followed by an intensive physiotherapy program designed to help the patient regain range of motion of the shoulder initially, and then strengthen the anterior muscle groups in hopes of decreasing the chances of redislocation.

Acute Posterior Dislocation of the Glenohumeral Joint (Fig. 2.26)

Posterior dislocation of the glenohumeral joint is relatively uncommon and unfortunately frequently missed on the initial eval-

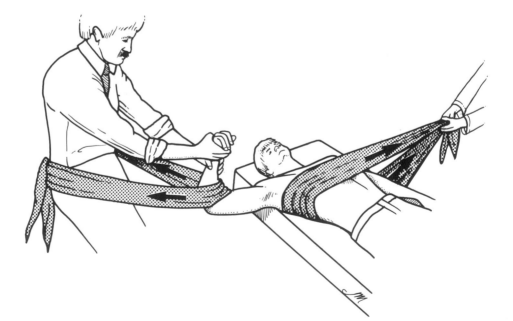

Figure 2.24. Closed reduction of a dislocated glenohumeral joint using the "double-looped sheet" method.

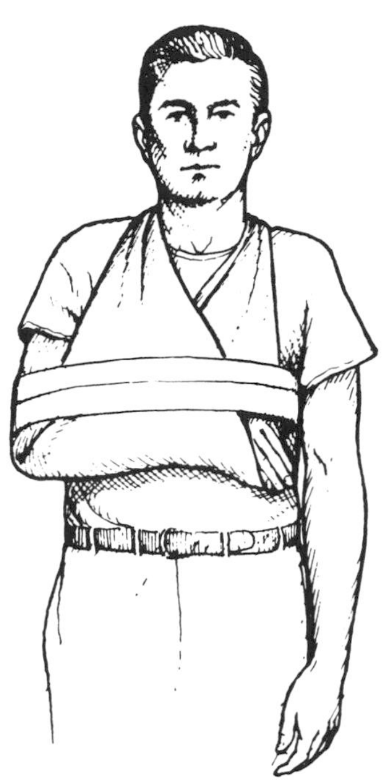

uation. It may be the result of either a direct or indirect force applied to the shoulder forcing the humeral head posteriorly out of the glenoid. Posterior dislocations are also frequently seen in individuals who have had a convulsion due to the severe associated contractions of the shoulder musculature.

Clinical Characteristics. The patient is in considerable distress and resists any attempt to move the shoulder. The arm is kept in a position of adduction and internal rotation. The coracoid process is abnormally prominent anteriorly, and swelling or a lump may be visible or palpable posteriorly. Three abnormalities often appear on the routine AP x-ray projection: the normal smooth, curved contour of the greater tuberosity laterally is absent due to internal rotation of the humerus; the normal parallelism between the humeral articular surface and the anterior glenoid rim is lost; the head of the dislocated humerus is displaced upward relative to the glenoid fossa. In addition to the AP projection, either an axillary or a lateral scapula view should be obtained in any

Figure 2.25. The conventional sling and swathe dressing for immobilization of the shoulder. (From Rockwood CA, Green DP, eds. Fractures in adults, vol 1. 2nd ed. Philadelphia: JB Lippincott Co, 1984:684.)

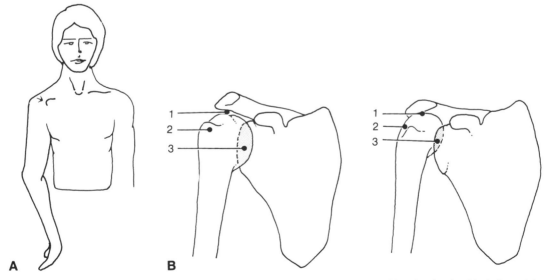

Figure 2.26. Posterior dislocation of the glenohumeral joint. *A,* patient's appearance. Note that the shoulder is flat and the coracoid process protrudes (arrow). *B,* three diagnostic features on the AP x-ray projection. *Left,* normal. *1,* upper border of the head of the humerus in normal position. *2,* normal contour reveals the greater tuberosity. *3,* half-moon crescent of projected overlap. *Right,* posterior dislocation. *1,* head of the humerus after dislocation, superior to normal position. *2,* internal rotation hides the greater tuberosity. *3,* half-moon crescent of projected overlap no longer apparent.

shoulder which has been injured. This will confirm the presence of a posterior dislocation.

Treatment. The same therapeutic principles described in the section on "Acute Anterior Dislocation of the Glenohumeral Joint" should be followed and the "looped sheet reduction maneuver" can be used. As traction is applied, the shoulder is gradually rotated externally and the humeral head pushed forward. X-rays in the AP and axillary or lateral scapula planes should be obtained after reduction to confirm that the dislocation has been reduced. A shoulder spica holding the arm in 20° of external rotation is then applied (Fig. 2.27). Consequently, an orthopaedic referral for application of the spica cast and subsequent care is usually most practical. As with acute anterior dislocations, patients over 40 years of age are immobilized 7 to 10 days for comfort, while patients under 40 years of age are immobilized for 6 weeks. When immobilization is discontinued, an intensive physiotherapy program is instituted to help the patient regain shoulder range of motion initially, and then strengthen the posterior muscle groups (the

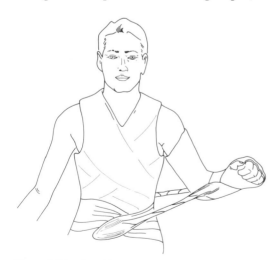

Figure 2.27. Shoulder spica used for immobilization after reduction of a posterior glenohumeral dislocation. Note that the shoulder is held in abduction and external rotation. (From Goss TP. Factors to consider in chronic symptomatic shoulder instability. Orthop Rev 1985;XIV(10):27–32.)

extensors and external rotators) in hopes of decreasing the chances of redislocation. If the shoulder is irreducible, referral to an orthopaedist is indicated.

FRACTURES OF THE CLAVICLE
Fractures of the Middle Third of the Clavicle

Most clavicular fractures occur through the middle third. The medial or proximal fragment is usually displaced upward because of the pull of the sternocleidomastoid muscle, and the lateral or distal fragment is usually displaced downward by the weight of the arm (Fig. 2.28A). Neurovascular injury is uncommon.

The figure-of-eight bandage (Fig. 2.28B) is the traditional method of treatment. Its primary intent is to reduce motion at the fracture site, thereby reducing the patient's discomfort. During the 1st week or 2 after injury, an arm sling may be added to support the weight of the arm and provide further pain relief. Although anatomic reduction of the fracture fragments is seldom obtained, these fractures almost always heal with full restoration of shoulder function and an acceptable cosmetic deformity. If a large gap is present at the fracture site after application of the figure-of-eight bandage, referral to an orthopaedist is indicated.

The figure-of-eight bandage is worn constantly for a period of at least 6 weeks (4 weeks for preadolescents). The patient is allowed to use the arm as symptoms allow, but strenuous activities are contraindicated. The fracture is considered to be healed at any time from 6 weeks onward, when adequate callus is visible on x-ray examination, when palpation of the fracture site is painless, and when the patient can move the arm fully without discomfort at the fracture site. After removal of the figure-of-eight bandage, the patient should be encouraged to gradually increase the functional use of the affected extremity while avoiding strenuous activities

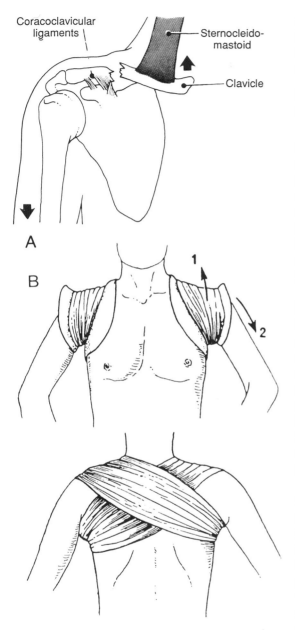

Coracoclavicular ligaments

Sternocleido-mastoid

Clavicle

A

B

Figure 2.28. A complete fracture of the middle third of the clavicle. *A*, forces causing displacement. *1*, the shoulder is held up, outward, and backward; *2*, the length and alignment of the clavicle are restored and maintained by the weight of the arms over the axillary pads. *B*, the figure-of-eight bandage used for immobilization. *1*, . . . pads (from DePalma AF. Surgery of the shoulder. 3rd ed. Philadelphia: JB Lippincott Co, 1983:351).

(sports, etc.) for an additional month. If one thinks that union is not proceeding satisfactorily, referral to an orthopaedist is indicated.

Fractures of the Lateral Third of the Clavicle

There are three types of lateral clavicular fractures (Fig. 2.29). In Type I fractures, the coracoclavicular ligaments remain attached to the proximal fragment. Consequently, displacement at the fracture site is within acceptable limits and figure-of-eight bandage immobilization is sufficient. The duration of immobilization and therapeutic principles are the same as those advised for fractures of the middle third of the clavicle.

In Type II fractures, the coracoclavicular ligaments are torn away from the proximal fragment. The proximal fragment is then drawn superiorly and posteriorly by the unopposed pull of the trapezius and sternocleidomastoid muscles, while the distal fragment is drawn down by the weight of the arm, creating a large gap at the fracture site. Surgical reduction and internal fixation of these fractures is necessary if union is to occur. These fractures, therefore, require orthopaedic referral for definitive care.

In Type III injuries, the articular surface of the distal clavicle is violated. These fractures are managed symptomatically with a figure of eight bandage and/or sling immobilization of the arm for discomfort, and gradual increase in functional use of the extremity as symptoms allow. Union usually occurs within 6 weeks. Symptomatic degenerative disease of the AC joint may occur at a later date. If sufficiently painful or disabling, surgical excision of the distal 0.5 inch of the clavicle is the treatment of choice.

Epiphyseal Separation at the Sternal End of the Clavicle

Patients younger than 25 years of age may suffer an epiphyseal separation when the medial end of the clavicle is subjected to

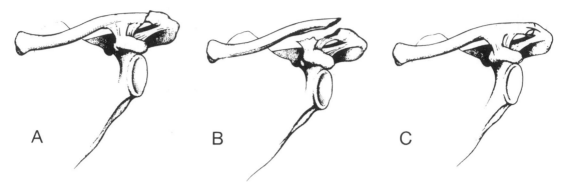

Figure 2.29.   Classification of fractures of the distal clavicle. *A*, type I (minimal displacement and intact ligaments). *B*, type II (significant displacement due to ruptured coracoclavicular ligaments). *C*, type III (intraarticular fracture). (From Rockwood CA, Green DP, eds. Fractures in adults, vol 1. 2nd ed. Philadelphia: JB Lippincott Company, 1984:708.)

significant direct or indirect forces (Fig. 2.30). This injury should not be mistaken for a sternoclavicular dislocation, which usually occurs in older patients. Treatment is identical to that described for the corresponding sternoclavicular dislocation (see section on "Sprains of the SC Joint" in this chapter).

Fractures of the Sternal End of the Clavicle

These fractures are more likely to occur after the age of 25 years, and are the result of forces similar to those that can dislocate the SC joint. Treatment is identical to that described for the corresponding sternoclavicular dislocation (see section on "Sprains of the SC Joint" in this chapter).

FRACTURES OF THE SCAPULA (FIG. 2.31)

Fractures of the body of the scapula usually demand little more than symptomatic care (use of an arm sling for comfort). One should look for and aggressively treat such serious associated injuries as multiple rib fractures resulting in a flail chest, hemothorax and/or pneumothorax, myocardial contusion, aortic tears, etc.

Fractures of the scapula may involve the articular surface of the glenoid. Undisplaced fractures are managed symptomatically with sling immobilization for discomfort and gradual increase in functional use of the shoulder as symptoms allow. Union occurs within 6 weeks. A displaced intraarticular glenoid fracture, however, should be re-

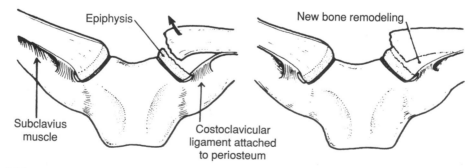

Figure 2.30.   Epiphyseal separation at the sternal end of the clavicle. (With permission from Rowe CR. Acromioclavicular and sternoclavicular joints. In: Rowe CR, ed. The shoulder. New York: Churchill Livingstone, 1988:317.)

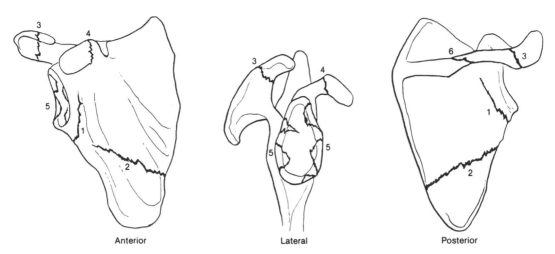

Anterior   Lateral   Posterior

Figure 2.31. Fractures of the scapula: *1,* Glenoid neck; *2,* body; *3,* acromion; *4,* coracoid process; *5,* glenoid fossa; *6,* spinous process. (From DePalma AF. Surgery of the shoulder. 3rd ed. Philadelphia: JB Lippincott Co, 1983:364.)

ferred to an orthopaedist since surgical reduction and internal fixation may be required.

Scapular fractures may also occur through the glenoid neck, acromion, and coracoid process. Unless deformity and displacement are severe, symptomatic sling immobilization is the treatment of choice with gradual increase in functional use of the extremity as symptoms allow. At 6 weeks, union is usually complete.

FRACTURES OF THE PROXIMAL HUMERUS

Fractures of the proximal humerus make up 4 to 5% of fractures in general and are more commonly seen in older individuals.

Clinical Characteristics

A significant force has been applied either directly or indirectly to the shoulder region and the patient localizes discomfort to the area. The shoulder is usually swollen, ecchymotic, and diffusely tender. Any attempt to move the shoulder causes increased pain. Neutral AP, transthoracic lateral, axillary, and lateral scapula views of the shoulder demonstrate the fracture.

Treatment

The proximal humerus is composed of four segments: the articular segment, the greater tuberosity, the lesser tuberosity, and the humeral shaft (Fig. 2.32A). Eighty percent of proximal humeral fractures are minimally displaced, i.e., none of the four major segments is displaced greater than or equal to 1 cm, nor rotated greater than or equal to 45°. Treatment consists of immobilization of the arm in a sling and swathe bandage for a total of 6 weeks. When the humerus moves as a unit (approximately 10 to 14 days), gentle dependent circular and pendulum range of motion exercises are begun. Moving as a unit means that when the arm is gently internally and externally rotated, one can manually feel the proximal humerus rotate correspondingly. At 4 weeks, passive/active-assistive shoulder range of motion exercises are instituted. At 6 weeks, union is generally complete, sling and swathe immobilization is discontinued, and active use is allowed. Physiotherapy continues on a daily basis until maximal range of motion and strength are regained. Fractures with moderate displacement (5 mm to 1 cm), moderate angulation (20° to 45°), and/or

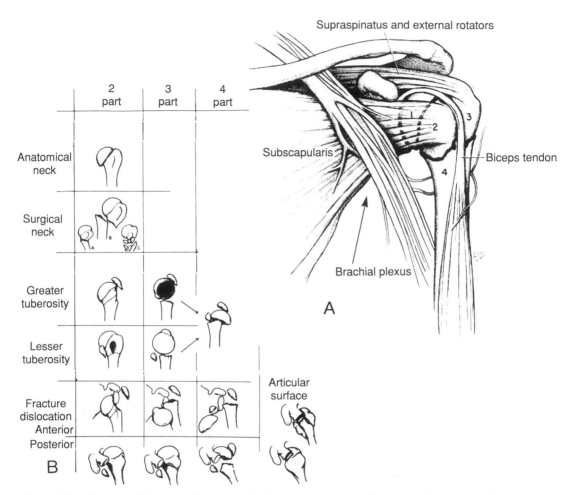

Figure 2.32. Fractures of the proximal humerus. *A*, the four major segments of the proximal humerus: *1*, articular segment; *2*, lesser tuberosity; *3*, greater tuberosity; *4*, humeral shaft. (From Neer CS II. Displaced proximal humeral fractures: I. Classification and evaluation. J Bone Joint Surg 1970;52A:1077–1089). *B*, the various types of significantly displaced fractures that can occur. (From Rockwood CA, Green DP, eds. Fractures in adults,; vol 1. 2nd ed. Philadelphia: JB Lippincott Co, 1984:678 and from Neer CS II. Displaced proximal humeral fractures: I. Classification and evaluation. J Bone Joint Surg 1970;52A:1077–1089).

comminution should be referred to an orthopaedist for initial management and subsequent follow-up.

Twenty percent of proximal humeral fractures involve significant displacement of one or more of the four major segments (Fig. 2.32*B*). Referral to an orthopaedist is indicated since surgery is often necessary. The blood supply to the articular segment comes in via the tuberosities. Consequently, if the articular segment is significantly separated from the tuberosities or vice versa, the articular segment has a 90% risk of undergoing avascular necrosis with subsequent collapse. Therefore, a primary prosthetic replacement is usually the treatment of choice. The rotator cuff inserts on the greater and lesser tuberosities. Consequently, if a fractured tuberosity is significantly displaced, a complete tear of the rotator cuff is present by definition. In addition, a significantly displaced tuberosity may fail to heal, or may interfere with glenohumeral range of motion. Therefore, a significantly displaced tuberosity needs to be surgically reduced anatomically and internally fixed, and the rotator cuff repaired. Finally, significant displacement of any of the major segments can result in a failure of the fracture to heal (a nonunion) or a healed fracture in abnormal position (a malunion) with resultant pain, cosmetic deformity, and/or limitation of glenohumeral range of motion in one or more directions. Here again, surgery may be required to avoid such an outcome.

Fractures involving the articular surface of the proximal humerus should be referred to an orthopaedist. If the articular surface is significantly disrupted, an open reduction and internal fixation or even a primary prosthetic replacement may be indicated to prevent later symptomatic degenerative joint disease.

Fracture-Dislocations of the Proximal Humerus

Fractures of the tuberosities may accompany dislocations of the shoulder but often return to normal position following reduction of the dislocation (see section on "Acute Dislocation of the Glenohumeral Joint"). If not, and for other displaced fractures of the major segments accompanying dislocations of the glenohumeral joint, referral to an orthopaedist is indicated. Surgical treatment is usually necessary and entails reduction of the dislocated humeral head, followed by reduction and stabilization of the associated fracture(s).

Fractures of the Proximal Humeral Physis

Fractures of the proximal humeral physis occur most frequently between the ages of 11 and 15 years, and males outnumber females by a three-to-one ratio. These fractures are usually the result of indirect trauma, but occasionally a direct blow or fall on the lateral aspect of the shoulder will be

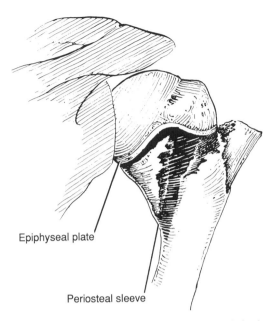

Epiphyseal plate

Periosteal sleeve

Figure 2.33. A fracture of the proximal humeral physis. (From Tachdjian MO. Pediatric orthopedics. Philadelphia: WB Saunders Co, 1972:1559.)

the mechanism of injury. The fracture may be displaced, angulated, or both (Fig. 2.33).

Clinical Characteristics. The patient is skeletally immature and has sustained an injury to the shoulder area. The patient is in considerable pain. Marked swelling and local tenderness are noted over the shoulder. The arm may be shortened and held in a varying degree of abduction and extension. There may be a prominence over the anterior aspect of the shoulder and the anterior axillary fold may be distorted with puckering. One may be able to feel false motion and crepitus over the fracture site. If displacement is slight, most of these physical findings will be absent. X-rays confirm the diagnosis.

Treatment. In infants and young children, displacement and angulation at the fracture site are difficult to determine radiographically since the epiphysis is mostly cartilage. Consequently, referral to an orthopaedist is indicated. When acceptable position has been achieved, the arm is immobilized in a sling and swathe or modified Velpeau bandage. Solid union occurs within 3 to 4 weeks, and most malalignments and angular deformities will correct themselves with growth and remodeling.

In children over 6 years of age and in adolescents, if there is no displacement or angulation, a sling and swathe or modified Velpeau bandage is applied. If displacement or angulation or both are present at the fracture site, referral to an orthopaedist is indicated since a closed reduction may be necessary. Solid osseous union generally occurs within 4 to 6 weeks, and growth and remodeling will correct most deformities.

FRACTURES OF THE SHAFT OF THE HUMERUS

Fractures of the shaft of the humerus may be transverse, oblique, comminuted, complete, or incomplete. They may also be open or closed. Alignment and apposition are usually satisfactory when the arm is dependent, but occasionally displacement and/or an-

gulation is unacceptable. Associated neurovascular injury is not uncommon. The radial nerve is particularly vulnerable due to its proximity to the humeral shaft (Fig. 2.34).

Clinical Characteristics

The injury is caused by a significant direct or indirect force applied to the humeral shaft. The arm is visibly swollen, frequently deformed, and extremely painful. When the fracture is complete, the arm is quite mobile and bony crepitus is felt with any manipulation of the arm. If the fracture is incomplete, the arm is exquisitely tender to local palpation. A few days after injury, ecchymosis and edema are quite visible over the dependent elbow and forearm areas. Anteroposterior and lateral x-rays of the arm confirm the presence of the fracture and define its configuration.

Treatment

Open fractures should be referred immediately to an orthopaedist for definitive care.

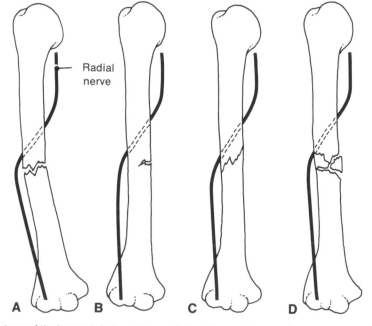

Figure 2.34. Fractures of the humeral shaft and the proximity of the radial nerve. *A*, transverse complete. *B*, transverse incomplete. *C*, oblique undisplaced. *D*, comminuted.

Regarding closed fractures, the presence of a strong radial pulse should be confirmed, and if absent, an immediate orthopaedic consultation should be obtained. Radial, ulnar, and median nerve function should be assessed next, and if evidence of peripheral nerve dysfunction is noted, the fracture should be splinted (as discussed below) and an orthopaedist consulted. The fracture is immobilized with two well-padded plaster splints (Fig. 2.35). The first is applied over the lateral aspect of the shoulder and upper arm, under the flexed elbow, and up the inner aspect of the arm to the axilla. A posterior splint is then added, running from the posterior aspect of the shoulder and upper arm, under the elbow, and along the ulnar aspect of the forearm to the metacarpophalangeal portion of the hand. The two splints are held in place with Ace bandages applied from the hand to the axillary aspect of the arm. The splints are allowed to set with the elbow in 90° of flexion and the forearm in neutral rotation. The arm is then allowed to hang dependently with either a sling or a collar and cuff for support. Usually the weight of the arm and the splints hanging in the dependent mode will effect an adequate reduction of the fracture. Post-splinting x-rays of the fracture site in the AP and lateral planes should be obtained and if the position is unsatisfactory (unacceptable displacement, distraction, and/or angulation), an orthopaedic consultation should be obtained. If the reduction is satisfactory, referral to an orthopaedist should be arranged for subsequent care.

If radial nerve function is lost following reduction of the fracture and splint immobilization, an orthopaedic consultation is clearly indicated. The radial nerve may be impaled by or caught between the fracture fragments during the maneuver, in which case immediate surgical exploration must be considered.

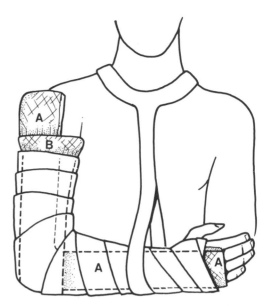

Figure 2.35. Immobilization of humeral shaft fractures using one long-arm posterior splint (*A*) and one medial-lateral splint (*B*). The arm is further supported by a sling or a collar and cuff dressing, and allowed to hang dependently.

Average healing time for these fractures is 8 weeks; however, delayed union and nonunion are not uncommon.

SUGGESTED READINGS

Bateman JE. The Shoulder and Neck. 2nd ed. Philadelphia: WB Saunders Co, 1978.

Crenshaw AH, ed. Campbell's Operative Orthopedics. St. Louis: The CV Mosby Co, 1987.

DePalma AF. Surgery of the Shoulder. 3rd ed. Philadelphia: JB Lippincott Co, 1983.

Evarts CM, ed. Surgery of the Musculoskeletal System. New York: Churchill Livingstone, 1990.

Neer CS II. Shoulder Reconstruction. Philadelphia: WB Saunders Co, 1990.

Post M. The Shoulder. 2nd ed. Philadelphia: Lea & Febiger, 1988.

Rockwood CA Jr, Green DP, eds. Fractures. 2nd ed. Philadelphia: JB Lippincott Co, 1984.

Rockwood CA Jr, Matsen FA III, eds. Philadelphia: WB Saunders Co, 1990.

Rowe CR, ed. The Shoulder. New York: Churchill Livingstone, 1987.

Tachdjian MO. Pediatric Orthopedics. 2nd ed. Philadelphia: WB Saunders Co, 1990.

CHAPTER 3

Elbow and Forearm

William J. Morgan, M.D.

Essential Anatomy

SKELETAL ANATOMY

The distal end of the humerus forms a complex articulation with the proximal radius and ulna to form the elbow joint (Fig. 3.1). The capitellum and trochlea form the lateral and medial articulating condyles of the humerus, respectively. These articulating condyles are rotated 30° anteriorly with respect to the long axis of the humerus. The capitellum is shaped like a sphere, providing axial rotation in its articulation with the radius. The trochlea has a grooved surface into which the proximal ulna fits to provide flexion and extension.

The anterior coronoid fossa and the posterior olecranon fossa are located just above the articular surface of the trochlea. These accommodate the coronoid in full flexion and the olecranon in full extension. The coronoid and olecranon fossae are bordered medially and laterally by the supracondylar bony columns, which end as the lateral and medial epicondyles.

There is approximately a 6° to 8° valgus tilt of the distal humeral articular surface. The long axis of the ulna is in valgus with respect to the long axis of the humerus. This angulation is called the carrying angle and shows some variation with respect to age and sex. The "normal" carrying angle is approximately 15°.

The proximal radius is a concave articular disc with articular cartilage covering approximately 240° of the outside circumference of the radial head. This provides for articulation with the capitellum and the proximal ulna in rotation. Distal to the radial head and proximal to the shaft of the radius is a narrowed portion called the neck of the radius. This area is stabilized by the annular ligament in rotation (Fig. 3.2). The radial tuberosity is the distal landmark for the neck of the radius, and is the site of attachment of the biceps tendon. The radial tuberosity also provides a valuable landmark in aligning midshaft fractures of the radius. Distally, the radius flares to form articulations with the carpus and the distal ulna. The radiocarpal joint is comprised of the scaphoid fossa adjacent to the radial styloid and the lunate fossa located distal and ulnarly. The concave semilunar facet is found on the distal ulnar surface of the radius and provides rotation about the ulna at the distal radioulnar joint (Fig. 3.3).

The proximal ulnar articulating surface is known as the sigmoid notch. This articulates with the trochlea of the humerus and is bordered posteriorly by the olecranon and anteriorly by the coronoid process. Just lateral to the sigmoid notch is a concave articulation of about 70° known as the lesser sigmoid notch. This forms the articulation of the circumference of the radial head in rotation. The lesser sigmoid notch is positioned perpendicular to the greater sigmoid notch.

The shaft of the ulna is somewhat narrowed compared with the proximal ulna, but distally flares to form the head of the ulna. This is comprised of the ulnar styloid and the

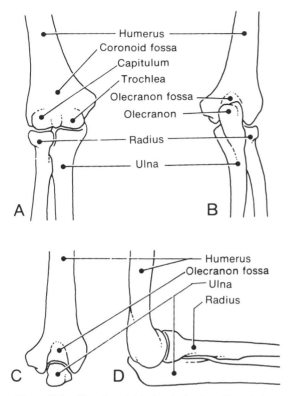

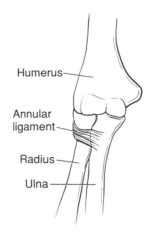

Figure 3.2.   Annular ligament.

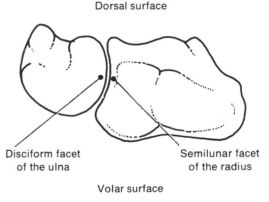

Figure 3.1.   The elbow joint. *A*, anterior view. *B*, posterior view *C*, posterior view, 90° of flexion. *D*, lateral view.

Figure 3.3.   Distal end of the radioulnar joint—forearm in midrotation.

convex distal ulna, which is covered with articular cartilage for 270° of its total circumference (Fig. 3.3). This articulation with the sigmoid notch of the distal radius allows for rotation of the distal radius around the ulnar head.

In full supination the radius and ulna are aligned in a somewhat parallel position and form a rectangle with respect to their proximal and distal articulations. In full pronation the distal radius rotates around the distal ulnar head, causing the radial shaft to cross over the anterior immobile ulnar shaft (Fig. 3.4).

LIGAMENTOUS AND CAPSULAR ANATOMY

The joint capsule makes its proximal attachments along the superior margin of the coronoid fossa anteriorly and along the superior margin of the olecranon fossa poste-

riorly (Fig. 3.5). The anterior capsule is somewhat thin and renders little stability to the elbow. The anterior capsule then makes its distal attachments along the articular margin of the trochlea medially and along the radial neck, blending into the annular ligament laterally. Posteriorly, the capsule makes its distal attachments to the medial and lateral margins of the trochlea.

The ligaments of the elbow are specialized thickenings of the capsule. The medial collateral ligament complex consists of three parts: the anterior bundle, posterior bundle, and transverse ligament (Fig. 3.5*B*). The anterior bundle makes up the major portion of

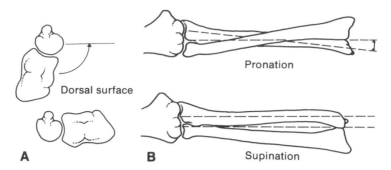

Figure 3.4. Movement of the radius and ulna during rotation of the forearm. *A*, semilunar facet of the distal end of the radius slides around the disciform facet of the distal end of the ulna. *B*, the ulna diverges 8° to 9° away from the longitudinal axis of the forearm during rotation from full supination to full pronation.

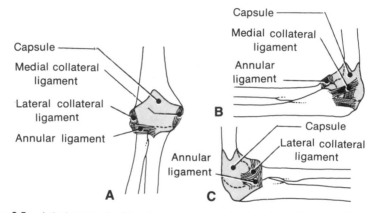

Figure 3.5. Articular capsule of the elbow joint. *A*, anterior view. *B*, medial view. *C*, lateral view.

the medial ligament complex. It takes its origin just inferior to the medial apophysis and inserts into the medial aspect of the coronoid process. The lateral ligament complex is made up of the radial collateral ligament and the lateral ulnar collateral ligament (Fig. 3.5C). The lateral ligament complex is not as well-defined as the medial complex and appears to be more of a capsular blend. It takes its origin from the lateral epicondyle apophysis and attaches to the annular ligament of the radius distally. The annular ligament has its origin and insertion on the anterior and posterior margins of the lesser sigmoid notch. It contains the radial head adjacent to the ulna, prevents anterior-posterior subluxation, and stabilizes the rotation of the radius upon the capitellum (Fig. 3.2).

The distal radioulnar joint is stabilized by the proximal aspect of the triangular fibrocartilage complex. This arises from the ulnar aspect of the lunate fossa of the distal radius and extends ulnarward to the base of the ulnar styloid. The dorsal and volar portions of the triangular fibrocartilage complex are thickened and form the poorly defined dorsal and volar radioulnar ligaments. The carpus is then stabilized to the distal radioulnar joint by the strong volar and weak dorsal perpendicular arms of the triangular fibrocartilage complex.

BURSAE AND MUSCLES

Twelve bursae have been reported to occur about the elbow joint, with three showing consistent clinical significance (Fig.

3.6). The olecranon bursa is situated posteriorly between the skin and the olecranon, and allows smooth gliding of the skin on the triceps tendon. The bicipitoradial bursa lies in the angle between the radial tuberosity and the insertion of the biceps tendon, and allows smooth gliding of the tendon on the surface of the bone. The radiohumeral bursa lies deep to the common extensor tendon attachments to the lateral epicondyle, inferior to the extensor carpi radialis brevis, and superficial to the radiocapitellar joint capsule. This allows for gliding of the extensor origin over the radiocapitellar capsule.

Many muscles take their origin and insertion about the elbow and forearm. On the anterior aspect of the elbow (Fig. 3.7), the deepest elbow flexor is the brachialis muscle. This muscle crosses the anterior capsule, with some fibers inserting into the capsule, and the final insertion of the brachialis tendon into the coronoid process. The biceps muscle overlies the brachialis and has two insertions. The bicipital aponeurosis, the lacertus fibrosis, inserts into the anterior medial muscle fascia of the proximal forearm. The distal biceps tendon then attaches to the posterior aspect of the radial tuberosity, acting as an elbow flexor and forearm supinator. Both the brachialis and biceps muscles are innervated by the musculocutaneous nerve. Also acting as an elbow flexor is the brachioradialis, which takes its origin along the lateral supracondylar region of the distal humerus and goes on to insert into the radial styloid. The extensor carpi radialis longus (ECRL) and brevis (ECRB) also take their origin from the lateral supracondylar ridge of the distal humerus, with the ECRB finding origin on the inferior surface of the lateral epicondyle. The extensor carpi radialis brevis is covered by the extensor carpi radialis longus at this level. The brachioradialis, ECRL, and ECRB make up the "mobile wad of Henry" and are innervated by the radial nerve proximal to its bifurcation.

The extensor digitorum communis takes its origin from the lateral epicondyle and is innervated by the deep branch of the radial nerve. The extensor carpi ulnaris takes its origin from two heads, the lateral epicondyle and the aponeurosis of the anconeus muscle. It is also innervated by the deep branch of the radial nerve. The supinator muscle is an important forearm rotator. It is a rhomboid-shaped muscle originating from the lateral aspect of the lateral epicondyle, the lateral collateral ligament, and the proximal ulna. It then runs obliquely to insert in the proximal one-third of the radius along its dorsal surface. Its innervation is derived from the posterior interosseous nerve as the nerve traverses through the substance of the muscle.

The triceps muscle takes its origin from three separate heads (Fig. 3.8), two of which arise from the posterior aspect of the hu-

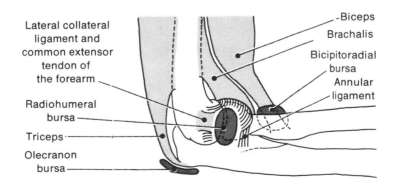

Figure 3.6. Three elbow bursae. The lateral collateral ligament and common extensor tendon have been reflected away to expose the radiohumeral bursa.

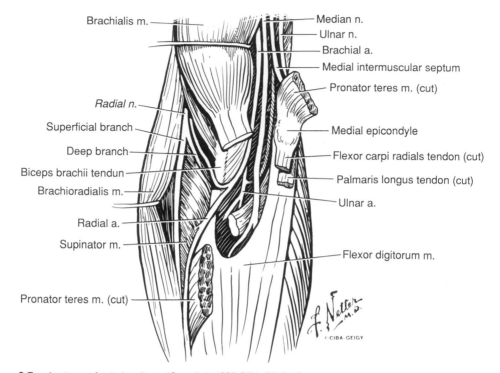

Figure 3.7. Anatomy of anterior elbow. (Copyright 1987 CIBA-GEIGY Corporation. Adapted with permission from the Ciba Collection of medical illustrations by Frank Netter, M.D. All rights reserved.)

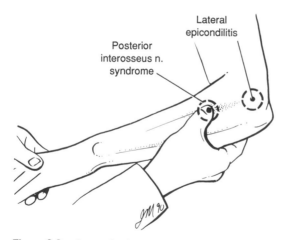

Figure 3.8. Areas of palpation to differentiate lateral epicondylitis from posterior interosseous nerve syndrome.

merus. The long head has its origin from the infraglenoid tuberosity of the scapula. The three heads then form a common expansion that inserts into the olecranon, thus acting as the primary elbow extensor. The triceps are innervated by the radial nerve. The anconeus muscle is a small oblique muscle running from the lateral epicondyle into the lateral aspect of the olecranon. Its function has been debated but it appears to act as a joint stabilizer.

The flexor pronator muscle group consists of the pronator teres, flexor carpi radialis, palmaris longus, flexor carpi ulnaris, and flexor digitorum superficialis (Fig. 3.7). They originate from the medial epicondyle and from the proximal ulna. The pronator teres inserts into the radius beneath the brachioradialis muscle at the junction of the proximal and middle thirds of the radius, thus acting as a strong pronator of the forearm. The pronator teres, flexor carpi radialis, palmaris longus, and flexor digitorum superficialis are innervated by the median nerve. The flexor carpi ulnaris muscle is innervated by the ulnar nerve. The flexor digitorum profundus muscle originates from the proximal ulna and does not cross the elbow joint. The muscle bellies contributing to the flexor digitorum profundus tendons to the index and long fingers are innervated by the median nerve, and those contributing to the ring and small fingers are innervated by the ulnar nerve.

INNERVATION AND BLOOD SUPPLY

The brachial artery enters the antecubital fossa medial to the brachialis muscle anteriorly and medial to the biceps tendon distally. It is crossed in the antecubital fossa by the median nerve and comes to lie lateral to the nerve. At the level of the radial head it bifurcates into the radial and ulnar arteries (Fig. 3.7). The radial artery then emerges from the antecubital space between the brachioradialis and pronator teres muscles, and continues down the forearm under the brachioradialis muscle. The ulnar artery emerges between the two heads of the pronator teres and runs distally down the forearm beneath the flexor carpi ulnaris muscle.

The median nerve accompanies the brachial artery into the antecubital fossa, after crossing to a position medial to the artery. At this point the median nerve passes under the bicipital aponeurosis and between the humeral and ulnar heads of the pronator teres muscle. Before diving beneath the flexor digitorum superficialis arch, the median nerve gives off the branch of the anterior interosseous nerve. The median nerve then runs distally in the forearm beneath the flexor digitorum superficialis muscle belly. The radial nerve emerges from the lateral intermuscular septum at the junction of the middle and distal thirds of the humerus. At the lateral elbow, the nerve lies between the brachialis muscle and the brachioradialis, ECRL, and ECRB muscle bellies. At the level of the radial head the nerve bifurcates, with the superficial branch continuing on down the forearm beneath the brachioradialis muscle belly. This branch supplies sensation to the dorsoradial aspect of the hand. At the

bifurcation, the deep branch or the posterior interosseous nerve, dives beneath the arcade of the Frohse into the muscle belly of the supinator from which it emerges distally. It then branches to innervate the extensor muscles of the fingers and thumb.

The ulnar nerve emerges from the medial intermuscular septum and runs along the muscle belly of the triceps and into the cubital tunnel, which lies just posterior to the medial epicondyle. It splits the two proximal heads of the flexor carpi ulnaris muscle and runs distally in the forearm between the flexor digitorum profundus and the flexor carpi ulnaris muscle bellies. The ulnar nerve's entrance into Guyon's canal is described in Chapter 4, "Wrist and Hand."

Nontraumatic and Overuse Disorders of the Elbow and Forearm

LATERAL EPICONDYLITIS

Lateral epicondylitis is an overuse syndrome of the upper extremity. Although called "tennis elbow," it is seen in many competitive athletes who use the upper extremity, e.g., tennis, baseball, and golf players. It is also a common complaint in those occupations requiring repetitious extension of the wrist or rotation of the forearm. It is frequently seen in carpenters, electricians, and others, and is a frequent source of workers' compensation claims.

The exact cause of lateral epicondylitis is unclear, but it occurs as an inflammatory process at the extensor origin at the lateral epicondyle, most specifically at the origin of the extensor carpi radialis brevis.

Clinical Characteristics

The patient with lateral epicondylitis presents with pain, generally felt at the lateral epicondyle, but if the problem is chronic, referred pain to the extensor surface of the forearm may be noted (Fig. 3.8). This pain is intensified by palpation over the lateral epicondyle, particularly along the anterior edge at the origin of the extensor carpi radialis brevis. There is full range of motion of the elbow and wrist without weakness, but the pain is exacerbated by resisted extension of the wrist or fingers. The pain may also be exacerbated by passively flexing the fingers and wrist with the elbow fully extended. In advanced cases there may be swelling and erythema about the lateral epicondyle. X-rays are usually normal, but calcific deposits may be noted adjacent to the lateral epicondyle in chronic cases.

Radial tunnel syndrome or posterior interosseous nerve syndrome is frequently misdiagnosed as lateral epicondylitis. Radial nerve entrapment may also occur coincident with lateral epicondylitis. The pain due to radial tunnel syndrome can generally be produced by resisted middle finger extension or forearm supination with the elbow extended. In radial tunnel syndrome there is also pain to palpation in the area between the mobile wad and the extensor digitorum communis just distal to the radial head (the area where the posterior interosseous nerve enters the supinator). Electromyographic studies are usually not helpful in the differentiation as there is a high incidence of false-negative results in radial tunnel syndrome. Other entities that may show similar presentations must be ruled out, including cervical spondylosis with cervical root compression and intraarticular abnormalities of the elbow.

Treatment

Treatment of lateral epicondylitis is related to the severity and chronicity of the problem at the time of presentation. In the acute onset with mild to moderate pain, nonsteroidal anti-inflammatory medications are recommended in conjunction with avoidance of aggravating activities and rest of the extremity. Immobilization of the wrist in a volar splint is helpful in alleviating repetitious flexion and extension activities of the wrist.

If this treatment is ineffective, a cortisone injection using 1 ml of 1% Xylocaine and 20 mg of triamcinolone is appropriate. This is injected in the area just anterior to the lateral epicondyle below the origin of the extensor brevis muscle. Care must be taken to avoid intradermal injections, and the patient must be warned of subcutaneous atrophy or pigmentation changes following injection of cortisone. No more than three injections are advisable. More recently, in an attempt to avoid these potential complications, steroid phonophoresis and steroid iontophoresis have been used successfully.

Once the acute inflammatory response has been controlled and the patient's pain has been relieved, a rehabilitation program should be instituted. The patient should be protected in the early parts of rehabilitation by the use of a counterforce brace, a canvas or Velcro strap that fits around the proximal forearm. A graduated exercise program is instituted, which includes specific rehabilitation exercises and the gradual resumption of the patient's usual activities. This is performed in conjunction with stretching exercises (Fig. 3.9). In cases of lateral epicondylitis related to sports activities, alterations in technique or equipment may be helpful in preventing recurrences. Should the patient's symptoms be recalcitrant to the above treatment or should a recurrence occur with resumption of the patient's usual activities, referral should be made to an orthopaedist for potential surgical treatment.

MEDIAL EPICONDYLITIS
Clinical Characteristics

Many athletes and laborers note the onset of pain on the medial aspect of the elbow overlying the medial epicondyle, similar to the onset of lateral epicondylitis. This appears to arise from repeated flexion activities of the wrist and fingers, thus initiating increased stresses at the flexor pronator origin.

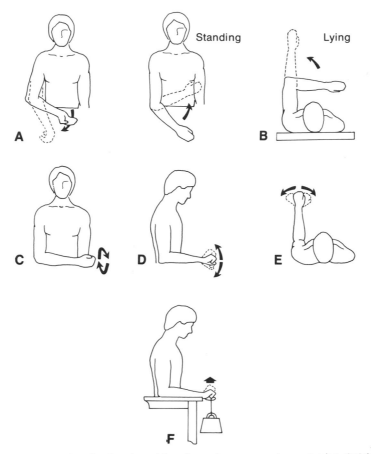

Figure 3.9. Rehabilitation exercises for disorders of the elbow. *A*, common extensor tendon stretching for mild tennis elbow. *B*, acute flexion-extension with and against gravity. *C*, unopposed forearm rotation. *D* and *E*, range of motion exercises for the wrist. *F*, common extensor strengthening exercise.

In the physical evaluation, one must differentiate medial epicondylitis from cubital tunnel syndrome (i.e., ulnar nerve entrapment at the elbow). In medial epicondylitis, pain is elicited by direct palpation of the bony prominence of the medial epicondyle. Pain is exacerbated by resisted flexion of the fingers and there may be swelling and erythema at the medial epicondyle. In a like manner, patients with cubital tunnel syndrome may present with medial elbow and forearm pain. In contrast to medial epicondylitis, there is a positive Tinel's sign over the ulnar nerve. The nerve may be able to subluxate. Paresthesias of the ulnar nerve may be elicited by prolonged elbow flexion in cubital tunnel syndrome. Electromyography may help in problematic clinical cases.

Treatment

The treatment for medial epicondylitis is similar to lateral epicondylitis, starting with rest and anti-inflammatory medication, then proceeding to steroid phonophoresis, local steroid installation (great care must be taken to avoid injection into the adjacent ulnar nerve), and orthopaedic referral in recalcitrant cases.

NONTRAUMATIC OVERUSE SYNDROMES OF THE ELBOW IN CHILDREN

Articular damage to the radiocapitellar and ulnohumeral joint can occur with repetitive stresses similar to those causing extraarticular pathology. In North America, this is frequently seen in adolescents involved in overhand throwing activities, particularly in Little League pitching.

Clinical Characteristics

Patients with the entity known as "Little League elbow" may present with lateral or medial elbow pain or a combination of the two. Little League elbow is the result of compressive forces at the radiocapitellar joint and distraction forces in the medial aspect of the elbow. This may result in articular damage to the capitellum, ligamentous instability of the medial elbow ligamentous complex, and tardy ulnar nerve palsy (Fig. 3.10). In this presentation it is important to examine radiographs, as findings relating to osteochondritis dissecans of the capitellum may be found. Osteochondritis dissecans of the capitellum clinically presents as pain and swelling over the lateral aspect of the elbow. With intraarticular injury the joint will usually be tender to axial compression or varus/valgus stresses while flexing and extending the joint. In severe cases, the patient may present with locking of the elbow due to fragmentation of the capitellum resulting in intraarticular loose bodies. X-ray evaluation will demonstrate apparent resorption and fragmentation of the capitellum.

Treatment of osteochondritis dissecans requires orthopaedic referral. Avoidance of stressful activities (e.g., pitching) is recommended in mild cases. In advanced cases, surgical intervention may be necessary.

Panner's disease or idiopathic avascular necrosis of the capitellum appears clinically and radiographically as osteochondritis dissecans but without an apparent stressful etiology. Treatment is as delineated above.

Traction injuries may also occur about the

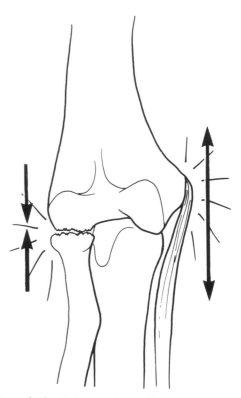

Figure 3.10. Pathogenesis of radiocapiteelum articular damage and medial ligamentous laxity in "Little League elbow." (Adapted from Pappas AM. Elbow problems associated with baseball during childhood and adolescence. Clin Orthop 1982;164:32, with permission of JB Lippincott Co, Philadelphia.)

elbow of a child due to overstress. These will often present as pain along the medial elbow, i.e., traction of the medial epicondyle, or pain at the posterior elbow, i.e., traction of the olecranon apophysis. Treatment should be geared to the severity of the injury. In mild cases immobilization for 3 weeks is recommended followed by a gradual rehabilitation program. If symptoms persist, the child has severe pain, or there are abnormalities on x-ray, the child should be referred for orthopaedic evaluation and treatment.

OVERUSE SYNDROMES IN THE FOREARM

It is unusual to encounter an inflammatory tenosynovitis in the forearm as there are no discrete tenosynovial compartments noted. One exception is the entity known as "intersection syndrome."

Clinical Characteristics

The symptoms of intersection syndrome are pain and swelling over the dorsoradial aspect of the distal forearm, in the area where the abductor pollicis longus and extensor pollicis brevis muscle bellies cross the extensor carpi radialis brevis and longus tendons. In advanced cases it may be associated with erythema and crepitus. It may also be associated with tenosynovitis of the second dorsal compartment.

Treatment

The initial conservative treatment consists of rest by immobilizing the wrist in a cock-up splint in approximately 15° of extension. Anti-inflammatory medication is useful, and in more advanced cases, steroid phonophoresis or corticosteroid injection into the area of tenderness may be helpful. In more advanced cases or those resistant to conservative therapy, referral to an orthopaedist for surgical decompression may be necessary.

BURSITIS

Many deep bursae about the elbow have been described, and these were reviewed in the "Essential Anatomy" section. In the past there was thought to be a strong association between radiohumeral bursitis and tennis elbow. Currently, radiohumeral bursitis is not thought to be a major contributor to tennis elbow and is itself a relatively rare entity.

Bicipital Radial Bursitis

Bicipital radial bursitis is an uncommon entity.

Clinical Characteristics. The patient presents with pain in the antecubital fossa radiating up the biceps tendon. Deep palpation of the radial tuberosity and the insertion of the biceps tendon reveals pain. Flex-

ion and supination against resistance will also aggravate the pain. X-rays are normal.

Treatment. Bicipital radial bursitis should be treated with rest and, in the acute stages, ice may be helpful. Anti-inflammatory medication should also be utilized. Short-term immobilization with an elbow splint, holding the elbow at 90° of flexion in neutral rotation, is indicated in severe cases. The patient must come out of the splint at least once or twice a day for range of motion of the elbow to prevent stiffness. The use of corticosteroid injections in this area is not advisable, as it may precipitate biceps tendon rupture. Those patients not responding to conservative treatment should be referred to an orthopaedist for further evaluation of a potential impending biceps tendon rupture.

Olecranon Bursitis

Olecranon bursitis is the most common superficial bursitis presenting about the elbow. The treatment of olecranon bursitis depends on its etiology, pathogenesis, and chronicity.

Clinical Characteristics. The onset of painless swelling of the olecranon bursa is usually the result of direct or indirect trauma. It results from repetitive stresses, such as "student's elbow" or "miner's elbow," or from direct contact, as in football players who play on artificial surfaces. Full range of motion of the elbow is usually present, but with a very swollen bursa flexion may be limited because of pain from compression of the distended bursa.

In those patients presenting with a painful olecranon bursitis, differentiation between inflammatory and septic causes must be made. Systemic inflammatory processes associated with olecranon bursitis include gout, hydroxyapatite crystal deposition, chondrocalcinosis, and rheumatoid arthritis. In cases of rheumatoid arthritis there may be a direct communication of the elbow joint with the bursa. To further make this differentiation, it is imperative that painful swelling of the olecranon bursa, particularly when associated with erythema, be aspirated. This should be done under sterile conditions as noted above. The correct diagnosis can be made by analyzing the fluid for leukocyte count, Gram stain, and culture and sensitivity testing. The fluid should also be analyzed for crystals in those cases where a crystalline inflammatory process is suspected.

Treatment.   Treatment of aseptic bursitis consists of anti-inflammatory medication, resting the elbow in a splint, and using compressive elastic wraps. Aspiration may be combined with the above treatment regimen for very swollen bursae. After sterile preparation, an 18-gauge needle is inserted into the olecranon bursa laterally (Fig. 3.11). A direct approach into the tip of the elbow may lead to a chronic sinus tract. On completion of the aspiration, a compressive dressing should be applied and the extremity rested in a splint. In traumatic olecranon bursitis, the future use of elbow pads may be helpful. Recurrences are treated as described above. In recalcitrant cases referral should be made to an orthopaedist for possible excision.

The treatment of olecranon bursitis associated with a systemic inflammatory process is directed at control of the underlying disease.

In cases of septic bursitis, treatment is initiated by aspiration and systemic antibiotics. Initial antibiotic treatment should be directed by the result of the Gram stain of the aspirate. Begin treatment with a broad-spectrum antibiotic. When the culture results are available, appropriate antibiotic modifications are made. Aspiration and irrigation are repeated on reaccumulation of the fluid. In cases that do not respond to aspiration, irrigation, and systemic antibiotics, referral to an orthopaedist should be made for incision, drainage, and possible bursectomy.

ENTRAPMENT NEUROPATHIES

Most entrapment and compression neuropathies about the elbow and forearm manifest themselves as pain and paresthesias in the hand. Some will also present as localized pain about the forearm and elbow itself. The following will be a review of radial and ulnar neuropathies about the elbow. Median nerve entrapment syndromes occur about the elbow, but will be discussed in Chapter 4, "Wrist and Hand," with carpal tunnel syndrome.

Radial Tunnel Syndrome

Radial tunnel syndrome is most frequently the result of a compression neuropathy of the posterior interosseous nerve at the arcade of Frohse as it enters the proximal border of the supinator muscle.

Clinical Characteristics.   The clinical presentation of this syndrome is most commonly that of aching pain along the extensor surface of the forearm and hand, as well as pain about the elbow, at the site of the posterior interosseous nerve entrapment. This proximal location often makes it difficult to differentiate it from the pain of tennis elbow. If fascicles of the superficial branch of the radial nerve are involved, there may be dysesthesias or decreased sensation along the dorsoradial aspect of the wrist and hand.

Diagnosis is often difficult to make and must be differentiated from tennis elbow or

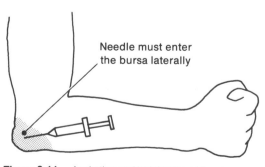

Needle must enter
the bursa laterally

Figure 3.11.   Aspiration and/or irrigation of the olecranon bursa space.

a cervical radiculopathy. Deep palpation approximately 4 cm distal to the lateral epicondyle between the heads of the extensor digitorum communis and extensor carpi radialis brevis muscle bellies elicits pain and paresthesias duplicating the patient's clinical presentation (Fig. 3.12). This pain should be out of proportion to palpation of the contralateral limb. Active supination from a fully pronated position may also duplicate the presenting pain. In severe cases of posterior interosseous nerve entrapment, weakness of finger extensors may be present and is diagnostic. Electromyography and nerve conduction studies have not been helpful in the diagnosis of radial tunnel syndrome because false-negative results occur frequently.

Treatment. Conservative treatment of radial tunnel syndrome involves avoidance of overuse activities. For example, excessive supination and pronation, as occurs with use of a screwdriver, may elicit these symptoms. Anti-inflammatory medication and short-term rest of the extensor muscles by a wrist splint may be helpful. If the symptoms persist after 2 weeks of conservative therapy or if weakness of the finger extensors is present, orthopaedic referral for probable surgical decompression is necessary.

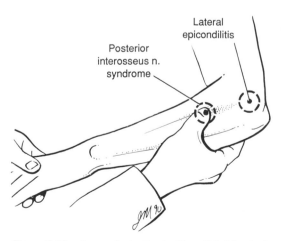

Figure 3.12. Areas of palpation to differentiate lateral epicondylitis from posterior interosseous nerve syndrome.

Wartenberg's Syndrome (Cheiralgia Paresthetica)

Wartenberg's syndrome (cheiralgia paresthetica) represents an entrapment of the superficial radial nerve in the distal forearm.

Clinical Characteristics. Pain localized to the dorsoradial aspect of the distal forearm with paresthesias in the distribution of the superficial branch of the radial nerve is characteristic of Wartenberg's syndrome. It may be iatrogenic or secondary to injury. The wearing of tight watchbands and bracelets has been associated with this syndrome.

Treatment. Treatment involves relieving any obvious extrinsic compressive devices and short-term wrist immobilization. In those cases where conservative treatment is ineffective, orthopaedic referral is necessary for surgical exploration.

Cubital Tunnel Syndrome

Entrapment of the ulnar nerve may occur in the cubital tunnel posterior to the medial epicondyle, more proximally at the intramuscular septum, and more distally between the two heads of the flexor carpi ulnaris muscle belly (Fig. 3.13).

Clinical Characteristics. Symptoms of ulnar nerve entrapment about the elbow generally are pain in the proximal ulnar aspect of the forearm and dysesthesias about the small and ulnar half of the ring fingers. Diagnosis is often made by palpation of the ulnar nerve at the medial epicondyle. There may be subluxation of the ulnar nerve over the medial epicondyle associated with pain and paresthesias. A positive Tinel's sign may be found at the cubital tunnel, proximally at the intramuscular septum, or more distally at the entrance of the ulnar nerve into the flexor carpi ulnaris muscle. Decreased sensation in the ulnar nerve distribution may be found and should be evaluated by moving two-point discrimination testing.

In more severe cases, intrinsic wasting of the hand may be present, and first dorsal in-

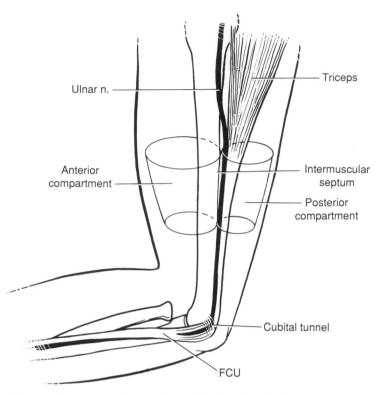

Ulnar n.

Triceps

Anterior compartment

Intermuscular septum

Posterior compartment

Cubital tunnel

FCU

Figure 3.13. Potential areas of ulna nerve entrapment around the elbow include: intermuscular septum, cubital tunnel and two heads of flexor carpi ulnaris muscle belly.

terosseous atrophy and a positive Froment's sign may be apparent. Froment's sign is a manifestation of weakness of the adductor pollicis (innervated by the ulnar nerve). When asked to pinch a piece of paper between the thumb and index finger (key pinch), the patient with adductor pollicis weakness will attempt to compensate by use of the flexor pollicis longus muscle (innervated by the median nerve). This will result in hyperflexion of the thumb interphalangeal joint (Fig. 3.14).

The paresthesias of cubital tunnel syndrome may be elicited or exacerbated by elbow flexion; this is a helpful diagnostic maneuver. Electromyography and nerve conduction studies are helpful in the diagnosis of cubital tunnel syndrome.

Treatment. Conservative treatment of cubital tunnel syndrome is usually ineffec-

tive. Persistent pain, paresthesias, and evidence of intrinsic muscle wasting indicate prompt orthopaedic referral for surgical decompression.

Traumatic Disorders of the Elbow and Forearm

FRACTURES AND DISLOCATIONS OF THE ELBOW AND FOREARM

Fractures and dislocations occurring about the elbow and forearm are common in children and adults. These represent severe and complex injuries, and frequently require orthopaedic referral. These injuries are plagued by the potential for severe and deforming complications. In the primary care setting, the initial recognition and treatment of these injuries may set the stage for a gratifying recovery or permanent disability.

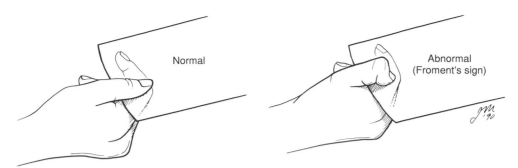

Figure 3.14.   Normal key pinch versus Froment's sign.

Most undisplaced fractures and simple dislocations about the elbow and forearm can be treated by the primary care physician. In this section, the author will describe most of the injuries and recommend a level of responsibility that the primary care physician should assume for each. Potential complications and the steps to avoid them in the initial treatment will be described.

Understanding the bony anatomy as well as the chronologic occurrence of the ossification centers about the elbow is imperative to the diagnosis and treatment of these injuries. The presence of an ossification center or the irregular appearance of such a center on x-ray may be misinterpreted as a fracture (Fig. 3.15).

Subluxation of the Head of the Radius

Subluxation of the radial head in children may be subtle in its presentation. This injury is a subluxation of the nonossified radial head from the capitellum and through the annular ligament (Fig. 3.16). It is most common in children between the ages of 2 and 3, and it is caused by abrupt axial forces on the radius, usually associated with a pronating force.

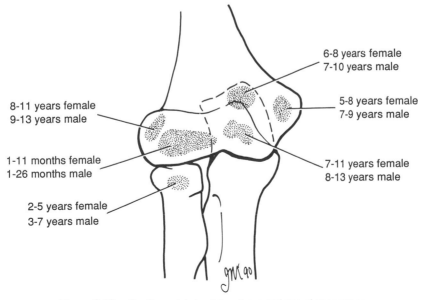

8-11 years female
9-13 years male

1-11 months female
1-26 months male

2-5 years female
3-7 years male

6-8 years female
7-10 years male

5-8 years female
7-9 years male

7-11 years female
8-13 years male

Figure 3.15.   Ossific nuclei about the elbow, and age of appearance.

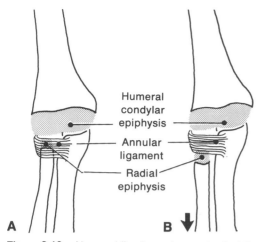

Figure 3.16. Nursemaid's elbow. *A*, normal articulation. *B*, radiohumeral subluxation.

The injury has many common names, including "pulled elbow" and "nursemaid's elbow." The latter name was derived from the frequent occurrence of subluxation of the radial head in children cared for by nursemaids. It is usually thought to have arisen from a sudden jerk on the extended arm of a toddler, such as pulling the child up over an obstruction in its path. The injury may also be caused by a fall as the toddler holds onto a suspending structure with one hand, again duplicating an axial force.

Clinical Characteristics. The history is usually consistent with an axial force on the toddler's arm. The toddler cries immediately and refuses to move the involved extremity. The clinical appearance of the arm is normal. The examiner who wins the trust of the child may note that gentle palpation localizes the pain to the radiocapitellar joint. X-rays are generally normal. Some subluxations of the radial head in children are reduced by the radiologic technologist when positioning the child's elbow in flexion and supination for a true lateral x-ray. Although many x-rays are normal, it is important to view an x-ray before attempting reduction to preclude the possibility of displacement of an intraarticular fracture. As radiographic changes in the child's elbow are often very subtle, it is recommended that comparison views of the unaffected elbow be obtained. While the diagnosis is strongly suggested by the parent's history, the definitive diagnosis is made by the maneuver that effects the cure.

Treatment. The child is usually more comfortable sitting in the parent's lap. The examiner must gain the child's confidence before attempting an examination and reduction. The examiner approaches the child slowly and face-to-face. The examiner then holds the elbow in one hand with the thumb overlying the head of the radius (Fig. 3.17). The elbow is slowly flexed while the forearm is rotated into full supination. Once the elbow has been flexed and supinated, the examiner may perceive a click at the radiocapitellar joint, signifying reduction. At this point the child generally no longer attempts to withdraw the arm and full flexion-extension of the elbow is possible. Following reduction, the child is quickly comfortable in resuming normal activities. At this point, re-

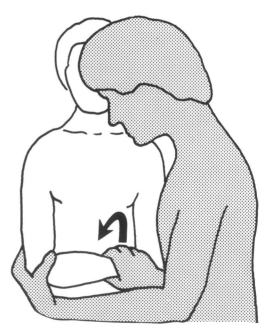

Figure 3.17. Reduction of nursemaid's elbow. Rotate from full pronation to full supination.

assurance to the parents that no permanent damage has been sustained and a simple explanation of the injury is all that is necessary. The child should not be immobilized or restricted in any way.

Supracondylar Fractures

Supracondylar fractures of the humerus are serious fractures occurring most frequently in children, usually between the ages of 5 and 8, with a peak at 6 years. The fracture is fraught with neurovascular complications and the possibility of permanent impairment and deformity. In undisplaced supracondylar fractures without evidence of neurovascular compromise, treatment by the primary care physician is indicated. In displaced supracondylar fractures or fractures associated with neurovascular compromise, immediate orthopaedic referral is mandatory. Appropriate splinting while awaiting orthopaedic evaluation will be reviewed. In the event of vascular compromise not controlled by elbow manipulation, further evaluation with arteriogram and vascular consultation must be obtained immediately.

Clinical Characteristics. Extension-type supracondylar fractures are the most common, accounting for 98% of supracondylar fractures (Fig. 3.18). The distal fragment is most often displaced in a posteromedial direction, though posterolateral displacement does occur. Flexion-type supracondylar fractures with anterior displacement are rare.

Consideration of elbow anatomy is helpful in predicting possible neurovascular compromise as well as planning the reduction maneuvers. In extension-type supracondylar fractures, the proximal humeral fragment may impale the anterior joint capsule, placing the median nerve and brachial artery at risk. In posteromedial displacement, the radial nerve is also at risk.

Vascular compromise may manifest as arterial rupture, venous rupture, arterial spasm, or compressive effects caused by hematoma or transudation obstructing venous outflow and, potentially, arterial inflow. Failure to institute immediate treatment may lead to compartment syndrome and ultimately to Volkmann's ischemic contracture. Therefore, in the event of a supracondylar fracture, the following neurovascular examination is imperative. Vascular pulses about the wrist must be palpable. If not immediately palpable and if the elbow is in a flexed position, extension may encourage return of the pulse. If the pulse is not palpable and nail beds are cyanotic, arterial disruption must be presumed and further evaluation and con-

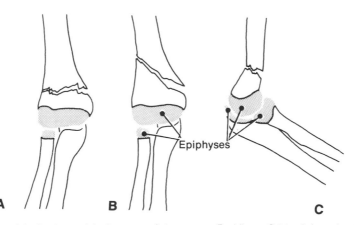

Figure 3.18.   Supracondylar fractures of the humerus. *A,* transverse. *B,* oblique. *C,* lateral view, showing most common angulation.

sultation must be instituted immediately. If this examination is also associated with marked swelling of the forearm and severe pain on extension of the fingers, associated compartment syndrome may be present and fasciotomy must be performed immediately. The median nerve can be evaluated by sensory check of the index finger and active wrist and finger flexion. If this motion and sensation are lacking, median nerve injury must be presumed. Decreased sensation along the dorsal web of the thumb and inability to extend the fingers at the metacarpophalangeal joints suggest injury to the radial nerve. Decreased sensation to the volar surface of the small finger or inability to actively adduct and abduct the straightened fingers suggests injury to the ulnar nerve.

Evidence of vascular or neural dysfunction is cause for immediate referral to an orthopaedist.

Treatment. All patients with displaced supracondylar fractures must be admitted to a hospital.

Emergency Treatment. Once the patient's neurovascular examination has been completed and found to be acceptable, the patient should be immediately splinted while awaiting referral to an orthopaedist or hospital admission. A posterior splint is applied to the elbow and secured with an elastic that does not cross the antecubital fossa. If there are good pulses and neurologic function is intact, the splint may be simply applied to the arm in the position in which it is resting. An area over the radial aspect of the wrist is left open for frequent inspection of the radial pulse. Flexing the elbow to apply this splint may cause obliteration of the pulse. The elbow should be extended until the radial pulse is palpable and the posterior splint applied in that position. Generally a splint applied with the elbow in approximately 30° of flexion is satisfactory until definitive treatment can be instituted (Fig. 3.19).

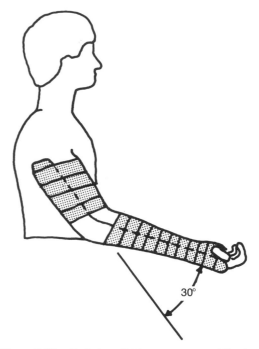

Figure 3.19. Posterior splint for emergency stabilization of elbow fractures and dislocations.

Reduction. While patients with nondisplaced fractures may be treated by the primary care physician, patients with displaced supracondylar fractures should be referred to an orthopaedist. Treatment of the displaced supracondylar fracture in a child by skeletal or skin traction was a popular method. It involves the insertion of a skeletal traction wire through the olecranon (Fig. 3.20). Overhead traction is preferred to control the swelling of the elbow. Although traction is a safe method of treatment, it requires frequent evaluation and a prolonged hospital stay. Also, while in skeletal traction, the 5- to 8-year-old child is constantly moving about, thus increasing the likelihood of malrotation or angulation of the fracture. This frequently results in a cubitus varus malunion. The preferred treatment for the displaced supracondylar fracture in a child is reduction under anesthesia and percutaneous pinning. This method decreases the hos-

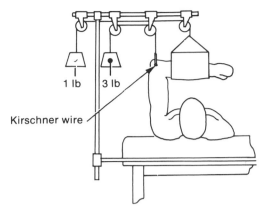

1 lb   3 lb

Kirschner wire

Figure 3.20. Traction reduction/immobilization of supracondylar fractures of the humerus.

pital costs and assures an anatomic reduction.

In an adult, displaced supracondylar fractures usually require open reduction and internal fixation.

Treatment after the Acute Phase. For a nondisplaced fracture or a fracture treated by percutaneous pinning, the patient is maintained in a posterior splint with the elbow in approximately 90° of flexion and the forearm in pronation. During the initial 1 to 2 weeks, frequent neurovascular checks are necessary until all swelling has decreased. Anteroposterior (AP) and lateral x-rays are taken weekly through the first 2½ weeks to ensure maintenance of reduction. After 2 weeks, a long-arm cast is applied, holding the elbow in 90° of flexion and the forearm in pronation. Casting is maintained

until x-rays demonstrate callus formation, usually within 6 weeks.

Rehabilitation. The goals of rehabilitation should be to restore a functional range of motion that is painless and associated with good strength. After cast removal, range of motion exercises in flexion, extension, supination, and pronation should be undertaken, and this can be followed by resistive exercises when motion is obtained. Full range of motion may not return. A lack of full extension by 10° to 15° is often noted. Passive painful stretching exercises are not indicated since they may increase the incidence of myositis ossificans.

Intraarticular Fractures of the Distal Humerus

Intraarticular fractures of the distal humerus occur in a variety of forms in the child and the adult. These may be fractures of the capitellum, intracondylar fractures, fractures of the trochlea, or comminuted "T" condylar fractures with a supracondylar extension (Fig. 3.21). In preschool children, many of the ossific nuclei above the elbow are undeveloped, and these fractures can be easily missed. A high degree of suspicion must be present when treating preschool children with limited elbow motion.

Clinical Characteristics. The injury usually results from a fall onto the outstretched arm or onto the elbow itself. Crepitation and pain with range of motion are present, and there is swelling about the

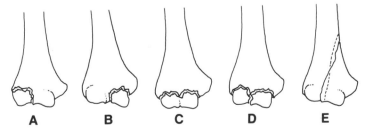

A   B   C   D   E

Figure 3.21. Fractures of the articular surfaces of the condyles, anterior view. *A,* fracture of the capitulum. *B,* fracture of the trochlea. *C,* transverse intercondylar fracture. *D,* T-shaped intercondylar fracture. *E,* spiral fracture.

elbow. In the adult, diagnosis from x-ray evidence is not difficult. In the child, however, only a small fleck of displaced bone may be apparent, but this suggests further displacement of the nonossified condyle. Highly suggestive of an intraarticular fracture is a positive fat pad sign (Fig. 3.22). This is caused by joint distention from the intraarticular hematoma displacing fat lining the inner surface of the brachialis muscle.

In the preschool child, none of these signs may be evident. The child with posttraumatic elbow pain should have a splint applied. Further diagnostic testing, such as arthrography, may be necessary. It is not recommended that the preschool child be immobilized awaiting a follow-up x-ray in 1 or 2 weeks. During that period of time, a displaced fracture could begin to heal in a malunited position.

Neurovascular examination should be performed and if any compromise is noticed, referral to an orthopaedist should be made immediately.

Treatment. *Undisplaced Fractures.* The undisplaced fracture can be treated definitively by the primary care physician by immobilization in a posterior elbow splint at 90° of flexion. Careful neurovascular checks should be made during the 1st week; thereafter the patient may be placed in a circular cast at 90° of flexion for an additional 3 to 5 weeks as dictated by x-rays and clinical examination. Rehabilitation as outlined above from supracondylar fracture should commence thereafter.

Displaced Fractures. Displaced intraarticular fractures require anatomic reduction, and therefore should be referred to an orthopaedist for operative reduction. The patient should be placed in a posterior splint for transport to the orthopaedist.

Fractures of the Medial Epicondyle

These fractures are thought to represent an avulsion injury by the flexor-pronator mass from its origin at the medial epicondyle.

Clinical Characteristics. The patient presents with posttraumatic pain, swelling, and tenderness over the medial aspect of the elbow. Undisplaced or minimally displaced fractures are defined as those displaced less than 1 cm from the anatomic position. Displaced fractures are defined as those displaced more than 1 cm from the anatomic position or displaced into the joint. Associated neurovascular compromise is usually manifested as an ulnar neuropathy, and the appropriate examination of the ulnar nerve should be performed when confronted with this injury. The degree of instability of the medial elbow must be ascertained. Gross instability may be apparent by a valgus resting posture of the elbow. If not, the elbow should be stressed in valgus by flexing the elbow approximately 20°, stabilizing the lateral elbow with one hand and pulling the forearm in a valgus direction with the other hand. As the normal ligamentous laxity varies from one individual to another, comparison with the unaffected elbow is necessary.

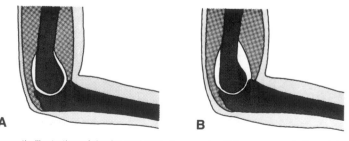

A   **B**

Figure 3.22. Diagrammatic illustration of the fat pad sign. *A,* normal soft tissue x-ray of elbow, lateral projection. *B,* soft tissue x-ray of elbow with fluid in joint, lateral projection.

Treatment. The treatment of the fracture is based upon the degree of displacement and the presence of instability.

Undisplaced or Minimally Displaced Fractures. The primary care physician can treat this fracture by immobilization in a splint or cast. As this injury is an avulsion injury by the flexor-pronator mass, it is best held reduced by flexion of the wrist and pronation of the forearm. During and after application of the immobilization device, frequent neurovascular examinations must be carried out.

Displaced Fractures. Those fractures displaced more than 1 cm or unstable to valgus stress require closed or open reduction. The primary care physician may attempt a closed reduction by manipulation of the medial epicondyle fragment with the elbow flexed, the forearm pronated, and the wrist flexed (Fig. 3.23). Closed reduction is often unsuccessful, and if so, referral to the orthopaedic surgeon should be made.

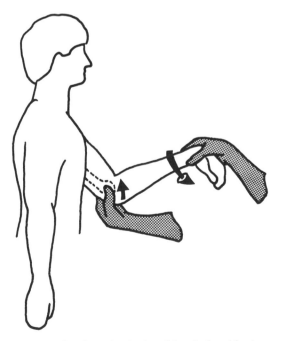

Figure 3.23. Closed reduction of the displaced fracture of the medial epicondyle.

Fractures of the Head and Neck of the Radius

Fractures of the radial head and neck occur frequently and are usually caused by a fall onto the outstretched hand, causing a valgus compressive force at the elbow.

Clinical Characteristics. Generally, these are manifested as radial head fractures in adults and as radial neck fractures in children (Fig. 3.24). The clinical examination usually reveals swelling about the elbow, limited motion, particularly in supination and pronation, and pain to palpation about the radial head. Radiographs should be obtained to define the fracture and the degree of displacement.

Treatment. *Undisplaced Fractures.* These fractures are best treated by splint or cast immobilization with the elbow in 90° of flexion and the forearm in full supination. In the child, these fractures should be immobilized for 4 to 6 weeks, followed by rehabilitation. In the adult, splint protection and early guarded mobilization (i.e., 1 week) with gentle flexion, extension, supination, and pronation are indicated to prevent joint contractures. Follow-up x-rays should be obtained within 1 week to document that displacement has not occurred with range of motion.

Partially Displaced Fractures of the Radial Neck. The degree of acceptable displacement in radial neck fractures is controversial. Children under 10 years of age will have a better result with mildly displaced fractures than children over 10 years of age and young adults. As a guideline, loss of apposition or angulation greater than 15° requires a closed reduction. In children, this should be performed under general anesthesia and full relaxation, particularly for fractures with angulation greater than 30°.

Under anesthesia, one operator grasps the upper arm for stability. The other operator extends the elbow and provides axial traction. Rotation of the forearm is performed with one hand while the radial head is pal-

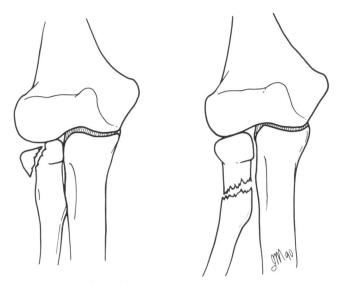

Fx. radial head vs. Fx. radial neck

Figure 3.24. Intraarticular radial head fractures are more likely to occur in adults; intraarticular radial neck fractures are more likely to occur in children.

pated with the thumb of the other hand. The prominent angulated radial head can be palpated laterally with the arm in mild supination. Once this is done, mild valgus stress is applied and manipulation performed on the radial head with a push from the operator's thumb. One guideline to adequacy of reduction under anesthesia is the finding of full supination and pronation of the forearm after reduction. Intraoperative radiographs are made to assess the adequacy of reduction. If reduction is noted to be adequate, the patient is placed in a posterior splint with the elbow at 90° of flexion and the forearm in mild supination. If reduction has not been achieved, the splint is applied and orthopaedic referral made.

Displaced Intraarticular Radial Head Fractures. These fractures must have anatomic reduction and should be referred to the orthopaedist for definitive evaluation and treatment. In totally displaced fractures of the radial head, particularly in children, there is a high association with elbow dislocation. In the child, spontaneous reduction of an associated elbow dislocation may occur, leaving the radial head displaced. In totally displaced or intraarticular fractures of the radial head, orthopaedic referral should be made for probable open reduction, internal fixation, or for excision.

Fractures of the Olecranon

Fractures of the olecranon are often caused by direct trauma to the elbow during a fall. They may also occur with avulsion of the olecranon by the triceps mechanism.

Clinical Characteristics. The patient presents with posttraumatic pain, swelling, and tenderness over the olecranon. Range of motion is usually limited. The ossification center for the olecranon appears at age 10 and is generally fused to the proximal ulna by age 16. There are reports of epiphyseal plates of the olecranon persisting into young adulthood. This should not be mistaken for a fracture of the olecranon, particularly in trauma cases. Persistent epiphyseal plates are generally bilateral, and contralateral elbow films should be obtained if questions arise.

Treatment. Treatment by the general practitioner depends on the degree of displacement and the location of the fracture.

Undisplaced fractures of the olecranon or avulsion fractures at the tip of the olecranon (Fig. 3.25) with minimal displacement may be treated in a long-arm cast with the elbow flexed 30° to 60°, determined by the patient's comfort. Immobilization should continue for approximately 4 weeks, at which time guided rehabilitation should be instituted. Radiographs should be repeated 1 week after the initial fracture to be sure that displacement has not occurred. In markedly displaced avulsion fractures of the tip of the olecranon or in intraarticular displaced fractures, a posterior splint holding the elbow at 30° should be applied and orthopaedic referral made for open reduction and internal fixation.

Fractures of the Coronoid Process

Fractures of the coronoid process are generally caused by an avulsion injury by the brachialis muscle at its insertion into the ulna.

Clinical Characteristics. The patient presents with swelling about the elbow and pain in the antecubital fossae. Care must be taken to evaluate the stability of the elbow as an associated elbow dislocation, and relocation must be ruled out. A sudden, strong, resisted contraction of the brachialis muscle may result in avulsion of the coronoid attachment. Radiographically, this fracture appears as a small chip on the lateral view (Fig. 3.26). Avulsion fractures of the coronoid process may be associated with more significant injuries, especially elbow dislocation, which will be reviewed later in this chapter.

Treatment. The elbow is flexed to 90°, and the radial pulse checked to be sure it is not diminished in flexion. The lateral radiograph is then obtained and position of the

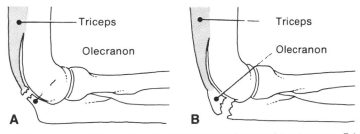

Figure 3.25.   Fractures of the olecranon. *A*, lateral view. Avulsion fracture of the tip of the olecranon. *B*, lateral view. Transverse fracture through the body of the olecranon.

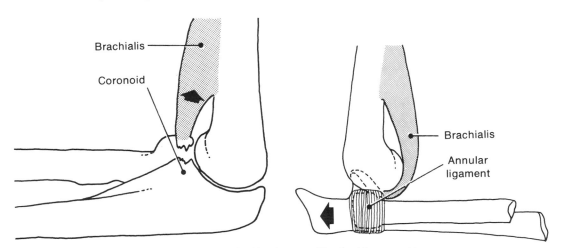

Figure 3.26.   Medial view. Avulsion fracture of the tip of the coronoid process.

fracture fragment is assessed. Continued displacement of the fracture fragment more than 5 mm indicates the need for orthopaedic referral. As noted above, this fracture can occur with an elbow dislocation and the dislocation may have been spontaneously reduced. In addition, on occasion the fracture fragments are not small and might include a significant amount of articular surface. These injuries should also be referred for orthopaedic evaluation and treatment. If the reduction is acceptable, the primary care physician should immobilize the elbow in 90° of flexion and in full supination. Immobilization should continue for 4 weeks, and guarded rehabilitation instituted, as outlined in the section on "Supracondylar Fractures."

Dislocations of the Elbow

Dislocations of the humeroradioulnar joint are rarely seen in skeletally immature children, and are more commonly seen in young adults. It generally is the result of a fall onto the outstretched hand with the arm in extension and adduction. Approximately 80 to 90% of elbow dislocations are posterior or posterolateral. Treatment of posterior dislocation will be discussed in this section. Anterior dislocation and divergent radial and ulnar dislocations are rare, and patients with these conditions should have a splint applied and be referred to an orthopaedist. Dislocation of the radial head associated with fractures of the ulna will be discussed later in this chapter.

Clinical Characteristics. Diagnosis of posterior dislocation of the elbow is generally obvious by the apparent deformity. The patient presents with significant swelling and pain about the elbow. Gross deformity of the elbow is usually apparent. The usual anatomic triangle, palpable posteriorly at the elbow, is made by the medial epicondyle, lateral epicondyle, and olecranon tip. This is distorted in posterior dislocation (Fig. 3.27). Radiographs should be obtained to rule out associated fractures. Diligent neurovascular examination should be undertaken before and after elbow reduction.

Treatment. Complete muscle relaxation is imperative in achieving a nontraumatic reduction. Depending on the age of the patient, time since dislocation, and degree of muscle spasm, the physician must choose general, regional, or intravenous sedation.

Many methods of elbow reduction have been described. Those involving countertraction in the axilla by use of a folded towel are not recommended because of the possibility of brachial plexus injury. In most instances, the primary care physician will not have the use of an experienced assistant and therefore the following simple method of reduction is suggested. Once adequate muscle relaxation has been obtained, the patient is

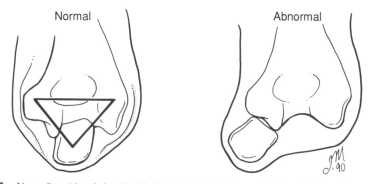

Figure 3.27.   Normally, a triangle is palpable between medial epicondyle, lateral epicondyle, and olecranon.

placed in the prone position and the forearm is hung from the side of the stretcher. Gentle downward traction is then applied at the wrist while the examiner guides the reduction of the olecranon with the thumb. Following reduction, the elbow should be flexed and gently extended through a full range of motion to assess the adequacy of reduction and to be sure there is nothing blocking motion within the joint. Postreduction x-rays should be obtained to rule out fractures that may not have been seen with the elbow dislocated and also to confirm that no bone injury occurred during reduction which may rarely happen. In addition, the x-ray is necessary to assess the quality of reduction of the elbow and any associated coronoid process fracture. If intraarticular fractures are noted or the coronoid fracture remains displaced, orthopaedic referral is recommended.

If the dislocation is associated with condylar fractures, immediate orthopaedic referral prior to reduction should be obtained. If there is associated neurovascular compromise of the elbow and orthopaedic assistance is unavailable, the primary care physician should attempt reduction as outlined above. If there is no neurovascular compromise, the elbow should be immobilized by a posterior splint, and the patient should be admitted to the hospital with close neurovascular observation until an orthopaedist is available. If the patient is not hospitalized, frequent neurovascular checks should be described to the family. The extremity should be elevated and ice packs applied.

Treatment following reduction depends on the stability noted during range of motion following reduction. In those dislocations that are stable through a full range of motion after reduction, early, guarded, gentle, active range of motion should be encouraged at 3 to 4 days, with splinting intermittently. At 3 weeks the splints are discarded and more aggressive, active range of motion is encouraged. There is no place for passive or forced manipulation following an elbow dislocation. If the elbow is unstable following reduction, the patient should be held in a long-arm splint for 3 weeks. Following this, active-assistive range of motion is begun in a protective splint within which elbow extension can be progressively increased.

The patient should be told at the time of dislocation that full range of motion following healing will in all likelihood not be recovered, especially full extension of the elbow. The potential to develop posttraumatic myositis ossificans should also be discussed.

Fractures of Both Bones of the Forearm

The radius and ulna comprise a parallelogram that includes the proximal and distal radioulnar joints. Therefore, a fracture of one bone of the forearm is often associated with disruption of either the distal or proximal radioulnar joint. These will be described in the sections on "Monteggia Fractures" and "Galeazzi Fractures."

Clinical Characteristics. The patient usually presents with posttraumatic pain, swelling, and variable deformity, depending on the degree of displacement. These injuries are almost always displaced to some extent. The patient has pain with any attempted motion of wrist or elbow. A careful evaluation of the neurologic status and vascular status should be performed.

Treatment. The treatment of fractures of both bones of the forearm is determined by the age of the patient and the location of the fracture (in the proximal, middle, or distal third of the forearm). In general, displaced fractures of both bones of the forearm in adults should be referred for orthopaedic evaluation and treatment because they usually require open reduction and internal fixation. In children, treatment depends on the age of the child and the location of the fracture. In general, the younger the child and the closer the fracture to the epiphyseal plate, the greater the amount of angulation that is acceptable. As a general guide, all deformities exceeding 10°, especially in the middle third of the forearm, should be corrected. The greater the residual angulation after healing, the greater the loss of supination and pronation of the forearm.

The position for reduction and the position of maintenance in a long-arm cast after reduction depend on the location of the fracture in the proximal, middle, or distal third of the forearm. Rotation of the proximal radius can be predicted by the position of the bicipital tuberosity on AP film of the proximal radius. The rotation of the forearm after fracture depends on the relationship of the site of the fracture to the insertion of the two supinators of the forearm, i.e., the supinator and the biceps tendon, and the two pronators of the forearm, i.e., the pronator teres and the pronator quadratus.

In fractures of the proximal third of the forearm, the proximal fracture fragment of the radius is controlled only by the supinator and the biceps tendon. The distal fragments are controlled by both the pronator teres and the pronator quadratus. Therefore, many fractures of the proximal third of the forearm are best reduced and held in supination (Fig. 3.28). This must be correlated radiographically by the location of the bicipital tuberosity and the alignment of the fracture.

Fractures of the middle third of the forearm are distal to the insertion of the pronator teres and therefore the action of the supinators is offset by the action of the pronator, thus holding the proximal fragments in neutral rotation (Fig. 3.29). These fractures are best held in a long-arm cast in neutral rotation. Once again, postreduction radiographic correlation must be ascertained.

Fractures of the distal third of the forearm are often stabilized by the broad origin and insertion of the pronator quadratus, and rotational deformities are unlikely. In these fractures, the action of the brachioradialis muscle on the radial styloid may contribute to angulation of the distal radial fragment.

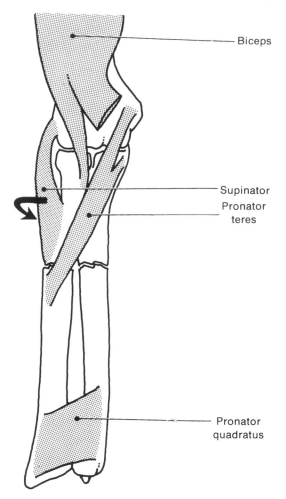

Figure 3.28. Second principle of treatment of forearm fractures. Proximal fragment of the radius supinates following fractures through the proximal third of the forearm, as the action of the supinator is unopposed.

These fractures should be held in slight pronation, wrist flexor, and ulnar deviation.

Undisplaced fractures of both bones of the forearm in the adult should be treated in a well-molded long-arm cast, taking advantage of the interosseous membrane to help hold the reduction (Fig. 3.29). The time of immobilization should be approximately 6 weeks, and this is modified based on the evidence of callus formation and clinical stability on follow-up examination. In fractures of the distal third of the radius and ulna,

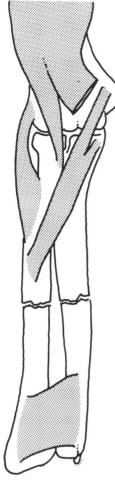

Figure 3.29. Third principle of treatment of fractures of the forearm. Proximal half of the radius remains in the neutral rotation following fractures through the middle third of the forearm, as the action of the pronator teres balances the action of the supinators.

conversion to a short-arm cast can generally be made at approximately 4 weeks. Repeat radiographs should be made after approximately 3 days and then 1 week to be sure of maintenance of reduction. Any displacement or angulation that takes place must be referred for orthopaedic follow-up. If no displacement occurs, the follow-up films should be made at 4 to 6 weeks.

In children, no more than 10° of angulation should be accepted. Some appositional

overlap may be accepted if there is no associated angulation. Once again, rotational alignment of the fragments must be appropriately checked.

Fractures of the distal third of the forearm may be held in slight pronation and wrist flexion, with three-point fixation within the plaster. Reduction of proximal and middle one-third fractures of both bones in children may be obtained by placing the child under anesthesia in finger trap traction to obtain length. Once length has been obtained, rotational control must be obtained and checked by x-ray. Once this is completed, a long-arm cast is applied and molded along the interosseous membrane as described in Figure 3.30. Radiographic follow-up should be obtained at 3 days, 7 days, 2 weeks, and 3 weeks.

Green-stick Fractures

Green-stick fractures may appear to have only angular deformity, but often have a rotational deformity as well. These should be reduced with gentle counterpressure, taking care to check both angulation and rotational deformities. Once reduction is obtained, a

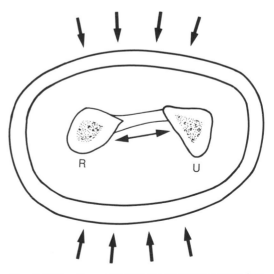

Figure 3.30. Proper AP mold in cast to help reduce forearm fracture via tension on interosseous membrane.

long-arm cast should be applied. Completion of the fracture is unnecessary, and may lead to further loss of rotational stability.

Plastic Bone Deformation

Occasionally a child will present with mild to moderate clinical deformity of the forearm following an injury. Pain is not usually extreme. X-rays reveal deformity of the radius and/or ulna, but no obvious fracture line. This represents plastic deformation of the bones. These patients should be referred for treatment.

Monteggia Fractures

The Monteggia fracture is a dislocation of the radial head that occurs in combination with fracture of the ulnar metaphysis or diaphysis. Because of the parallelogram, mechanics of the radius and ulna working through the distal and proximal radial ulnar joints, an isolated fracture of the ulna is often associated with displacement of the radial head. The most common pattern of the Monteggia fracture is anterior dislocation of the radial head with fracture of the ulnar diaphysis or metaphysis. Lateral or anterolateral dislocation of the radial head also occurs, with posterior radial head dislocation being uncommon.

Clinical Characteristics. The patient presents with posttraumatic pain, swelling, and deformity of the elbow and forearm. Depending on the type of injury, the tenderness is located in the ulnar metaphysis or diaphysis, and displacement of the radial head may be palpable. Any attempt to rotate the forearm or otherwise move the elbow is painful. Neurologic examination should be performed. Injury to the deep branch of the radial nerve is the most common neurologic injury.

As noted above, the forearm represents a parallelogram with ulna, radius, and distal and proximal radioulnar articulations. Therefore, in an isolated fracture of the ulna,

further investigation of the wrist and elbow is imperative to rule out articular disruptions.

Treatment. These injuries should be splinted and referred for orthopaedic evaluation. Closed treatment can be successful in children; however, operative treatment is usually necessary in adults.

Galeazzi Fractures

The Galeazzi fracture is a fracture of the distal shaft of the radius which occurs in combination with dislocation of the distal radial ulna joint. The joint disruption occurs because of the same "parallelogram effect" that operates in the Monteggia fracture, which causes radial head dislocation with fracture of the ulna.

Clinical Characteristics. The patient presents with posttraumatic pain, swelling, and deformity of the distal radius and wrist. Subluxation or dislocation of the distal ulna may be evident with prominence of the distal ulna dorsally. Range of motion of the wrist is limited and painful.

X-rays reveal the deformity. The subluxation of the distal ulna is best seen on a true lateral x-ray. Comparison views of the contralateral wrist are often necessary to make a diagnosis with certainty.

Treatment. These injuries require open reduction, internal fixation, and should be splinted and subsequently referred to the orthopaedist.

COMPARTMENT SYNDROME

Compartment syndrome and Volkmann ischemic contracture may be a complication of elbow and forearm fractures. In the past, Volkmann ischemic contracture was a far too common, unfortunate result of fractures about the elbow in children, particularly supracondylar fractures. This results from prolonged ischemia of the forearm musculature with muscle necrosis, and ultimately replacement by fibrous tissue. This results in a severe deformity of the hand and wrist with paralysis. The key to avoiding Volkmann ischemic contracture is recognizing arterial injury and compartment syndrome early and providing immediate, nonoperative or operative intervention. The primary care physician is in the best position to observe the early manifestations of this syndrome, when it is reversible.

Clinical Characteristics

The patient may present with an arterial injury caused by open laceration or to arterial disruption secondary to a severely displaced fracture or dislocation. These patients will have a cool, pale extremity with altered pulse. The patient may also present with a closed blunt injury with or without fracture. In these patients, a high index of suspicion must be maintained.

Early signs of a compartment syndrome will be manifested by pain on passive stretch of the muscles in that compartment. There will also be tense swelling. A patient with an impending compartment syndrome of the volar forearm compartment will experience significant pain on passive extension of the fingers. Later (and often too late) findings will include paresthesias, numbness, and muscle weakness. The pathophysiology of compartment syndrome is discussed in more detail in Chapter 8.

Treatment

Effective treatment of ischemia from arterial injury and for compartment syndrome is based on early recognition. Therefore, in supracondylar, elbow, or forearm fractures or dislocation, the following principles should be observed. In acute fractures, meticulous neurovascular examination should be undertaken to ascertain the presence of adequate distal pulses. Nail beds are checked for adequate capillary refill as well as the lack of cyanosis. Neurologic examination should be done to establish any neu-

rologic injury. Initial immobilization should be in the form of splints, which can accommodate swelling and provide access for further examination. In displaced fractures about the elbow, immediate application of a cylindrical cast is ill-advised. Frequent neurovascular checks should be made in the first 1 to 2 days following the fracture. As stated above, early muscle ischemia is manifest by complaints of pain out of proportion to the underlying injury. The pain is exacerbated by passive stretch of ischemic muscle. Frequent passive manipulation of the fingers both in flexion and extension may indicate an early compartment syndrome if this is associated with extreme pain.

If any of these physical findings are present, immediate relief of external pressures must be provided by splitting dressing and bivalving casts. In the supracondylar fracture, if relief is not achieved by these means, the elbow should be extended. If pain and swelling continue, the possibility of compartment syndrome is considered and immediate orthopaedic consultation should be obtained for possible fasciotomies. If arterial injury is diagnosed, orthopaedic and/or vascular referral is made immediately.

MYOSITIS OSSIFICANS

The formation of heterotopic bone is, unfortunately, a common complication of trauma to the elbow. It is most often associated with extensive damage to the brachialis muscle. Formation of heterotopic bone can cause bridging across the elbow joint and frank ankylosis.

Pathogenesis

Many factors have been implicated in the pathogenesis of myositis ossificans, but it is primarily a result of the initial soft tissue injury. Excessive force used in reducing a fracture or dislocation about the elbow, leading to increased soft tissue damage, may be contributory. Aggressive rehabilitation, particularly passive stretching exercises, may be another contributory factor.

Prevention

The following recommendations are made to avoid this complication. In the early rehabilitation of elbow fractures, active and active-assistive range of motion exercises that are not painful should be performed. Painful passive stretching should be avoided. A high index of suspicion should be maintained in patients who have prolonged tenderness and pain about the elbow and difficulty in regaining motion. In these patients a slow rehabilitation program should be maintained with careful radiographic monitoring. More immobilization may be indicated. It is important to note that the radiographic evidence of developing myositis ossificans is not usually present for 3 to 4 weeks following the injury and consequently the clinician must have a high index of suspicion based on the clinical presentation. In patients where x-rays do show progressive myositis ossificans, it is best to immobilize the elbow in approximately 45° of flexion and refer the patient for further evaluation and treatment to the orthopaedic surgeon.

Recently, indomethacin has been utilized in the prophylaxis of myositis ossificans in severe elbow injuries. The recommended dose is 25 mg three times a day. This medication is suggested only for those patients who do not have a contraindication to its use.

In early rehabilitation, active-assistive range of motion exercises that are painless should be performed. Painful passive stretching may increase the incidence or severity of myositis ossificans. A high index of suspicion should be maintained in patients who have prolonged tenderness about the elbow and difficulty in regaining motion. Patients with these clinical presentations should have a slow rehabilitation with careful radiographic monitoring. If there is radiographic evidence of worsening myositis ossificans, immobilization in a position of function (i.e., approximately 45° of elbow flexion) has been suggested. Patients with established or progressive myositis ossificans should be referred for orthopaedic evaluation, as future excision may be indicated.

SUGGESTED READINGS

Bora FW Jr, ed. The pediatric upper extremity. Philadelphia: WB Saunders; 1986.

Green D, ed. Operative hand surgery. New York: Churchill Livingstone; 1988.

Stern P, ed. Hand clinics—difficult fractures of the hand and wrist. Philadelphia: WB Saunders; 1985.

Strickland J, ed. Hand clinics—flexor tendon surgery. Philadelphia: WB Saunders; 1985.

Taleisnik J, ed. The wrist. New York: Churchill Livingstone; 1985.

Zook E, ed. Hand clinics—the perionychium. Philadelphia: WB Saunders; 1990.

CHAPTER 4

Wrist and Hand (Including Upper Extremity Nerve Injuries)

Thomas F. Breen, M.D.

This chapter will be devoted to frequently encountered pathology in the hand and wrist as well as compressive neuropathies of the hand and forearm.

Essential Anatomy

X-RAY ANATOMY

Figure 4.1 shows the anteroposterior (AP) and lateral radiographs of the hand. These are the basic screening x-rays for the workup of any hand or wrist problems. Specific x-ray views and supplementary imaging studies will be discussed when appropriate in each section.

BONES OF THE WRIST

The wrist is a series of complex joints with multiple bones and articulations, including the distal radius and ulna. The anatomic limits of the carpus are often defined as extending from the distal articular surface of the radius to the carpometacarpal joints. Because fractures of the distal radius have such a direct effect on wrist function, the wrist is defined as starting 3 cm proximal to the radial carpal joint extending distally to the carpometacarpal joint.

The carpus consists of eight bones with multiple concave and convex articular surfaces allowing for complex arcs of motion in multiple planes without sacrificing stability. The radiocarpal joint is a biconcave articular surface, triangular in shape with its apex toward the radial styloid. The radiocarpal articulation is composed of two fossae, the radioscaphoid and radiolunate. The joint surface is directed in a palmar and ulnar direction of 11° and 22°, respectively. This is important when treating distal radius fractures and will be discussed later.

The ulnar side of the wrist has no direct bony articulation between the distal ulna and the carpus. Rather, the ulnar side of the carpus is supported in a sling-like fashion by the triangular fibrocartilage complex, which lies interposed between the distal ulna and triquetrum, allowing for an increased arc of pronation and supination of the forearm at the distal radioulnar joint.

The majority of wrist flexion and extension occurs at the radiocarpal joint with a small amount at the midcarpal joint, defined as the articulation between the lunate and capitate as well as the triquetrum and hamate. Clinically, this area of the wrist is a common source of wrist ligament instability, degenerative joint disease, and chronic wrist pain.

The carpometacarpal joints have relatively little motion. They are not common sites of clinical problems except for the thumb metacarpotrapezial joint, which is the site of frequent fractures (such as Bennett's and Rolando's fractures, discussed later). The thumb metacarpotrapezial joint is the joint in the body that most frequently develops degenerative arthritis because of its high joint reaction forces and wide arc of motion in multiple planes. It is composed of two orthogonal saddle-shaped bones that permit a wide range of motion, facilitating complex thumb function.

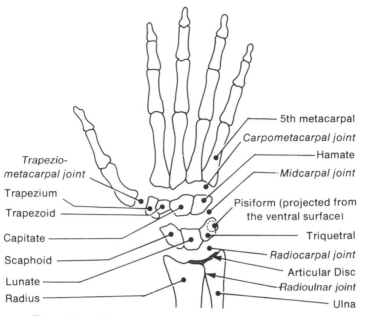

Figure 4.1.   Schematic drawing of hand and carpal bony anatomy.

The scaphoid bone is the most important bone in the wrist, providing a stabilizing bridge or link between the proximal carpal row (lunate and triquetrum) and distal carpal row (trapezium-trapezoid-capitate and hamate). It is also the most frequently fractured bone in the adult wrist. The diagnosis of a scaphoid fracture is sometimes difficult to make but is one that is essential for proper treatment because of its precarious blood supply which predisposes it to develop avascular necrosis or nonunion after fracture.

The lunate has a proximal convex surface that articulates with the lunate fossa of the distal radius and a distal concave articular surface, which articulates with the head of the capitate. Radially, the lunate articulates with the scaphoid where trauma to the scapholunate interosseous ligament results in painful radial wrist instability. Ulnarly, the lunate articulates with the triquetrum, the site of ulnar-sided wrist pain and carpal instability secondary to attenuation of the lunotriquestral ligament. The lunate, like the scaphoid, has a precarious vascular supply,

predisposing it to idiopathic avascular necrosis, known as Kienböck's disease.

The triquetrum articulates with the lunate radially, the hamate distally, the pisiform palmarly, and the triangular fibrocartilage complex proximally. Trauma to the triangular fibrocartilage complex is a common cause of ulnar-sided wrist pain.

The hamate is a member of the distal carpal row articulating with the triquetrum, lunate, and the fourth and fifth metacarpals. The hook of the hamate extends in a palmar direction constituting the medial wall of the carpal tunnel. The hook may be fractured and this can be the source of "occult" wrist pain.

The pisiform is the smallest bone of the wrist. It is the only carpal bone with a tendon insertion. It is a sesamoid bone within the substance of the flexor carpi ulnaris tendon, articulating with the triquetrum dorsally, and is frequently affected by degenerative arthritis.

The trapezoid, in the distal carpal row, is the only bone that articulates with a single metacarpal (index metacarpal). It also articulates with the scaphoid, trapezium, and capitate.

The capitate is the center of wrist rotation. It articulates with the second, third, and fourth metacarpals distally, the trapezoid radially, and the hamate ulnarly. Proximally, the capitate articulates with the lunate and is the major articulation of the midcarpal joint, where instability and ligamentous disruption commonly occur.

LIGAMENTS OF THE WRIST

The purpose of the wrist ligaments is to provide interosseous stability to an inherently unstable bony arrangement. The ligaments are divided into dorsal and palmar contributions. The key ligaments responsible for stability are the palmar ligaments, which are more stout and morphologically distinct than their dorsal counterparts. Palmarly, the major ligaments are the radiocapitate, radiolunotriquetral, and radioscaphoid ligaments (Fig. 4.2).

Distally, the most important palmar intrinsic wrist ligament is the capitotriquetral ligament, which is primarily involved with stabilizing the distal to the proximal carpal row. The radial collateral ligament and ulnar collateral ligament are specialized condensations of the wrist capsule and do not appear to be true wrist ligaments.

Dorsally, the ligaments are less strong and distinct structures. The main contributor is the dorsal radiocarpal ligament. The remaining dorsal ligament is the scapholunate interosseous ligament. This is a short, stout, triangular ligament which is commonly injured in dorsiflexion wrist sprains (Fig. 4.3).

The clinically important ligaments are palmar and they function to stabilize the proximal carpal row to the distal radius. There are fewer ligaments stabilizing the distal to proximal row (midcarpal joint) and hence this joint is a source of symptomatic wrist instability.

BIOMECHANICS OF THE WRIST

The wrist can be thought of as a central flexion-extension link composed of the radius, lunate, and capitate. Since no extrinsic tendons from the forearm musculature insert onto any carpal bone (except the flexor

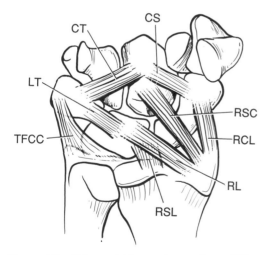

Figure 4.2.   Palmar wrist ligamentous anatomy. *RCL,* radiocollateral; *RSC,* radioscaphocapitate; *RL,* radiolunate; *LT,* lunotriquetral; *RSL,* radioscapholunate; *CS,* scaphocapitate; *CT,* capitotriquetral; *TFCC,* triangular fibrocartilage complex. (Adapted from illustration by Elizabeth Roselius, copyrighted 1988. Reprinted with permission from Taleisnik J. The wrist. New York: Churchill Livingstone, 1985:14.)

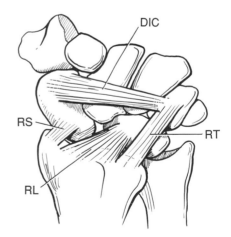

Figure 4.3.   Dorsal wrist ligamentous anatomy. *DC,* dorsal complex; *RS,* radioscaphoid; *RL,* radiolunate; *RT,* radiotriquetral. (Adapted from illustration by Elizabeth Roselius, copyrighted 1988. Reprinted with permission from Taleisnik J. The wrist. New York: Churchill Livingstone, 1985:23.)

carpi ulnaris on the pisiform), motion across the wrist is initiated at the base of the metacarpals where the tendons insert. Flexion and extension forces are transferred across the inherently unstable proximal and distal carpal bones, which would tend to collapse with any force transferred across them. Stability is afforded by the scaphoid, which bridges these two intercalated segments. As the wrist is dorsiflexed or palmar flexed, the scaphoid moves in a synchronous direction, allowing motion but maintaining a stabilizing bridge across both links of the intercalated chain. With radial and ulnar deviation, similar changes occur between the scaphoid and the proximal and distal links.

CARPAL TUNNEL

This is a very common site of hand and wrist pathology. It is a closed tunnel on four sides with three sides composed of the carpal bones and the roof (palmar surface) formed by the flexor retinaculum extending from the hook of the hamate and pisiform ulnarly to the trapezium and scaphoid radially. The contents of the carpal tunnel are the nine extrinsic flexor tendons (eight flexor profundus and superficialis tendons and one flexor pollicis tendon) and the median nerve. The ulnar nerve and artery, radial artery, flexor carpi ulnaris, flexor carpi radialis, and palmaris longus lie outside the carpal tunnel (Fig. 4.4).

FLEXOR TENDON SYSTEM

The wrist flexors (flexor carpi radialis and flexor carpi ulnaris) insert at the base of the index and little metacarpals, respectively. The extrinsic flexor tendons to the digits all course through the carpal tunnel. The flexor pollicis longus tendon, the deepest and most radial tendon within the tunnel, inserts onto the base of the distal phalanx of the thumb. The flexor digitorum superficialis tendons are the most superficial tendons in the carpal tunnel and palm. At the level of the proximal

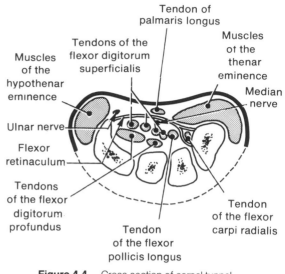

Figure 4.4.   Cross-section of carpal tunnel.

phalanx of each digit, the superficialis tendon divides and splits into two slips which insert along the palmar aspect of the middle phalanx. The flexor digitorum profundus, which lies deep to the flexor digitorum superficialis, emerges between the two slips of the superficialis, inserting at the base of the distal phalanx.

The flexor tendons in each digit travel in a fibroosseous tunnel between the metacarpal neck and the distal interphalangeal (DIP) joint. This fibroosseous tunnel serves a dual purpose, providing nutrition to the tendon by synovial diffusion and mechanical stability by a series of pulleys or thickenings of the sheath.

The median nerve, which courses deep to the transverse carpal ligament, lies just ulnar to the flexor carpi radialis and radial to the palmaris longus. The ulnar nerve lies dorsal to the flexor carpi ulnaris and does not enter the carpal tunnel. The ulnar artery courses radial to the ulnar nerve. The radial artery runs just radial to the flexor carpi radialis tendon, then travels dorsally through the base of the anatomic snuff-box.

EXTRINSIC EXTENSOR TENDONS

The extensor tendons pass over the dorsum of the wrist, arranged in six separate compartments (Fig. 4.5). The first dorsal compartment contains the abductor pollicis longus and the extensor pollicis brevis. The second extensor compartment contains the tendons of the extensor carpi radialis longus and the extensor carpi radialis brevis. The third dorsal wrist compartment contains the extensor pollicis longus, which passes around Lister's tubercle of the dorsal distal radius. The fourth extensor compartment is comprised of the four extensor digitorum communis (EDC) tendons to each digit and the extensor indicis proprius (EIP) tendon to the index finger, providing independent extension. The fifth dorsal compartment contains the extensor digiti minimi (EDM) tendon. This tendon provides independent

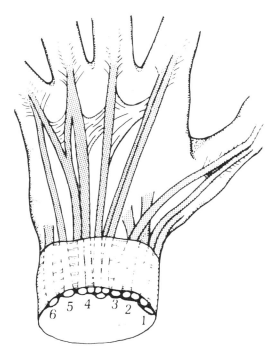

Figure 4.5. Dorsal extensor compartments of the hand. (From The hand: examination and diagnosis. 2nd ed. New York: Churchill Livingstone, 1983:17. Reprinted with permission of the American Society for Surgery of the Hand.)

extension to the little finger. The EIP and EDM lie to the ulnar side of their respective EDC tendons. The sixth dorsal compartment contains the tendon of the extensor carpi ulnaris, which inserts at the base of the fifth metacarpal.

INTRINSIC MUSCULATURE OF THE HAND

Unlike the extrinsic muscles, the intrinsic muscles of the hand are defined as those that have both their origins and insertions within the hand. These are the thenar, interosseous, lumbrical, and hypothenar muscles. The thenar muscles lie on the radial palmar side of the hand covering the thumb metacarpal. The components of the thenar muscle group are the abductor pollicis brevis (APB), opponens pollicis (OP), flexor pollicis brevis (FPB), and adductor pollicis muscles. The APB, OP, and FPB pronate and oppose the thumb and are median-innervated, while the adductor pollicis adducts the thumb and is innervated by the ulnar nerve.

The lumbrical and interosseous muscles flex the metacarpophalangeal (MCP) joints and extend the interphalangeal (IP) joints of each finger. There are two groups of interosseus muscles, four dorsal and three palmar, both innervated by the ulnar nerve. While each contributes to MCP joint flexion and IP joint extension, the palmar layer adducts and the dorsal layer abducts the digits.

There are four lumbrical muscles. They are unique in that they have no bony origin. They originate from their respective flexor digitorum profundus tendons in the palm, coursing to the radial side of the MCP joints. Like the interosseous muscles, the lumbricals flex the MCP joints and extend the IP joints. In most instances, the radial two lumbrical muscles are innervated by the median nerve and the ulnar two by the ulnar nerve.

The hypothenar muscle group is comprised of the abductor digiti minimi (ADM), flexor digiti minimi (FDM), and opponens digiti minimi (ODM). The ADM originates from the pisiform bone and inserts onto the ulnar side of the base of the proximal phalanx of the little finger. The FDM arises from the hamate and transverse carpal ligament and inserts with the abductor digiti minimi on the proximal phalanx. The ODM lies deep to these muscles. The hypothenar muscles abduct and supinate the little finger.

DORSAL EXTENSOR APPARATUS

Special mention is made of the dorsal extensor apparatus of the digit because of its complex anatomy and the many hand problems that are associated with it (Fig. 4.6). The dorsal extensor apparatus of the digit has contributions from both the extrinsic extensors (EDC, EIP, EDM) as well as the intrinsic extensors (lumbricals and interossei). Extension of the MCP joint is through the sagittal band, which is a sling enveloping the MCP joint. It is through this sling that the extrinsic extensor extends the MCP joint. The lumbrical and interosseous form the oblique and transverse fibers of the intrinsic apparatus. The transverse fibers act to flex the MCP joint and the oblique fibers act to extend the IP joint. The central continuation of the extrinsic extensor forms the central slip, which inserts at the base of the middle phalanx and is the extrinsic contributor to IP joint extension. The lateral bands course distally and fuse to form the terminal extensor tendon which inserts at the base of the distal phalanx, functioning as the prime extensor of the DIP joint.

COMPARTMENTS AND SPACES OF THE PALM

There are distinct compartments and potential spaces within the palm. Infections of the hand are common and knowledge of the compartment anatomy will aid in detection and treatment.

There are three distinct compartments (Fig. 4.7). The hypothenar and thenar compartments lie on either side of the central compartment. The central compartment houses the flexor tendons of the digits and common digital nerves, as well as the superficial palmar arch.

Infections in the hand usually are confined to one of these three compartments and most often do not violate their boundaries. Infections in the digital flexor tendon sheaths can penetrate into the central com-

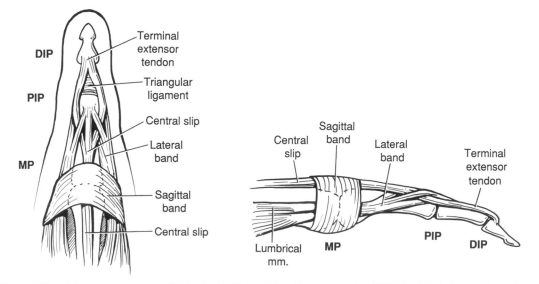

Figure 4.6.   Extensor anatomy digit. (Illustration by Elizabeth Roselius, copyrighted 1988. Reprinted with permission from Green DP: Operative hand surgery. 2nd ed. New York: Churchill Livingstone, 1988.)

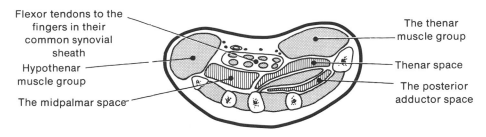

Figure 4.7. Compartments of the hand.

partment. Infections within the sheath of the flexor pollicis longus of the thumb are usually confined to the thenar compartment, which is clinically evident dorsally in the first web space. Most early infections will lie in the subcutaneous fascia and loose connective tissue; however, when inadequately treated or discovered late, these infections can spread into the synovial and deep fascial spaces of the hand.

Nontraumatic Conditions of the Wrist and Hand

MEDIAN NEUROPATHY OF THE FOREARM AND HAND

Carpal Tunnel Syndrome

The anatomy of the carpal tunnel was discussed at the beginning of this chapter. Any process that increases the pressure within the carpal tunnel, such as a tumor, ganglion, synovial proliferation, or simple edema, can result in median nerve dysfunction. The median nerve at the wrist is 94% sensory and only 6% motor. Therefore, dysfunction at the wrist is usually manifested by sensory changes. Chronic or severe median nerve compression will manifest both sensory and motor changes.

Clinical Characteristics. The carpal tunnel is the most common site in the upper extremity for median nerve compressive neuropathy. Patients will complain of pain, paresthesias, numbness, and/or a "pins and needles" sensation in the median nerve distribution of the hand, classically described in the thumb, index, middle, and radial aspect

of the ring finger. However, symptoms may be isolated to one or two digits. Patients may also experience nocturnal paresthesias and complain that they awaken in the middle of the night with these symptoms and have to "hang the hand over the bed and shake it" to obtain relief. There is an increased incidence of carpal tunnel syndrome in patients with diabetes, thyroid disease, amyloidosis, and rheumatoid arthritis.

Examination will reveal a Tinel's sign, which is performed by percussing the median nerve at the level of the palmar wrist, resulting in an uncomfortable or painful tingling sensation distally into the thumb, index, or middle finger. Maintaining the involved wrist in a palmar-flexed position also will frequently reproduce symptoms. This is known as a Phalen's sign. Recent studies have shown that the Phalen's sign is a more specific predictor of carpal tunnel syndrome than is a positive Tinel's sign. The earliest objective sensory finding seen in a patient with carpal tunnel syndrome is diminished vibratory sensation. This can be tested with a 256-cycle tuning fork. More severe median nerve involvement at the carpal tunnel will result in an abnormal two-point sensory discrimination. The examination of the patient with carpal tunnel syndrome should always include motor testing of the median-innervated thenar musculature. Weakness and/ or atrophy is a sign of significant compression, and usually warrants immediate decompression and no trial of conservative nonoperative therapy.

The workup of carpal tunnel syndrome

also should include an electrodiagnostic study. The patient with a prolonged distal motor latency at the wrist should be suspected of having a carpal tunnel syndrome. Radiographic examination of the patient with a suspected carpal tunnel syndrome is rarely helpful.

Treatment. Once the diagnosis has been made and substantiated, the patient without thenar atrophy can be treated initially with conservative therapy. This includes resting splints with the wrist in neutral flexion, which minimizes the carpal tunnel pressure and often gives temporary relief. These splints are most effective at night while sleeping; however, many patients will use them during the day.

If the patient has persistent symptoms even with the splint and his symptoms are less than 6 months old, consideration can be given to injection of the carpal tunnel with 1 ml of soluble steroid such as dexamethasone and 1 ml of 1% Xylocaine without epinephrine. Using a 25-gauge needle, injection is 1 cm proximal to the distal wrist flexion crease between the flexor carpi radialis and palmaris longus. The needle enters the skin at a 45° angle and is advanced 1 cm where it pierces the transverse carpal ligament. This is depicted in Figure 4.8. After penetration of the transverse carpal ligament, the needle is then advanced approximately 1 cm further. If at this time the patient describes any median nerve distribution paresthesias, the

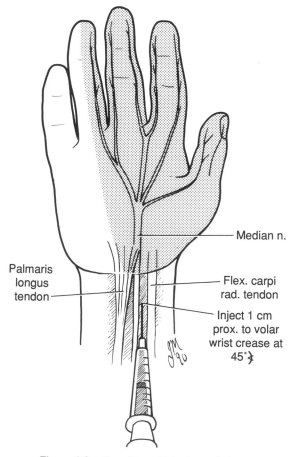

Figure 4.8. Carpal tunnel injection technique.

needle should be withdrawn and redirected in a slightly more superficial angle. Injection is given into the space of the carpal tunnel, not into the nerve or tendon. After the patient is injected, the wrist is splinted in a neutral wrist splint for 3 weeks.

If the carpal tunnel symptoms progress or do not improve over the span of 6 weeks, surgical referral is indicated for decompression of the carpal tunnel. If upon initial workup there is evidence of thenar muscle weakness and/or atrophy, conservative therapy is not warranted and immediate referral to an orthopaedic surgeon is indicated.

Pronator and Anterior Interosseous Nerve Syndrome

The workup of a patient with pain and paresthesias in the median nerve distribution should include an examination of the entire median nerve to rule out a more proximal site of compression. Although compression at the carpal tunnel is the most common site for median nerve dysfunction, there are two sites more proximal in the forearm where the median nerve can be compressed and result in symptoms that very closely resemble carpal tunnel syndrome.

The median nerve can be compressed at the level of the pronator teres along the volar forearm just distal to the elbow where the median nerve travels between the two heads of the pronator teres. The symptoms are purely sensory and identical to a carpal tunnel syndrome. Suspicion should be directed to the pronator tunnel when the examination and workup are not suggestive of carpal tunnel syndrome and symptoms persist. There will often be tenderness over the median nerve at this level as well as a positive Tinel's sign. The workup of a patient with suspected pronator syndrome should include electromyography, and the neurologist should specifically look for compression more proximally at the pronator tunnel in addition to the carpal tunnel. Treatment of this entity includes long-arm posterior

splinting with the elbow in 90° of flexion and midposition rotation. Most symptoms will resolve within 6 to 8 weeks. Persistent symptoms or progressive symptoms are an indication for referral for operative decompression.

The anterior interosseous nerve syndrome is a specific compression of the anterior interosseous nerve branch of the median nerve. This occurs just distal to the pronator teres where the nerve branches from the median nerve. The patient will usually present with few sensory changes but rather weakness or paralysis of the flexor pollicis longus and/or flexor digitorum profundus of the index and middle fingers. Patients will complain of weakness, especially with pinching maneuvers, and have tenderness at the level of the anterior interosseus nerve origin. This lies on the volar aspect of the forearm along the midline approximately 8 cm distal to the elbow flexion crease where the nerve travels under the proximal muscle origin of the flexor digitorum superficialis. As with the pronator syndrome, the anterior interosseous nerve syndrome can be splinted in a long-arm posterior splint maintaining the elbow in 90° of flexion and the forearm in neutral rotation. Most of these symptoms will resolve in 6 to 8 weeks. If weakness and/or paralysis continue, referral should be made for decompression.

COMMONLY SEEN SOFT TISSUE AFFLICTIONS OF THE HAND AND WRIST
De Quervain's Syndrome

De Quervain's syndrome is a stenosing tenosynovitis of the first dorsal compartment over the radial styloid, which houses the abductor pollicis longus and extensor pollicis brevis tendons. It is commonly seen in patients who use their hands and thumbs in a repetitive fashion. The dorsal sensory branch of the radial nerve passes directly over these inflamed tendons. If the inflammation is severe enough, the dorsal sensory branch of the radial nerve can become irritated and the patients may also complain of pain and paresthesia-like sensation radiating distally into the thumb and over the dorsum of the hand and index finger.

Clinical Characteristics. On examination, the patients will have tenderness to palpation over the area of the first dorsal compartment which lies at the radial styloid. They will have a positive Finklestein's sign. This maneuver is performed by having the patient make a fist with the thumb tucked underneath the digits, followed by a manual ulnar deviation of this fisted hand. Radiographs should be obtained to rule out fracture of the radial styloid or bony protuberances which may be causing a mechanical irritation of the first dorsal compartment contents.

Treatment. After the diagnosis has been made, initial treatment is conservative. This involves injection of the first dorsal compartment with a solution of 0.5 ml of soluble steroid and 1 ml of 1% plain Xylocaine using a 25-gauge needle. The site of injection is depicted in Figure 4.9. After injection, the thumb and wrist are placed in a thumb spica splint made of plaster or thermoplastic. The splint is worn continually for 3 weeks and then discontinued. If after this time the patient is still symptomatic, surgical referral should be made for possible decompression of the first dorsal compartment.

Stenosing Tenosynovitis of the Flexor Tendons (Trigger Finger/Trigger Thumb)

The fibroosseous tunnel and thickenings that constitute the flexor tendon pulley system have been described at the beginning of this chapter. The most proximal portion of the fibroosseous tunnel (A-1 pulley) is the site for a very common entity called a trigger finger or a trigger thumb.

Clinical Characteristics. Irritation or inflammation of the fibroosseous tunnel and tendon system may result in a nodule on the flexor digitorum superficialis tendon which prevents smooth gliding within this fibroosseous tunnel. As the nodule enlarges and the inflammation and edema increase, the tendon may actually catch on the most proximal portion of this A-1 pulley, causing a locking of the finger in flexion. This catching of the flexor tendon will produce a sensation of snapping, and will often elicit pain in the palm at the level of the A-1 pulley, which may radiate along the digit up to the level of the proximal interphalangeal (PIP) joint. Triggering can also occur in the thumb at the level of the thumb A-1 pulley and involves the flexor pollicis longus tendon.

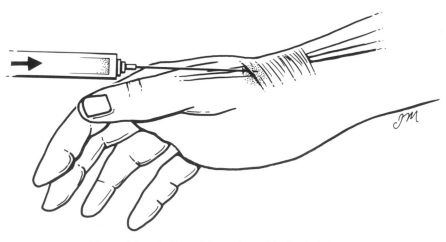

Figure 4.9.   De Quervain's syndrome injection technique.

Treatment. If the symptoms have been present for less thàn 3 months, conservative therapy may be considered. An injection is given into the fibroosseous sheath at the level of the A-1 pulley, using a solution of 0.5 ml of soluble steroid and 1 ml of 1% plain Xylocaine (Fig. 4.10). Injection is into the fibroosseous tunnel and not the flexor tendon. The patient is then encouraged to move the tendon, bathing the flexor tendon. This local deposition of anti-inflammatory medication will diminish tenderness and synovial edema, allowing a smoother excursion of the flexor tendon. If symptoms persist for 2 weeks after injection, or if symptoms have been present for more than 3 months, referral should be made for division of the A-1 pulley under local anesthesia.

Congenital Trigger Thumb. Occasionally a young child or infant will be seen with a congenital trigger thumb. The child will have a small nodule on the palmar surface of the flexor pollicis longus which catches on the proximal edge of the A-1 pulley. The etiology of this is unclear, and is usually not amenable to injection therapy. This should be referred to a hand surgeon for definitive operative care.

Ganglion Cyst

Clinical Characteristics. The most common mass seen in the hand is the ganglion cyst. They typically occur in one of four locations: (*a*) on the dorsal aspect of the wrist, emerging from the scapholunate joint capsule; (*b*) on the radial volar aspect of the wrist, from either the tenosynovium of the radial wrist flexors or the joint capsule of the wrist; (*c*) on the dorsal aspect of the hand, emerging from the sheath of the extensor tendons to the fingers; (*d*) on the palmar aspect of the fingers, usually near the MCP joints. Ganglions in this location often present as hard nodules and may seem bony to the patient. These cysts classically contain a thick, gelatinous material secondary to concentration of the synovial fluid contents. They are often painless and cause no functional limitation, and can simply be observed. If the cysts become large, however, they can be painful or patients may complain of the appearance. These are relative indications for surgical excision. The size of the ganglion cyst will often change.

Treatment. If the cyst is small, aspiration of the cyst contents with a large-bore needle is indicated. A small amount of soluble steroid can be injected into the cyst after aspiration to facilitate cyst wall sclerosis. Besides relieving the distention of the cyst and flattening the contour of the hand, the wall of the cyst may scar enough to obliterate the lumen and prevent recurrence. Because of the cyst's long stalk, which usually origi-

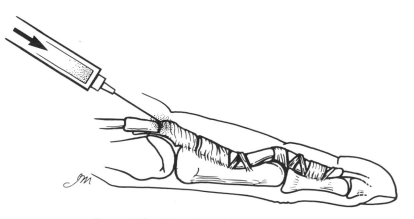

Figure 4.10. Trigger finger injection technique.

nates from one of the carpal joints, recurrence is common. If there is pain, the cyst is large, or there is a question of etiology, surgical excision should be considered and orthopaedic referral made. Meticulous dissection is needed to fully excise the entire cyst as well as its stalk down to the wrist joint.

Mucous Cysts

Mucous cysts are cysts that occur on the dorsal aspect of the distal phalanx of the digits secondary to mucoid degeneration of the deep fascia, usually associated with osteoarthritic dorsal spurring of the DIP joint.

Clinical Characteristics. The cyst, which is often painful, protrudes between the proximal nail fold and the attachment of the terminal extensor tendon of the DIP joint. Pressure on the germinal matrix of the nail by the cyst may result in abnormal nail production manifested by longitudinal grooving. Unlike the ganglion cyst, mucous cysts usually do not spontaneously remit.

Treatment. Local care of these cysts by percutaneous draining or unroofing and cauterizing almost always results in a recurrence and occasionally infection. Definitive removal requires a meticulous surgical excision and often excision of overlying skin that has become attenuated. Because of these surgical considerations, mucous cysts should be referred to a hand surgeon for definitive treatment.

Dupuytren's Contracture

The palmar fascia of the hand may undergo a nodular, hypertrophic degeneration of uncertain etiology which can result in flexion contractures of the MCP and occasionally PIP joints, known as Dupuytren's contracture.

Clinical Characteristics. Degeneration usually begins in the distal palm as a palpable nodularity of dense fascia which often becomes adherent to the overlying skin. This can result in puckering of the skin at the level of the distal palm. As the degenerative pro-

cess continues it extends distally into the digit, resulting in contracture of the involved fascia, flexing the MCP joint and/or PIP joint. This occurs more commonly in the ulnar half of the palm and ring and little fingers. Dupuytren's contracture is more commonly seen in patients of northern European descent and is associated with Peyronie's and Lederhosen disease.

Treatment. Treatment of Dupuytren's contracture is surgical. Simple palmar nodularity can be observed and may not progress beyond this point. Developing flexion contracture in the digit should alert the practitioner to the potential need for surgical excision. Flexion contractures beyond 30° at the MCP joint or *any* flexion contracture of the PIP joint is an indication for referral to a hand surgeon for definitive surgical care.

Human and Animal Bites

Human bites most often result in a laceration to the dorsum of the hand secondary to a blow by the fist to the mouth of another individual. This will often result in a laceration at the level of the MCP joint. Because of the mixed flora and virulent anaerobic organisms in the mouth, these injuries should be treated as emergencies. It is common to have associated intraarticular penetration by the tooth, resulting in a deep inoculation of microbes. Extensor tendon lacerations frequently occur with these injuries.

Human bite injuries should be treated with aggressive surgical debridement and vigorous irrigation. The wounds should be left open and dressed. The hand should be splinted and the patient treated with intravenous antibiotics covering *Streptococcus*, *Staphylococcus*, and anaerobic organisms, especially *Eikenella corrodens*. The antibiotic coverage should be a penicillin and a broad-spectrum cephalosporin. These injuries are best treated on an inpatient basis for wound care and intravenous antibiotic therapy. Duration of hospital care is dependent on the magnitude of the wound. Intravenous antibiotic prophylaxis for 48 hours followed by a 2-week course of oral antibiotics will usually suffice. Evidence of intraarticular involvement or signs of infection should be cause for immediate transfer to an orthopaedic surgeon. It is important to splint and elevate the involved hand. This can be done with a palmar forearm-based splint, maintaining the wrist in neutral position with the MCP joints flexed to 70° and the IP joints in extension (Fig. 4.11). If there is any doubt regarding the severity of a human bite injury to the hand, prompt referral should be made.

Domestic animal bites can produce rapidly developing cellulitis and lymphangitis. The usual pathogens are *Pasteurella multocida* (a Gram-negative coccus), *Staphylococcus,* and anaerobes. The antibiotics of choice are penicillin and a cephalosporin. Recommendations regarding irrigation, debridement, splinting, elevation, and the need for intravenous antibiotics are the same as those for human bite wounds.

These wounds should not be sutured primarily. They should be left open and loosely packed to facilitate any drainage. All wounds should be cultured for both aerobic and anaerobic organisms at the time of presentation.

ACUTE INFECTIONS
Paronychia

A paronychia is the most common infection seen in the hand and involves the soft tissue fold around the fingernail (Fig. 4.12). The infection is usually secondary to the in-

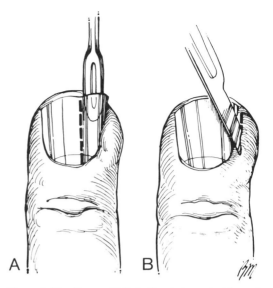

Figure 4.12. Parenychial infection drainage incisions. *A,* elevation and removal of lateral one-third of the nail plate. *B,* longitudinal incision of abscess. (Illustration by Elizabeth Roselius, copyrighted 1988. Reprinted with permission from Green DP. Operative hand surgery. 2nd ed. New York: Churchill Livingstone, 1988:1029.)

troduction of *Staphylococcus aureus* into the paronychial tissues by either a hangnail, manicure instrument, or tooth.

Clinical Characteristics. This infection causes exquisite tenderness. During the early stages, the presentation is usually a tender cellulitis with no obvious abscess formation.

Treatment. If seen in the early stages, a paronychia can be treated with warm saline soaks, oral antibiotics (a first-generation cephalosporin), splinting, and elevation of the affected digit. If an abscess is present and is superficial, it can be treated by opening the thin layer of tissue over the abscess with a

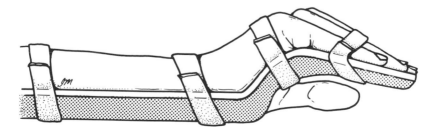

Figure 4.11. Forearm-based resting splint.

sharp blade. This can often be done without anesthesia; however, if anesthesia is necessary, a routine digital block will suffice.

If larger, more extensive lesions are found, such as a large abscess or one that has traveled to the other side of the nail, referral should be made for surgical care. This involves a complete unroofing of the paronychia and occasional removal of a portion of the nail. The wound is then cultured, irrigated, and packed with plain gauze to facilitate drainage, followed by primary intravenous antibiotic therapy. The packing is removed 2 to 3 days later and warm saline soaks are started, which will often be adequate to eradicate the infection. It is critical when unroofing the abscess that the blade be directed away from the nail bed to keep from damaging the nail-producing matrix underneath the nail plate (Fig. 4.12).

Felon

A felon is a subcutaneous abscess involving the distal pulp of the digit. Because of the dense collection of fibrous septa that are normally found in the pulp, the infection is particularly resistant if inadequately treated. The multiple septa divide the pulp into many small compartments and unless drainage is meticulous and complete, there will often be a residual focus of infection left behind.

Clinical Characteristics. A patient with a felon will usually present with a swollen, cellulitic, exquisitely tender mass on the palmar aspect of the fingertip, involving the entire pulp. The progression of the infection is quite rapid and the patient will present quite early because of the exquisite tenderness and pain. The abscess can often break down the vertical septa within the pulp and extend to the distal phalanx, producing an osteomyelitis, or penetrate the skin superficially. Untreated felons can also involve the neurovascular bundles and obliterate the terminal portions of the digital vessels, resulting in a slough of the distal portion of the

finger. Extension can also progress to the flexor tendon sheath or the DIP joint.

Treatment. Because of all of these potential sequelae, prompt care of the felon is essential. The sole treatment for a felon is surgical drainage, which usually can be done in the emergency department by the primary treating physician using distal block anesthesia. There is usually a palpable and clinically apparent fluctuance in the pulp within 48 hours of onset. The incisions for drainage are depicted in Figure 4.13. Whatever the choice of incision, it is imperative to avoid injury to the digital nerve and vessels. The flexor sheath should not be violated. To ensure adequate drainage, all vertical septa should be divided. The cavity is then irrigated with 2 liters of normal saline using a 50-ml syringe with an 18-gauge flexible catheter on the end. After irrigating the wound, a loose, plain gauze pack is placed in the cavity and the hand placed in a compressive bulky dressing with a plaster splint

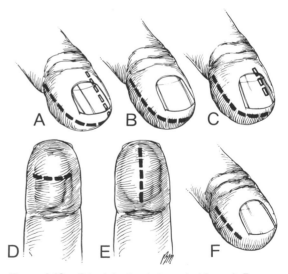

Figure 4.13.   Felon infection drainage incisions. *A–F*, accepted inscisions for drainage of felon abscess. *D* and *E*, should be avoided because of sensitive scar potential. (Illustration by Elizabeth Roselius, copyrighted 1988. Reprinted with permission from Green DP. Operative hand surgery. 2nd ed. New York: Churchill Livingstone, 1988:1031.)

to rest the extremity. After 36 hours, the packing is removed and warm soaks can be started. The wound is never sutured closed and is allowed to heal by secondary intention. After initial cultures have been obtained, the patient is started on intravenous cephalosporin antibiotic therapy for 48 hours, followed by 2 weeks of oral antibiotic therapy.

Herpes Simplex Whitlow

Special mention is made of this critically important entity. The primary care physician must make the differential diagnosis between a bacterial paronychia or felon and the herpetic whitlow. The herpetic whitlow is a viral infection caused by the herpes simplex virus. It is seen frequently in small children and dental or medical personnel. The recognition of this infection is important because it is treated nonoperatively, unlike the surgical drainage necessary for routine pyogenic infections.

Clinical Characteristics. The affected finger is painful with secondary erythema, vesicles, or bullae present, but overall the tenderness is less than with pyogenic infections. The fluid in the vesicles may be clear or turbid but not purulent. The lesions become encrusted over time and the superficial epidermis can desquamate.

Treatment. The process is usually self-limiting and usually resolves in 3 to 4 weeks. The vesicles can be cultured if seen early. The diagnosis is made on clinical impression and a high index of suspicion. When a patient presents with symptomatic erythema and swelling of the distal digits along with small vesicles or bullae, it is extremely important to consider this diagnosis. Incising this aseptic (nonpyogenic) area is contraindicated because of the possibility of secondary bacterial infection. Showering of virions to the blood stream with secondary viral encephalitis has been described. If there is any question of the diagnosis of distal fingertip infection, whether a pyogenic infection or

herpetic whitlow, prompt referral to a hand surgeon is appropriate.

Traumatic Disorders of the Wrist and Hand

LIGAMENTOUS SPRAINS TO THE WRIST AND CARPAL INSTABILITY

These injuries can range from a mild sprain, treatable with simple immobilization for 2 weeks, to severe ligamentous disruption of the wrist with concomitant fracture, nerve dysfunction, or compartment syndrome. Although these injuries are relatively common and can usually be treated conservatively, it is important to understand the pathomechanics of these injuries so that the pathologic anatomy can be appreciated and proper treatment instituted. Unrecognized ligamentous injuries can lead to chronic carpal instability. The treatment of these chronic instabilities is more difficult and less predictable than the proper primary treatment of the acute injury.

Most severe wrist ligament injuries can be categorized as some form of perilunate dislocation. A dorsiflexion injury to the wrist with ligamentous disruption will generally force the carpal bones dorsally out of their normal relationship to the radius and ulna, leaving only the lunate normally articulated with the radius (Fig. 4.14). As one can see in Figure 4.15, these injuries occur in a predictable fashion about the lunate, hence the term perilunate disassociation. The most common injuries are to the ligaments stabilizing the lunate and scaphoid, causing an abnormal relationship between these two bones. As the severity of the injury increases, the ligament disruption proceeds in a clockwise direction around the lunate, causing dissociation not only between the lunate and scaphoid but also the lunate and capitate and lunate and triquetrum. The most severe of these injuries is a complete lunate dislocation where the lunate dislocates into the carpal tunnel. Many ligamentous in-

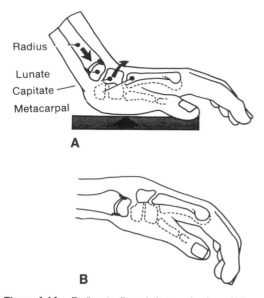

Figure 4.14. Perilunate dissociation mechanism of injury. A, fall on outstretched extended wrist. B, resultant dorsal subluxation of carpals with lunate remaining colinear with radius.

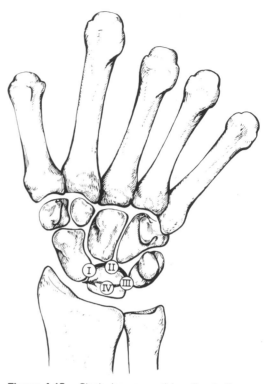

Figure 4.15. Clockwise sequential perilunate ligamentous disruption. (From Mayfield JK. Wrist ligamentous anatomy and pathogenesis of carpal instability. Orthop Clin North Am 1984;15(2):214. Reprinted with permission of WB Saunders Co, Philadelphia.)

juries seen in the emergency department will be some variation of the perilunate dislocation.

When working up a patient with acute wrist pain, it is critically important to obtain good AP and lateral radiographs of the hand and wrist in neutral position (i.e., without any ulnar-radial deviation or palmar dorsiflexion of the hand or wrist). This may require supervision.

Several measurements should be made on these radiographs and compared with accepted normal values and with the contralateral wrist if outside the normal range. The first is the scapholunate angle seen on the lateral x-ray, depicted schematically in Figure 4.16. The normal range is from 40° to 60°. With a dorsiflexion wrist ligamentous injury (perilunate dissociation) the derangement will allow the scaphoid to palmar flex, assuming a more vertical position. This would result in an increased scapholunate angle. The second important angle on the lateral x-ray is the radiolunate angle. The

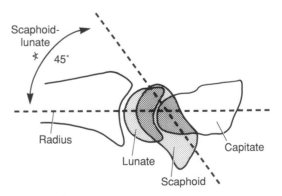

Figure 4.16. Critical radiographic angles assessing perilunate instability. (Adapted from Linscheid RL, Dobyns JH, Beabout JW, et al. Traumatic instability of the wrist. J Bone Joint Surg 1972;54A:1614.)

longitudinal axes of both of these bones should be collinear (with the accepted norm from 0° to 11°, as depicted in Fig. 4.16). Third, the angle between the lunate and capitate should be measured. Again, this should be collinear. When these angles fall outside the normal range, it should alert the practitioner to possible ligamentous disruption. On the AP radiograph, the scapholunate interosseous space should be measured. The accepted amount of space between the scapholunate is 2 to 3 mm. Distances greater than this should alert the practitioner to possible ligamentous injury. If the above abnormalities are noted, referral to an orthopaedist is indicated. Surgical treatment may include closed reduction and percutaneous pinning or open reconstruction.

The x-ray evidence of carpal instability may be subtle. When the instabilities occur in association with fractures of the distal radius or carpus, it is common to focus on the fractures and miss an associated ligamentous injury. Consequently, it is essential to carefully assess x-rays for any evidence of wrist instability. This is most commonly seen with scaphoid, triquetrum, radial styloid, and intraarticular distal radius fractures.

ASSOCIATED MEDIAN NERVE INJURIES

It is also important to recognize the potential for median nerve injury with fractures and dislocations of the wrist. Patients with these injuries present with pain and paresthesias in the median nerve distribution associated with an acute injury. Although this is usually transient, it needs to be addressed promptly with reduction and stabilization. Median nerve symptoms occur more frequently with severe ligamentous disruptions in the wrist and should alert the practitioner to the potential severity of the injury. Once these injuries have been recognized, simple splinting with a palmar-based plaster splint maintaining the wrist at neutral, combined with elevation to minimize swelling, is necessary prior to referral. This referral should

be made immediately because of the difficulty in treating these injuries after swelling has set in.

One particular ligamentous injury to the wrist mentioned earlier is the lunate dislocation. It is readily recognized on the lateral x-ray as a dislocated lunate lying in the carpal tunnel palmarly. This dislocation occurs with extremely high energy force to the dorsiflexed wrist. The median nerve is often contused or even disrupted. The patient will present with extreme pain in the wrist and a palpable mass on the palmar aspect of the wrist. Examination of AP and lateral radiographs of the wrist will reveal the palmarly dislocated lunate.

This severe injury is an indication for primary reduction by an orthopaedic surgeon or, if none is available, the primary care practitioner. Reduction without delay will minimize swelling, relieve the pressure on the median nerve, and make transport to the orthopaedic surgeon much easier for the patient. Reduction should be done with intravenous regional anesthesia (Bier's method) supplemented with parenteral analgesia and sedation. There are many techniques to reduce the palmar dislocation of the lunate; however, the easiest is with the hand suspended in finger traps. The initial maneuver is to dorsiflex the wrist to its maximal extent. With the patient's wrist dorsiflexed, push distally and dorsally on the lunate. With the wrist distracted, the lunate can be manipulated over the palmar edge of the radius and can be felt to engage this articulation. Once this is felt, the hand and wrist are palmar flexed while continuing thumb pressure on the lunate. The reduction occurs with an audible snap. After the reduction has been accomplished, the wrist should be splinted in a long-arm posterior splint, maintaining the elbow at 90° with the wrist in neutral rotation. Radiographs should be obtained to document relocation and the patient should be referred immediately to an orthopaedic surgeon. Prior to the referral, median nerve function should be reassessed and documented.

FLEXOR AND EXTENSOR TENDON INJURIES

Injuries to the Flexor Tendons and Neurovascular Bundles

Diagnosis. All flexor tendon lacerations should be referred to a hand surgeon for primary repair. Referral should be prompt because of the necessity for primary repair within the first 10 days. The challenge for the primary care practitioner is to recognize the injury and make the proper diagnosis. In examining for lacerations of the flexor digitorum superficialis (FDS), flexor digitorum profundus (FDP), and flexor pollicis longus (FPL), the most important part of the examination is the systematic assessment of all flexor tendons in the hand and the overall posture of the resting hand. Specific examination for the FDS, FDP, and FPL is illustrated in Figures 4.17 to 4.19. The presenting resting posture of the hand will often give a clue to the lacerated structures. The normal cascade of the digits is depicted in Figure 4.20. Lacerations of the FDP and/or FDS tendons will alter this normal cascade and should be compared with the contralateral

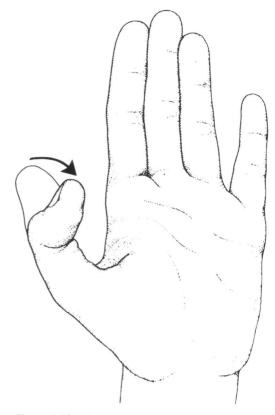

Figure 4.18. Examining for flexor pollicus longus integrity. (From The hand: examination and diagnosis. 2nd ed. New York: Churchill Livingstone, 1983:13. Reprinted with permission of the American Society for Surgery of the Hand.)

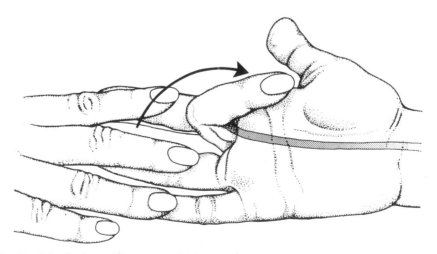

Figure 4.17. Examining for flexor digitorum superficialis integrity. (From The hand: examination and diagnosis. 2nd ed. New York: Churchill Livingstone, 1983:15. Reprinted with permission of the American Society for Surgery of the Hand.)

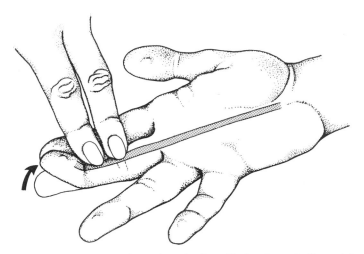

Figure 4.19. Examining for flexor digitorum profundus integrity. (From The hand: examination and diagnosis. 2nd ed. New York: Churchill Livingstone, 1983:14. Reprinted with permission of the American Society for Surgery of the Hand.)

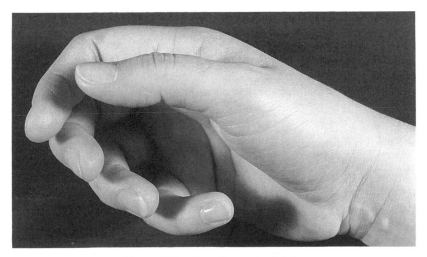

Figure 4.20. Normal cascade of digits.

hand. A single intact flexor tendon in one digit can still give a flexion posture to the hand and may mask a laceration of the remaining tendon in the digit to the casual observer.

Frequently, lacerated flexor tendons are associated with injuries to the digital nerves and arteries. It is important to assess the overall viability of the digit. A digit that is avascular distal to the laceration is an acute emergency and the patient should be re-ferred to an orthopaedic surgeon immediately. The involved finger with a suspected flexor tendon laceration should be examined closely for digital nerve involvement. This is best done testing for two-point discrimination at the tip of the finger. The normal two-point discrimination at the tip of the finger should be 4 to 5 mm on either side of the fingertip and should be compared with the uninvolved fingers. An abnormal two-point discrimination should alert the practitioner to possible digital nerve injury. Because of the relationship of the nerve and the artery in the digit (artery is dorsal to the nerve in the digital vascular bundle), digital artery disruption is usually accompanied by digital nerve laceration. Excessive bleeding from the laceration may indicate a digital artery injury. No attempt should be made to insert clamps into the wound to control the bleeding. Prolonged digital pressure with a compressive bandage over the site will usually take care of most bleeding problems.

Consideration should also be given to the possible partial flexor tendon lacerations. A partial laceration often will not exhibit an abnormal cascade of the resting hand. Although function of the suspected flexor tendon will be intact grossly, there will be considerable discomfort when the patient is asked to flex the involved DIP or PIP joint. There will also be tenderness at the site of the partial laceration. Partial flexor tendon lacerations should be treated by the practitioner as complete lacerations and referred to a hand surgeon.

Treatment.   After the injured structures have been well-delineated, the skin laceration can be sutured primarily after wound irrigation and installation of either 1% plain Xylocaine digital block or local anesthetic at the site of the wound. After the wound is closed with 4-0 nylon simple sutures, the hand should be placed in a dry sterile dressing, protected with a dorsal splint maintaining the wrist in 25° of palmar flexion with the MCP joints of the involved digits at 70° of flexion with the IP joints extended.

Extensor Tendon Injuries

Unlike flexor tendon injuries, extensor tendon injuries are more amenable to treatment by the primary care practitioner. All extensor tendon lacerations need to be surgically repaired. However, because of the extensor tendon's superficial location on the dorsum of the hand, combined with little retraction of lacerated ends, the tendon

stumps are often visible within the laceration. If there has been retraction of the tendon ends, exploration is needed to locate them and this is an indication for referral to an orthopaedist. If the extensor tendon ends are exposed in the wound, however, primary repair can be performed in the emergency department utilizing nonabsorbable suture such as 4-0 nylon. This can be performed utilizing a modified Kessler stitch as outlined in Figure 4.21. After repair, the wrist should be immobilized in 25° of dorsiflexion. This will enable the MCP joints to be placed in 70° of palmar flexion with the IP joints extended, reducing postoperative joint stiffness while still protecting the repair (Fig. 4.11). There is never an indication for splinting the wrist in neutral and the MCP and PIP joints in extension. Extensor tendon repairs should be protected for 4 weeks. After 4 weeks of immobilization the splint can be removed and therapy started with active and active-assistive range of motion of the wrist, MCP, and IP joints. Extensor tendon injuries from the level of the MCP joint distally should be referred to a hand surgeon for definitive repair. If a laceration of a portion of the extensor tendon over the MCP joint or dorsal digit is suspected, the skin laceration can be sutured primarily after adequate local or digit block anesthesia, splinted, and referred. Tendon avulsions on both the flexor and extensor side will be discussed in the next section.

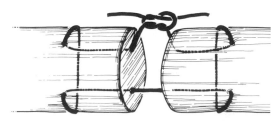

Figure 4.21.   Modified Kessler tendon core suture. (Illustration by Elizabeth Roselius, copyrighted 1988. Reprinted with permission from Green DP. Operative hand surgery. 2nd ed. New York: Churchill Livingstone, 1988:1943.)

LIGAMENTOUS INJURIES AND TENDON AVULSIONS IN THE DIGIT

Mallet Finger

The mallet finger is a common avulsion injury of the terminal extensor tendon of the DIP joint.

Clinical Characteristics. This injury occurs when there is an acute, forceful passive flexion of the DIP joint with concomitant active extension of the joint. This results in a droop or extension lag of the DIP joint (Fig. 4.22). The abnormal posture of the digit will be quite obvious to the examiner, and there will be no active extension of the joint. Tenderness over the dorsum of the DIP joint will be noted. Radiographic examination is essential to rule out a bony avulsion, which is best seen in the lateral view.

Treatment. It is critical to assess any degree of subluxation of the DIP joint, which accompanies bony avulsion. Subluxation of the joint, usually in a palmar direction, is an indication for prompt referral for operative treatment. Most mallet fingers, however, are amenable to closed conservative treatment, including those that are associated with bony avulsion. Conservative treatment consists of maintaining the DIP joint in extension for 6 weeks while bony union occurs or a midsubstance disruption heals. It is important to reinforce the need for *continuous*

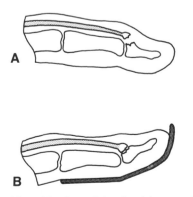

Figure 4.22. Mallet finger deformity. *A,* bony avulsion of terminal extensor tendon. *B,* reapproximation of bony fragment using extension splint.

splinting of the DIP joint in extension. There are a variety of splints that can be placed either on the dorsal or palmar aspect. Commercially available plastic splints that come in a variety of sizes can be used. These are used to splint the finger on the palmar aspect maintaining the DIP joint in extension. In splinting the mallet finger, it is important to keep the PIP joint free, which will help maintain a supple finger. Any extension lag after 6 weeks of splinting should be resplinted for an additional 4 weeks. If after that time there is still an extension lag, the patient should be referred to a hand surgeon for possible operative intervention.

Boutonnière Deformity

The boutonnière deformity of the digit is second only to the mallet finger in the incidence of tendon disruptions in the digit.

Clinical Characteristics. The posture of the boutonnière deformity, depicted in Figure 4.23, is flexion of the PIP joint combined with a hyperextension deformity of the DIP joint. This injury is usually secondary to a blow to the end of the finger resulting in a rupture of the central slip at the base of the middle phalanx. Also disrupted is the triangular ligament, the dorsal stabilizer of the lateral bands, resulting in palmar subluxation of the lateral bands that converts these structures from extensors of the PIP joint to flexors of the PIP joint. This results in a loss of extensor power at the PIP joint and a relative increase at the DIP joint, creating a secondary hyperextension deformity. When these injuries are seen acutely, there is tenderness at the central slip insertion and an inability to extend the PIP joint, with a loss of active flexion at the DIP joint.

Treatment. Treatment should consist of splinting the PIP joint in extension while leaving the MCP joint and DIP joint unsplinted (Fig. 4.24). The splint should be worn for 6 weeks. As with the mallet finger, this is not a part-time splinting regimen and should be worn continuously.

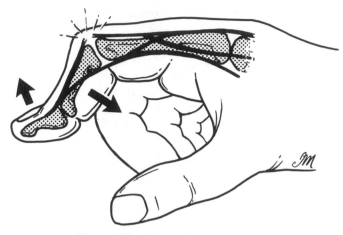

Figure 4.23. Boutonnière finger deformity.

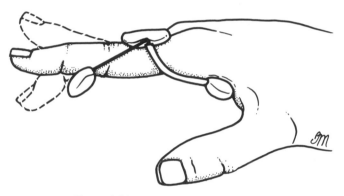

Figure 4.24. Boutonnière extension splint.

Chronic mallet and boutonnière deformities often have secondary stiff PIP and DIP joints. Because these deformities are not usually fully passively correctable, they are not amenable to splinting regimens. Chronic mallet and boutonnière deformities should be referred to a hand surgeon for more specific dynamic splinting and possible surgical correction. These deformities are also seen as sequelae of rheumatoid arthritis. Although the pathologic anatomy is similar, there are some subtle differences. The indications for primary surgery are greater when associated with rheumatoid arthritis. The patient should be referred initially to a hand surgeon for definitive care.

Swan Neck Deformity

Swan neck deformity (depicted in Fig. 4.25) occasionally is seen as an acute injury; however, it is more commonly seen as a late sequela of a chronic untreated mallet finger or in the patient with rheumatoid arthritis. It is also seen in the digit with a chronic post-traumatic absence of the flexor digitorum superficialis tendon. The deformity is a hyper-extension deformity at the PIP joint with an extension lag and/or flexion contracture of the DIP joint. The swan neck deformity, unlike the mallet or boutonnière deformity, is an indication for primary referral to a hand surgeon.

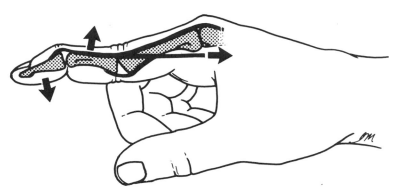

Figure 4.25. Swan neck deformity anatomy.

Gamekeeper's Thumb

Gamekeeper's thumb (often called skier's thumb) is a traumatic disruption to the ulnar collateral ligament complex of the thumb MCP joint.

Clinical Characteristics. This injury often occurs after a fall on the thumb with a hyperextension and hyperabduction force. This results in ulnar laxity of the MCP joint and often dorsal subluxation of the joint secondary to palmar plate involvement. Ulnar collateral ligament integrity is essential for a strong pinch and, if chronically lax, the patient will complain of weakness in activities such as opening a car door, a jar, or turning a key. In the acute setting the patient will have swelling, ecchymosis, and tenderness along the MCP joint. Ninety-five percent of ligamentous injuries to the MCP joint of the thumb are to the ulnar collateral ligament and 5% to the radial collateral ligament. Radiographic examination is essential. If the ligamentous injury is through the midsubstance of the ligament, the x-rays will show only soft tissue swelling and possible joint subluxation. Frequently, however, there is bony avulsion of the ulnar collateral ligament insertion at the base of the proximal phalanx.

Treatment. If the bony fragment is more than 1 mm displaced or involves more than 10% of the articular surface, operative intervention and primary repair are indi-cated and referral should be made to a hand surgeon. If, however, the fragment is anatomically aligned or displaced less than 1 mm (Fig. 4.26), this can be treated conservatively with a well-molded short-arm thumb spica cast for 6 weeks.

If radiographs show no bony involvement, the degree of laxity should be assessed with stress radiographs of the thumb MCP joint, which are critical in determining whether or not operative intervention is indicated (Fig. 4.27). Laxity of the ulnar collateral ligament of the thumb greater than 35° on an AP radiograph or laxity greater than 15° relative to the contralateral thumb are indications for surgery and referral. If the laxity falls within these limits, the injury can be treated with a thumb spica cast for 6 weeks.

Avulsion of the Flexor Digitorum Profundus Tendon

Avulsion of the distal osseous insertion of the flexor digitorum profundus tendon at the base of the distal phalanx is a common injury seen in sporting activities. This occurs most often in the ring finger, and is secondary to a player catching his fingertip in the jersey of an opposing player. There is a sudden hyperextension force of the DIP joint against the actively flexed DIP joint, resulting in an avulsion of the FDP insertion from the base of the distal phalanx.

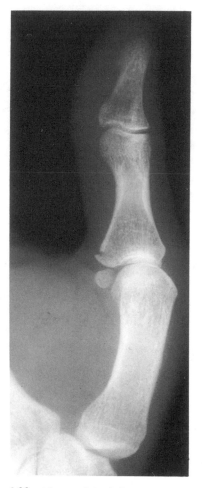

Figure 4.26. Ulnar collateral ligament avulsion from metacarpophalangeal joint of thumb (gamekeeper).

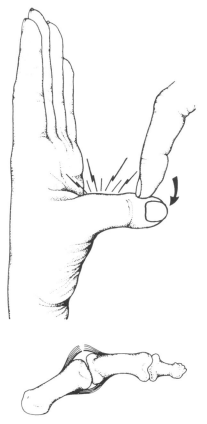

Figure 4.27. Midsubstance tear of ulnar collateral ligament from metacarpophalangeal joint of thumb. (From The hand: examination and diagnosis. 2nd ed. New York: Churchill Livingstone, 1983:62. Reprinted with permission of the American Society for Surgery of the Hand.)

Clinical Characteristics. The patient will present with an inability to actively flex the DIP joint and will have considerable discomfort over the area of the FDP insertion. Depending on the degree of retraction of the tendon, the tenderness over the stump may range from the level of the distal digital crease proximally to the palm. With a midsubstance rupture of the tendon, retraction of the proximal stump can occur to the level of the palm. Radiographs are essential in assessing this injury, since often the avulsion will have a bony component and the fleck of bone will be seen on the lateral x-ray.

Treatment. These injuries should be treated like flexor tendon lacerations: splinted as described and referred to a hand surgeon for definitive surgical treatment.

FINGERTIP INJURIES

Injuries to the fingertip are among the most common hand injuries that the primary care practitioner will see. Often there is injury to the nail bed and associated distal phalanx fracture. As with any injury to the digit, examination requires a systematic evaluation of the flexor and extensor tendons and the radial and ulnar neurovascular bundles, and an overall assessment of the viability of the tip. Most of these injuries occur from the level of the nail fold distally, which would preclude any surgical revascularization or reimplantation.

Digital Tip Amputations

Fortunately, the majority of these injuries do not cause a devascularization of the tip. The main concerns are (*a*) soft tissue coverage of the tip, (*b*) bony stabilization, and (*c*) repair of nail bed injuries. Treatment consists of suture repair of pulp and nail bed lacerations. If there is soft tissue loss to the fingertip, the configuration of the remaining tip often will dictate suitable options for closure. Fingertip amputations with soft tissue loss can be divided into three different configurations, as depicted in Figure 4.28. In Figure 4.28*A*, there is vertical loss of soft tissue. Without shortening the distal phalanx, these are difficult to close primarily and often are treated with dressing changes and allowed to granulate in secondarily. If consideration is given to restoring the length and contour of the fingertip, the patient should be referred to a hand surgeon. The configuration in Figure 4.28*B* shows greater soft tissue loss on the dorsum than on the palmar side. As one can visualize, with this type of configuration, closure will be easier with this than with the vertical loss. Closure can be accomplished with various palmar-based flaps brought up to the dorsum or it can be treated in a closed nonoperative fashion. At this level there is often exposed bone, and bone

shortening will be necessary to facilitate soft tissue closure. The configuration depicted in Figure 4.28*C* shows that there is more soft tissue loss on the palmar side. Palmar-based flaps obviously will not be suitable in this particular situation and other options such as thenar flaps or flaps from distant sites would be necessary to gain primary soft tissue closure.

With fingertip amputations, a smooth and well-padded tip is desired for good functional restoration. In addition, inadequate soft tissue support of the nail bed will lead to abnormal nail growth around the tip known as a parrot-beak deformity. It is therefore important to maintain soft tissue support as much as possible. Generally speaking, soft tissue loss of 1 cm^2 or less will heal very well by secondary intention if no local flap coverage or primary suture repair is possible. If this course of treatment is followed, simple dressing changes will suffice. This is an especially useful strategy to employ when treating minor soft tissue loss of the digital tip in children. Considerable contouring of the tip can be expected in the pediatric setting.

Digital Tip Crush Injuries

The majority of fingertip injuries are not amputations of the tip but rather lacerations or crush injuries. Most of these soft tissue lacerations can be sutured primarily. Often the tip injury will be quite distressing for the patient because of the less than acceptable

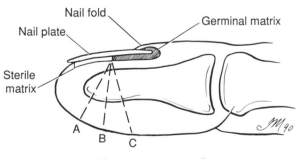

Figure 4.28.   Nail anatomy. *A–C,* see text.

initial cosmetic appearance. However, with healing and maturation, fingertip injuries tend to contour quite nicely and most often will end up with a good cosmetic result.

When a fingertip crush injury is seen in the emergency department, close inspection should be made of the nail bed. The nail bed can be divided into two parts, the germinal matrix and the sterile matrix. This is depicted in Figure 4.28. Lacerations of the germinal and/or sterile matrix should be recognized and sutured primarily with 6-0 absorbable suture, enhancing chances for a normal nail growth. Severe crush injury to the fingertip with an intact nail plate should not lead the examiner to assume that there is no nail bed injury. A significant crush injury to the fingertip requires nail plate removal to inspect the germinal and sterile matrix. After inspection and repair of any matrix lacerations, the nail plate should be replaced into its original bed underneath the proximal nail fold to prevent adhesion formation. Small holes can be made in the nail plate with a portable cautery or heated paper clip to facilitate any drainage from the subungual area. If the nail plate is unavailable, a substitute can be inserted in its place in the form of a nonadherent dressing or piece of foil from a suture pack.

Very few fractures of the distal phalanx need to be internally fixed. With sutured soft tissue and an intact nail bed or repaired nail bed, there will often be adequate support to the fracture and only external splinting will be necessary. Splinting for fingertip injuries is necessary more for soft tissue support and protection than for bony immobilization. These injuries are quite painful and splinting will give some protection against the inevitable bumping of the tip during healing. Virtually all fingertip injuries can be treated with digital block anesthesia utilizing 1% plain Xylocaine.

Pediatric Fingertip Injuries

While the adult guidelines for treatment of fingertip crush injuries apply to children,

the treatment of fingertip amputations varies somewhat. Soft tissue loss to the fingertip in children can almost always be treated conservatively without flap coverage or skin grafting. Children do quite well with regeneration, granulation, and ultimate contouring of the finger with loss not exceeding 1 cm^2. Not infrequently, a small child will be brought in with a tip amputation secondary to various home accidents. If the tip is brought in, it can be sutured on primarily as a composite graft after cleansing and will often do quite well. Activity and discontinuance of splinting should depend on the extent of soft tissue healing and the lack of pain, not the x-ray appearance, as x-rays will often show little healing of the distal phalanx fracture. If the injury is isolated to the fingertip, it is important to mobilize the remaining joints of the hand to minimize stiffness during recovery. Splinting for protection is confined to the DIP joint and soft tissue tip. If the loss of tissue is greater than 1 cm^2, referral to a hand surgeon should be considered. Because of the extensive nature of these injuries, these patients, both adults and children, should be covered prophylactically with a first-generation cephalosporin for 1 week.

GUIDELINES FOR THE CARE OF AMPUTATION OF DIGITS OR THE HAND

The success of digital and hand replantation has increased dramatically in recent years with the improvements in microvascular techniques. Consequently, any patient with an amputated thumb, digit, or multiple digits should be considered as a candidate for possible replantation.

After the overall stability of the patient has been secured, treatment of the amputated part as well as the stump is undertaken. One of the most important factors in the success or failure of replantation is the warm ischemia time of the amputated part. This must be minimized. The amputated part should be kept cold to reduce the metabolic demands of the part and slow cell necrosis.

It is critical, however, not to freeze the part as cells and fluid will crystallize and preclude a successful revascularization. The simplest way to maintain the digit cold is to place the amputated part in a cellophane bag filled with normal saline. Direct submergence within the saline for a period of time will not have an adverse effect on the soft tissues. This bag, with the amputated part, is placed in an ice chest to provide rapid cooling without inadvertent freezing (Fig. 4.29). This setup can be transported with the patient to a medical center that is equipped to perform microvascular surgery.

The finger or hand stump should be wrapped in sterile gauze dressings with compression as necessary to slow any bleeding. Arterial bleeding can usually be easily controlled with a compressive dressing. If the bleeding is uncontrollable, a tourniquet can be applied as long as it is diligently monitored by a physician. The tourniquet should be released every 15 minutes to ensure that the extremity remains well perfused. The ultimate decision regarding suitability of the patient and/or amputated part for replantation should be made by the microvascular team.

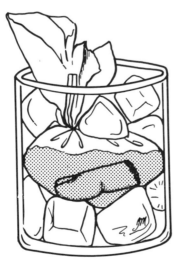

Figure 4.29. Amputated part—preservation and transport.

FRACTURES OF THE HAND AND WRIST

Fractures of the hand and wrist are the most common hand problems seen by the primary care practitioner. This section will cover the most commonly seen fractures in the hand and wrist, including intraarticular and extraarticular fractures of the distal radius.

While some fractures are amenable to initial and definitive care by the primary practitioner, certain fractures should be referred directly to the orthopaedic surgeon. Emphasis over the last 15 years has been on a more aggressive surgical approach to many of these fractures, providing accurate fracture healing and early motion, which facilitates rehabilitation and functional recovery.

Extraarticular Distal Radius Fractures

Colles' Fracture. Extraarticular distal radius fractures are the most commonly seen fractures of the wrist and hand, occurring secondary to falls on the outstretched arm and hand. The fracture configuration is dependent on the position of the hand at the time of impact. The most common mechanism of injury is a fall on the dorsiflexed hand resulting in a Colles' fracture of the distal radius. This fracture is seen most often in the elderly and osteoporotic patient. By definition, a Colles' fracture is extraarticular and occurs 2.5 to 3 cm proximal to the articular surface of the distal radius (Fig. 4.30).

Clinical Presentation. Because this fracture occurs with the hand dorsiflexed, the distal fracture fragment is angulated dorsally and may be displaced dorsally and radially as well. The ulnar styloid may or may not be

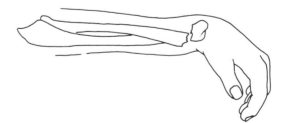

Figure 4.30. Colles' fracture of distal radius.

fractured. The displacement produced by this fracture has been called a "silver fork" deformity because of the gross appearance of the hand and wrist. The patient presents with swelling and often ecchymosis, if some time has passed since the injury occurred. Because of the nature of the injury as well as the angulation and displacement of the proximal fragment in the volar direction, careful examination should be made of the integrity of the median nerve as this can be injured secondary to bony fragments or traumatic swelling around the carpal tunnel.

X-ray Appearance. Routine AP and lateral radiographs will show the characteristic fracture through the metaphysis of the distal radius. There is dorsal displacement of the distal fragment with frequent comminution and intraarticular extension. The fracture fragments can be impacted, adding to the difficulty of an adequate reduction. Anteroposterior and lateral tomograms can be obtained to more accurately delineate the fracture configuration.

Treatment. Although the majority of Colles' fractures can be treated conservatively with closed reduction and casting, there are indications for more aggressive intervention. When the fracture has extensive comminution and/or impaction that cannot be reduced and controlled adequately with closed methods, open reduction and internal fixation or external fixation may be indicated. These techniques permit more precise fracture fragment alignment, increased stability, and early functional rehabilitation of the hand and elbow.

The mildly comminuted extraarticular distal radius fracture with dorsal angulation can usually be treated with closed reduction and casting. These fractures can usually be handled in the office or emergency department setting with adequate anesthesia, either a hematoma or regional (Bier's) block. Although some practitioners utilize intravenous analgesia and sedation with agents such as meperidine and diazepam, it is risky

in the elderly patient and not always as effective as either of the above methods. A hematoma block can easily be given using 1% or 2% Xylocaine injected into the hematoma around the fracture site. Precise location can be documented by aspiration of the syringe, noting the withdrawal of blood from the fracture site. Injection of 5 ml of local anesthesia into the hematoma will give adequate anesthesia for most of these fractures. Frequently muscle relaxation of the extremity is necessary for an adequate closed manipulation. This can be achieved with an intravenous regional block. If this is done correctly, it is a safe and very effective anesthesia. The specific technique is discussed in Chapter 11.

Once the arm is anesthetized, the reduction is performed by one of two methods, either manual traction and manipulation or manipulation following weighted hand suspension using finger traps. With both techniques the critical factor is distraction of the fracture fragments followed by precise manual manipulation.

The most commonly used technique is countertraction of the proximal forearm as depicted in Figure 4.31. This is followed by an exaggeration of the dorsal angulation (Fig. 4.32). After adequate distraction and exaggeration of the deformity, the distal fragment is reduced in a dorsal and ulnar direction as depicted in Figure 4.33. Traction is necessary to distract and disimpact the fracture fragments. While the reduced fracture is held in position, a short-arm cast is applied, leaving the MCP joints free. The reduction is then checked with an x-ray in the cast.

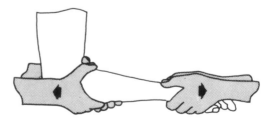

Figure 4.31. Colles' fracture reduction technique.

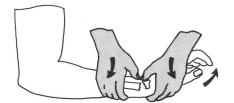

Figure 4.32.   Colles' fracture reduction technique.

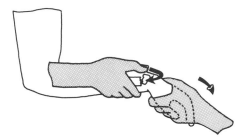

Figure 4.33.   Colles' fracture reduction technique.

When utilizing finger traps and counterweights, as depicted in Figure 4.34, adequate anesthesia and relaxation are necessary for patient tolerance. The patient is instructed to lie supine on a bed or stretcher with the shoulder and affected arm just at the edge. The shoulder should be abducted 90° and the elbow flexed 90°. The forearm is then

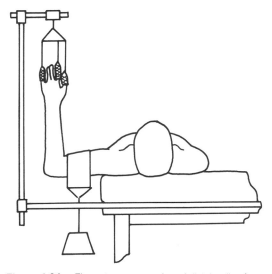

Figure 4.34.   Finger trap suspension of distal radius fracture.

suspended by finger traps attached to the thumb and index finger. Leave the middle, ring, and little fingers free to facilitate an ulnar deviating force to the hand and wrist, which results in a more anatomic realignment of the fracture fragments. Depending on the degree of impaction, counterweights can be used with a sling over the proximal arm; however, this is often unnecessary. When counterweights are used, weights ranging from 5 to 10 pounds will suffice. After suspending the arm for approximately 10 minutes, the fracture is reduced in the same fashion as depicted in Figures 4.31 and 4.32. After reducing the fracture, a plaster short-arm cast is applied, leaving the MCP joints free. The arm can then be removed from the traps and radiographs obtained to document the reduction.

As with all fractures of the distal radius, three radiographic criteria should be reviewed to assess the adequacy of reduction. These are the radial styloid height and inclination (Fig. 4.35), both seen on the AP film, and distal radius articular tilt (Fig. 4.35), seen on the lateral film. The most critical of these parameters is the articular tilt seen on the lateral view. The normal tilt is 11° palmar. Any tilt less than neutral, i.e., any dorsal tilt, should not be accepted and is an indication for referral.

The duration of immobilization is usually 5 to 8 weeks. It is beneficial to remove the cast as soon as the fracture is stable, minimizing the almost invariable loss of some wrist motion which will occur following these fractures. Because the fractures occur more commonly in the elderly, hand therapy will often be necessary after the cast is removed to maximize motion and function.

There has been some debate regarding the benefits of a short-arm versus long-arm cast for adequate immobilization of this fracture. In the elderly, a long-arm cast can be quite debilitating and most fractures can be treated with a short-arm cast. If the reduced fracture cannot be stabilized with a short-

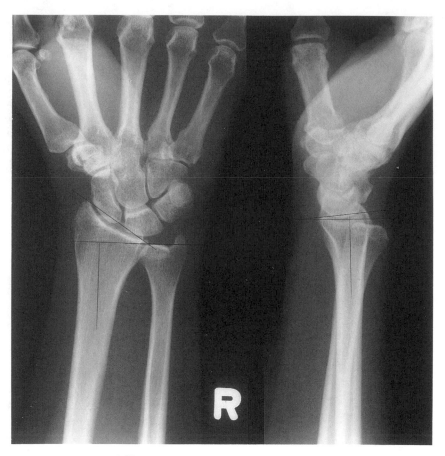

Figure 4.35. Radiographic parameters of reduction adequacy.

arm cast, then more aggressive intervention such as external fixation is indicated to maintain reduction while allowing mobilization of both the hand and elbow.

Smith's Fracture. This fracture, less common than the Colles' fracture, is often called a reverse Colles' fracture. It occurs when an individual falls on the outstretched arm while the wrist is palmar flexed (Fig. 4.36), resulting in a palmar-angulated distal fragment. Like the Colles' fracture, it is a fracture of adults, especially in the elderly and osteoporotic patient.

Clinical Characteristics. The patient presents with swelling and pain at the wrist with tenderness. There may be ecchymosis. The hand appears to be displaced in a pal-

mar direction relative to the forearm. There may be prominence of the distal ulna.

X-ray Appearance. Routine AP and lateral radiographs of the wrist will show the characteristic volar displacement of the dis-

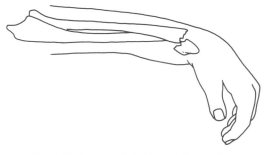

Figure 4.36. Smith's fracture of distal radius.

tal metaphyseal fragment with the characteristic fracture through the distal radial metaphysis. The angulation and displacement are essentially the opposite of the more commonly seen Colles' fracture. These fractures are often comminuted and impacted. Anteroposterior and lateral tomograms are helpful in delineating the details of the fracture if this is not clear on the plain radiographs.

Treatment. The anesthesia and distraction techniques are the same as those described for the Colles' fracture. Because the mechanism of injury is different, the reduction technique is the opposite of the Colles' fracture. The reduction is accomplished by manipulating the distal fragment posteriorly and the proximal fragment anteriorly. The wrist is then immobilized in a neutral position in a well-molded long-arm cast. Radiographic examination is necessary after the fracture reduction, and the same criteria for acceptable reduction as the Colles' fracture are used. The indications for orthopaedic referral are also the same.

Barton's Fracture. The Barton's fracture, depicted in Figure 4.37, has the same pathomechanics as the Smith's fracture. Unlike the Colles' or Smith's fracture, however, it is intraarticular with a large palmar fragment. Hence, the reduction must be anatomic, often requiring open reduction and internal fixation for accurate realignment and fixation. Displaced Barton's fractures should be referred after splinting to an orthopaedist for definitive care.

Although the Colles', Smith's, and Barton's fractures are most often seen in the middle-aged and elderly patient, comminuted intraarticular distal radius fractures are being increasingly seen in the young active patient. These should not be confused with the fractures described above. Intra-articular distal radius fractures in young individuals are the result of high-energy trauma often secondary to motor vehicle accidents or falls from heights. These fractures, which have a concomitant large zone of injury to the perifracture soft tissues and marked displacement, are treated with open reduction and internal fixation, bone grafting, and/or external fixation. Nondisplaced fractures can be managed by the primary care physician with a long-arm cast. Many of these fractures will appear relatively anatomically aligned on plain radiographs. These should be viewed critically and tomograms utilized if there is any question as to the degree of joint incongruity, impaction, or displacement.

Carpal Fractures

Fractures of the carpal bones, unlike the extraarticular distal radius fractures in the elderly, are more commonly seen in the adolescent and young adult, occurring secondary to a fall on the dorsiflexed hand and wrist. Radiographs initially may be negative, but if the clinical suspicion is sufficient, follow-up x-rays are mandatory to definitively rule out a fracture that may become radiographically demonstrable after a short period of time (approximately 2 weeks) due to early resorption or subsequent displacement at the site. With any fracture workup within the carpus, wrist instability, subluxation or dislocation of neighboring carpal bones must be ruled out. Because of the potential morbidity of carpal fractures and associated carpal instabilities, early follow-up with an orthopaedist is warranted. Surgery is frequently required to restore proper alignment and stability.

Scaphoid Fractures. The scaphoid is the most frequently fractured carpal bone.

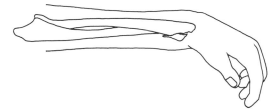

Figure 4.37. Barton's fracture of distal radius.

This usually occurs secondary to a fall on the outstretched, dorsiflexed hand and wrist. The scaphoid may be fractured at one of three points: the tuberosity, waist, or proximal pole (Fig. 4.38). Because of the precarious vascular supply to the scaphoid, avascular necrosis and/or nonunion of the fracture should always be anticipated and discussed with the patient. Although this is a recognized problem with scaphoid fractures, approximately 90% of these fractures will heal well when properly treated. The more proximal the fracture the greater the incidence of vascular compromise to the scaphoid and hence potential for nonunion and/or avascular necrosis of the proximal fragment. Because of these complications, it is essential that the fracture fragments be adequately aligned.

Clinical Characteristics.   There will be a history of falling on the extended arm with the wrist dorsiflexed with subsequent severe wrist pain, particularly on the radial side. The entire wrist may be somewhat tender but the anatomic snuff-box (the region of the wrist on the radial aspect delineated by the extensor pollicis longus and extensor pollicis brevis tendons) will be exquisitely tender. Anteroposterior, lateral, and oblique x-rays of the wrist should be obtained. The oblique or scaphoid view may show a fracture line not always visible on the AP and lateral views. Not infrequently, fractures of the scaphoid will be undetectable during the first few days following injury. Therefore, when a scaphoid fracture is clinically suspected and initial x-rays fail to confirm the diagnosis, the patient should be treated as if there was a fracture and immobilized for 2 weeks, with repeat x-rays obtained at that time. If the x-rays at that time are still inconclusive and clinically the patient still is suspected of having a scaphoid fracture, then a bone scan can be obtained to definitively rule this out.

Treatment.   The natural tendency is for the distal fragment to become palmar flexed. This is seen on the AP film as a foreshortened scaphoid and the classic "humpback" deformity with volar angulation on the lateral x-ray. If the fracture is allowed to heal with this deformity, posttraumatic arthritis and carpal instability may result. Consequently, adequate reduction is necessary. A palmar-to-dorsal pressure on the distal pole of the scaphoid reduces the distal fragment on the proximal fragment. The wrist is then immobilized in a short-arm thumb spica cast to the tip of the thumb, immobilizing the MCP as well as IP joint. If more than 1 mm of displacement shows up on either the AP or lateral postreduction x-ray, the patient should be referred to an orthopaedist for possible open reduction and internal fixation. This fracture requires meticulous follow-up care with serial x-rays. Adequate alignment of the fracture fragments will most often lead to a satisfactory result; however, acceptance of a less than satisfactory reduction will predispose the patient to developing a nonunion or malunion with potential debilitating sequelae.

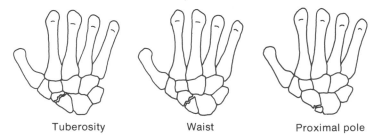

Tuberosity   Waist   Proximal pole

Figure 4.38.   Scaphoid fracture (as labeled in text).

Because these fractures heal slowly, the treating physician should counsel the patient that prolonged immobilization for 10 to 12 weeks may be necessary to obtain union. If after 10 weeks of immobilization there is still a lack of adequate radiographic evidence for union, the fracture may be considered a delayed union but not necessarily a nonunion. At this point the patient should be referred to an orthopaedist for further care, which may necessitate continued immobilization or surgical intervention, including bone grafting and/or internal fixation.

Hamate Fractures. Although not as serious an injury as the scaphoid fracture, fractures of the hamate can be debilitating.

Clinical Characteristics. Fractures of the hamate, especially the hook that protrudes into the palm, can be a source of considerable pain. This is most often secondary to racquet sports, construction injuries using a jack hammer, or falls on the outstretched wrist. The patient will present with pinpoint tenderness over the hook in the palm. Radiographic examination including AP and lateral views often will be inconclusive, but the fracture can be delineated with a carpal tunnel view. Further workup includes tomograms and/or bone scan if the diagnosis is uncertain.

Treatment. If a fracture of the hamate is documented, simple immobilization with a short-arm cast for 4 to 6 weeks will usually heal the fracture. Occasionally, the fracture will fail to heal and will develop a painful nonunion. If this happens, the patient should be referred to an orthopaedist for simple excision of the fracture fragment, which usually relieves the symptoms.

Metacarpal and Phalangeal Fractures

Fractures of the metacarpal and phalanges are common injuries. They can be the result of blunt trauma, or twisting or torquing forces and often are associated with dislocations of the MCP or PIP joints. Most of these fractures go on to primary union without difficulty. However, because of intrinsic and extrinsic muscle forces, these fractures may be displaced, angulated, or malrotated resulting in malunions, which can adversely affect hand function. Because of this, more emphasis has been given recently to surgical treatment of displaced fractures with open reduction and internal fixation, which allows better control of displacement and immediate institution of hand therapy. This minimizes the risk of tendon adhesion, ligament shortening, and capsular contraction which can occur rather early with hand fractures treated with prolonged immobilization.

Fractures of the Bases of Metacarpals Two through Five and/or Subluxation of Their Articulations with the Carpus. A direct blow can fracture the base of any metacarpal. A torquing dorsiflexion force to the hand and wrist can either fracture the bases of the fourth and fifth metacarpals or subluxate their articulation with the capitate and hamate. These injuries occur frequently. Subluxation of the index and middle metacarpals at their articulation with the trapezoid and capitate, however, are relatively rare injuries. Unless a high index of suspicion is maintained these injuries can be taken for carpal sprains and, if neglected, may result in chronic painful and stiff hand and wrist secondary to instability and posttraumatic arthritis.

Clinical Characteristics. The patient will present with tenderness localized to the base of the injured metacarpal. Often there is a bony prominence in the region of the base of the injured metacarpal. X-rays are obtained in the AP, lateral, and oblique planes. These will demonstrate the fracture of the involved metacarpal or subluxation at the carpometacarpal joint. If there is any doubt, lateral tomograms or computerized tomography can be utilized.

Treatment. The majority of these injuries can be treated in a closed fashion. When a reduction is necessary, adequate anesthesia can be obtained by utilizing a hematoma block, a regional peripheral nerve block, or an intravenous regional anesthesia (Bier's) block.

Nondisplaced fractures of the base of the metacarpals should be immobilized with a short-arm cast. Usually the digits do not need to be mobilized. Displaced fractures are reduced by traction with local pressure over the prominent proximal end of the distal metacarpal fracture. The injuries usually reduce quite easily but they can be unstable. If any instability is noted after reduction, these patients should be referred to an orthopaedic surgeon. Patients with these injuries should be followed closely and reexamined and have x-rays within 7 days. If there is subsequent redisplacement of the fracture fragments, the patient should be referred to an orthopaedic surgeon for consideration for open reduction and internal fixation.

Subluxations of the metacarpals with their carpal articulations generally occur dorsally and are usually quite easily reduced by pushing in a dorsal-to-palmar direction directly over the dorsum of the subluxated metacarpal while applying straight traction to the affected ray. After reduction, the wrist is placed in a short-arm cast with the wrist in slight dorsiflexion. It is essential that any recurrence of dorsal instability be detected with serial x-rays and close follow-up. If stability is maintained, these injuries should be immobilized for 4 to 6 weeks. Any resubluxation will require orthopaedic referral.

Fractures of the Thumb Metacarpals.
Hyperabduction and hyperflexion of the thumb are the usual mechanisms for these injuries. Most common are the extraarticular transverse fracture of the thumb metacarpal, and the Bennett's and Rolando's fractures (intraarticular fractures of the thumb metacarpal).

Clinical Characteristics. Pain at the radial aspect of the wrist should alert the practitioner to suspect, in addition to these inju-

ries, trauma to the trapezium, scaphoid, or radial styloid. Anteroposterior and lateral radiographs of the thumb are essential in making the correct diagnosis. The Robert's view, which is an AP view of the hyperpronated hand and wrist, will give an unobstructed view of the trapezium metacarpal joint and further aid in the accurate delineation of the fractures.

Treatment of Extraarticular Fractures. Extraarticular fractures of the thumb metacarpal are very amenable to closed reduction and cast immobilization. Because of the wide arc of motion of the thumb, especially at the trapezial metacarpal joint, a less than anatomic alignment of the metacarpal fracture will not significantly alter the ultimate functional result. After adequate anesthesia either by hematoma block or intravenous regional anesthesia, gentle longitudinal traction on the thumb either manually or by suspension in finger traps, and gentle manipulation of the fracture is followed by thumb spica cast. Angulation up to 15° can be tolerated with no loss of function. If an adequate reduction cannot be obtained or maintained, then referral to an orthopaedist is indicated.

Treatment of Intraarticular Fractures. Bennett's fractures, because they are intraarticular, demand an accurate reduction (Fig. 4.39). The displacement of the fracture is actually the main metacarpal segment which is displaced in a dorsal and radial direction by the pull of the abductor pollicis longus. The small intraarticular fragment on the ulnar side of the metacarpal base is held in its anatomic position by the palmar oblique ligament with reduction performed by realigning the thumb metacarpal to this small fragment. Because this fracture is frequently unstable following reduction and casting, it should be treated primarily with closed reduction and percutaneous pinning for stability, and thus should be primarily referred to an orthopaedist.

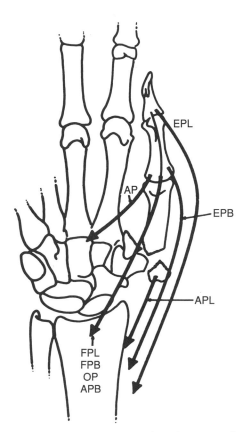

EPL

AP

EPB

APL

FPL
FPB
OP
APB

Figure 4.39. Bennett's fracture of thumb metacarpal and deforming forces. (Adapted from Breen TF, et al. Intra-articular fractures of the basilar joint of the thumb. Hand Clin 1988;4(3):496. Reprinted with permission of WB Saunders Co, Philadelphia.)

Dislocations of the Thumb Carpometacarpal Joint

Dislocations of the base of the thumb are relatively easy to reduce by gentle traction on the thumb and manipulation of the base of the thumb metacarpal in a palmar-ulnar direction. These dislocations are unstable because of capsular incompetence and lax supporting ligamentous structures that are disrupted by definition, hence these dislocations, once reduced, should be referred to an orthopaedist for percutaneous pinning.

Dislocations of the MCP, PIP, and DIP Joints

Although any MCP joint can be dislocated, the thumb appears to be the most vulnerable.

Clinical Characteristics. These dislocations are almost always dorsal, i.e., the phalanx is dorsal to the metacarpal. The mechanism of injury is a hyperextension force to the MCP joint. The articular surface of the proximal phalanx is displaced dorsally and proximally. A rent in the capsule allows dorsal migration of the proximal phalanx or a tear through the volar plate of the MCP joint allows palmar migration of the metacarpal head.

Treatment. Fortunately, the thumb MCP joint dislocation is relatively easy to reduce. Gentle traction is utilized on the digit. After gentle traction on the digit, pressure is applied to the dorsum of the digit near the base of the proximal phalanx. This pressure is directed in a palmar and distal fashion. As the base of the proximal phalanx is brought just distal to the articular surface of the metacarpal, the digit will begin to relocate. It is imperative that collateral stability be assessed after reduction. Because of the frequency of associated collateral ligament injury, immobilization of the digit with the MCP joint flexed 50° is needed not only to prevent hyperextension of the digit but to allow for collateral ligament healing. Immobilization can be with either a forearm-based thumb spica splint or cast. Protected motion can be started in therapy after 4 weeks of immobilization. If unable to reduce these dislocations closed, do not persist with more vigorous traction and reduction forces. Prompt referral to an orthopaedic surgeon is warranted for open reduction.

The mechanism of injury and reduction techniques for MCP dorsal dislocations of the index, middle, ring, and little fingers are the same as for the thumb. Treatment with forearm-based splint immobilization, maintaining the MCP joint in 50° of flexion for 4 weeks will usually provide stability (Fig. 4.40). Not infrequently, these dislocations will be impossible to reduce closed because of soft tissue interposition and should be primarily referred to an orthopaedic surgeon for open reduction.

Fractures of the Metacarpal Shaft

Clinical Characteristics. These fractures may be transverse, oblique, or spiral. Transverse fractures usually result from a direct blow to the dorsum of the hand. The oblique and spiral fractures usually result from a fall on the palmar or dorsal surface of the metacarpal heads or from an axial load such as punching with a closed fist. Displacement of metacarpal diaphyseal fractures is almost invariably an apex dorsal angulation, secondary to the force of the interosseous muscles. Oblique and spiral fractures tend to shorten and override more than transverse fractures. It is also important to recognize rotational malalignment as the distal fracture fragment rotates relative to the proximal fragment. These deformities must be corrected when assessing the adequacy of the closed reduction.

Treatment. Many of these fractures can be treated conservatively. Nondisplaced transverse fractures can be treated nonoperatively and supported with an outrigger splint, as depicted in Figure 4.40, which should be worn for 4 weeks, followed by a removable splint in the same hand position, with gentle active and active-assistive range of motion therapy to the wrist, MCP, and PIP joints. It is imperative when treating this fracture conservatively to closely monitor the fracture alignment with serial radiographs to detect any displacement. The patient should be reexamined within 7 days after initial splinting to detect any changes in alignment. If the fracture does displace with more than 1 mm of shortening, 10° of dorsal angulation, the patient should be referred to an orthopaedist for consideration of open reduction and internal fixation.

Transverse fractures that are angulated and displaced should be reduced. Dorsal angulation can cause a cosmetic deformity as well as palmar hand pain, secondary to a palmarly displaced metacarpal head, which can be quite uncomfortable for the patient when gripping objects tightly. Because of these problems, dorsally angulated fractures need to be reduced as anatomically as possible.

When treating these fractures, the physician should always examine very closely for rotational malalignment. Although it is important to examine the digits from end on with the fingers extended for any gross evidence of malalignment, examination with the fingers flexed into the palm will make small malalignment more readily noticeable. The amount of angulation acceptable when treating these fractures conservatively depends on the particular metacarpal involved.

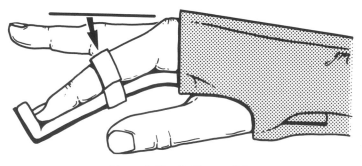

Figure 4.40. Outrigger splint.

A good rule of thumb for residual dorsal angulation of metacarpal shaft fractures is 10° for the index finger, 15° for the middle finger, and 20° for the ring and little fingers. The ring and little metacarpals are more mobile than the index and middle fingers because of their mobile carpometacarpal articulations and will tolerate more angulation. Shortening more than 1 mm or any rotatory malalignment should not be automatically accepted, and a reduction should be attempted.

When the alignment does not fall within these limits, reduction under intravenous regional anesthesia should be performed, using straight traction on the involved digit with direct pressure in a dorsal-to-palmar direction over the apex of the fracture angulation. Once the fracture is reduced, a short-arm cast is applied with the wrist in neutral position or slightly dorsiflexed with an incorporated aluminum outrigger splint for 4 to 5 weeks. The fracture should be followed weekly with serial x-rays to rule out any displacement. Redisplacement after closed reduction or an inability to obtain initial fracture reduction within the limits outlined are indications for referral to an orthopaedist for surgical intervention.

Metacarpal fractures associated with significant soft tissue injury to skin, subcutaneous tissue, or flexor and extensor tendons should be referred directly to an orthopaedist for possible operative intervention. Open reduction and rigid internal fixation of these fractures will facilitate fracture healing and better treatment of the associated soft tissue injuries.

Spiral or oblique fractures tend to shorten and malrotate more frequently. These fractures, though they initially may be anatomically aligned, will frequently shorten and displace because of the force of the interosseous muscles. If these fractures are nondisplaced, they can be treated with simple immobilization with a forearm-based resting splint, as with the metacarpal fractures described above. These fractures, however, do require close follow-up because of their propensity to displace. Radiographs of these fractures should be made within 7 days for assessment of stability. If there is evidence of shortening of 1 mm or more, or evidence of digit malrotation on clinical examination, the patient should be referred to an orthopaedist for possible open reduction and internal fixation.

Fractures of the Metacarpal Neck

Clinical Characteristics. Fractures of the metacarpal neck result from punching with a closed fist in a manner that applies force to the dorsal aspect of the MCP joint. The MCP joint is displaced palmarly with the apex of angulation directed dorsally and usually impacted. Most commonly affected are the ring and little fingers.

Treatment. Because of the overall mobility of the ring and little finger metacarpals, these fractures tend to do well when treated conservatively as they can tolerate a less than anatomic union. Metacarpal neck fractures of the index and middle fingers should be addressed by an orthopaedic surgeon because malalignment of the fracture is less well-tolerated by these digits. Nondisplaced metacarpal neck fractures of the index and middle finger and those with angulation less than 10° can be treated with a simple forearm-based resting splint or cast with finger extension. Fracture angulation greater than 10° is an indication for referral. As with any hand trauma, AP and lateral radiographs are an essential component of the workup.

Fracture reduction requires either a hematoma block or intravenous regional anesthesia. When reducing fractures of the metacarpal neck, it is important to first disimpact the fragments. Disimpaction can be accomplished by flexing and distracting the MCP joint manually to 90° and gently manipulating the proximal phalanx in a radial-ulnar direction to disimpact the fracture fragments. Once the fracture has been disimpacted, the MCP joint can be extended and the fracture reduced by applying direct pressure with the thumb in a dorsal-to-palmar direction on the apex of the angulated fracture (Fig. 4.41). Fracture reduction with this maneuver will not succeed unless the fracture has been fully disimpacted.

Once reduced, the fracture should be immobilized in a forearm-based ulnar gutter splint which is well-molded over the area of the fracture. The MCP joint is kept in 70° of flexion and the PIP joint is extended. This will minimize joint stiffness during this period of immobilization lasting 4 weeks. As swelling subsides, the splint can loosen and the fracture may displace. Consequently,

close follow-up is necessary (within the 1st week), and remanipulation or referral is indicated for any subsequent displacement. After 4 weeks of immobilization, radiographs should be obtained out of plaster. If the fracture appears radiographically healed with no tenderness over the fracture site, then mobilization of the MCP and PIP joints can be commenced.

Phalangeal Fractures and Fracture-Dislocations of the PIP and IP Joints

Fractures of the phalanges are common injuries. Fractures of the proximal and middle phalanges are usually secondary to hyperextension or hyperabduction forces.

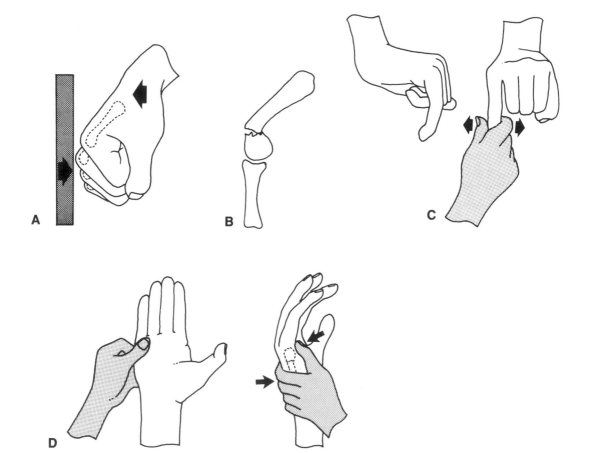

Figure 4.41. Boxer fracture of fifth metacarpal and reduction technique. *A*, mechanism of injury; *B*, dorsal angulation; *C*, disimpaction of fragments; *D*, reduction maneuver.

They frequently involve the PIP and MCP joints, and phalangeal fractures that extend into the joint surface often indicate an actual fracture-dislocation. This must be kept in mind when evaluating these injuries, which will be discussed later in this chapter.

Distal Phalangeal and DIP Joint Injuries. Fractures of the distal phalanx are usually the result of a crush-type injury. Often these fractures have associated extensive soft tissue injuries to the tip and/or nail bed. These specific fingertip injuries have been covered in an earlier section. Avulsion fractures of the terminal extensor tendon (mallet finger) have also been discussed. Fractures of the distal phalanx usually are very slow to show radiographic evidence of healing.

Very few fractures of the distal phalanx require more than protective splinting. The fracture should be treated symptomatically and splinted until there is no further fracture tenderness. Isolated fractures of the distal phalanx can be treated with splints that immobilize the DIP joint and leave the PIP joint free, minimizing stiffness.

Middle Phalangeal and PIP Joint Injuries. Fractures of the middle phalanx can be treated utilizing the same guidelines as those for fractures of the metacarpal shaft. Fractures of the middle phalanx are often associated with a crush-type injury with significant soft tissue involvement. When there is accompanying soft tissue injury and dorsal extension apparatus involvement, it is imperative that the fracture alignment be anatomic and stable, allowing for proper wound care and early motion. The threshold for referral to an orthopaedic surgeon should be low.

One particular fracture of the middle phalanx that needs to be highlighted is the commonly seen fracture of the palmar base (Fig. 4.42). This is an intraarticular fracture that is the result of a hyperextension and/or dorsal dislocation of the PIP joint, commonly seen in athletic activities. It is essentially an avulsion injury of the distal insertion of the pal-

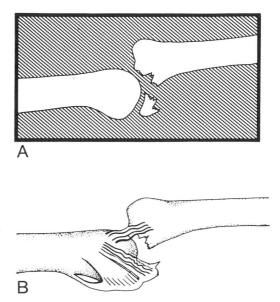

Figure 4.42. Volar plate avulsion of proximal interphalangeal joint. *A*, fracture of volar base middle phalanx with joint subluxation. *B*, volar plate attachment to fragment and tear of collateral ligament. (Adapted from The hand: examination and diagnosis. 2nd ed. New York: Churchill Livingstone, 1983:57. Reprinted with permission of the American Society for Surgery of the Hand.)

mar plate. This will often lead to joint instability and dorsal subluxation, even after reduction of a dislocated joint. This injury should be recognized early and treated promptly, minimizing the chances of a chronically stiff or unstable PIP joint.

If the fracture fragment involves less than 40% of the articular surface seen on the lateral radiograph, the injury can frequently be treated in a conservative fashion. Treatment should allow protected early motion while maintaining a well-reduced joint. This can best be accomplished with dorsal extension block splinting, depicted in Figure 4.43. Because of the initial dorsal joint subluxation, the reduced joint is more stable in flexion. Flexion of these PIP joints will also reapproximate the avulsed palmar plate. The initial position of the PIP joint should be the maximum extension that still maintains both a congruent PIP joint as well as apposition of the palmar fracture fragment. This should be

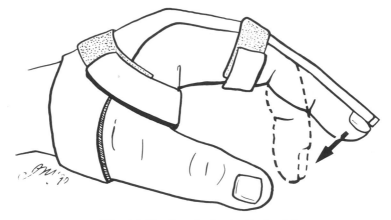

Figure 4.43. Dorsal extension block splint.

documented with radiographs while in the splint. Once the dorsal extension block splint is applied and in place, active flexion of the PIP joint and extension of the joint within the confines of the extension block is encouraged. The follow-up is augmented with serial x-rays. On a weekly basis, the splint is altered to allow 10° more extension. After a change in the splint allowing more extension, a congruent joint is documented with a lateral radiograph. If congruency is lost, the digits should be maintained in the previous degree of flexion. Once the PIP joint has been brought out to full extension over the course of 4 to 5 weeks, the splint can be discontinued and gentle strengthening exercises can be started.

The keys to proper treatment of this fracture are (*a*) closed treatment for injuries involving less than 40% of the articular surface; (*b*) dorsal extension block splinting, maintaining a congruent joint and apposition of the palmar plate or fracture fragment; (*c*) gradual extension of the splint, allowing more extension of the PIP joint on a graduated basis over 4 to 5 weeks; (*d*) when utilizing the dorsal extension block splint, immobilization of the MCP joint to prevent flexion, so that the forces can be directed at the PIP joint while in the splint; and (*e*) referral of injuries involving more than 40% of

the articular surface or joint subluxation to an orthopaedist for possible surgical treatment.

Lesser injuries of the PIP joint are seen that do not begin with a frank dislocation. Forces that laterally angulate, hyperextend, or hyperflex the joint may injure the capsule or its collateral ligaments. This is the classic "jammed" finger seen in sports. It is important to examine the collateral ligaments to assess any degree of instability. Because the PIP joint is essentially a hinge joint, there should be no more than 10° of laxity in either radial or ulnar directions with lateral stress. If there is tenderness about the joint with no gross instability, subluxation of the joint, or fracture, this injury can be treated with buddy taping to an adjacent finger for stability for 2 to 3 weeks. Range of motion within the confines of the buddy taping is allowed. If there is gross instability and/or avulsion fracture of the collateral ligaments seen on the AP radiograph with displacement greater than 1 mm, referral to an orthopaedic surgeon is indicated.

Proximal Phalangeal and MP Joint Injuries. As with metacarpal shaft fractures, fractures of the proximal phalanx can occur in a variety of configurations. Transverse, oblique, or spiral fractures often lead to angulation and/or shortening with a potential for rotational deformity. Proximal phalanx fractures tend to be palmarly angulated because of the pull of the intrinsic tendons. Similar fracture treatment guidelines are advised for the proximal phalanx fracture as for the metacarpal shaft fracture. Because of the close adherence of the dorsal extensor apparatus at the level of the proximal phalanx, proper treatment of these fractures is essential to minimize extensor adhesions and a subsequently stiff finger. Because of the functional benefits of early mobilization, many surgeons feel that surgical treatment of displaced fractures is indicated. Rigid stabilization with precise rotational control of the digit permits early mobilization. Unless the fracture is anatomically aligned by closed reduction or is a nondisplaced fracture, consideration should be given to referral to an orthopaedic surgeon for possible open reduction and internal fixation. If the fracture is anatomically aligned, continued conservative therapy is indicated. Immobilization should be with a forearm-based splint with the affected digit immobilized to the tip of the finger. The MCP joint

should be in 70° of flexion and the IP joints extended. Immobilization should be for 4 to 5 weeks with supervised hand therapy instituted as soon as the fracture will allow, i.e., when there is no further fracture tenderness. Rigid internal fixation of these fractures allows virtually immediate postoperative mobilization.

Because many of these injuries are associated with a severe crushing force, many proximal phalanx fractures are comminuted and unstable. These should be referred promptly to an orthopaedic surgeon for either internal or external fixation.

SUGGESTED READINGS

Bora FW Jr, ed. The pediatric upper extremity. Philadelphia: WB Saunders Co, 1986.

Green D, ed. Operative hand surgery. New York: Churchill Livingstone, 1988.

Stern P, ed. Hand clinics—difficult fractures of the hand and wrist. Philadelphia: WB Saunders Co, 1985.

Strickland J, ed. Hand clinics—flexor tendon surgery. Philadelphia: WB Saunders Co, 1985.

Taleisnik J, ed. The wrist. New York: Churchill Livingstone, 1985.

Zook E, ed. Hand clinics—the perionychium. Philadelphia: WB Saunders Co, 1990.

CHAPTER 5

Thoracic and Lumbosacral Spine

M. Timothy Hresko, M.D.

Essential Anatomy

An understanding of the structural characteristics of the thoracic and lumbosacral spine is fundamental to an understanding of spinal trauma and back pain syndromes. This material will be presented in four subsections:

1. The bone structure and clinical importance of the functional units of the thoracic and lumbosacral spine.
2. The ligaments of the thoracic and lumbosacral spine.
3. The muscles of the spine.
4. The distribution of nerve roots L-3 through S-1.

FUNCTIONAL UNITS
Thoracic Vertebrae (Fig. 5.1)

The bodies of the thoracic vertebrae are heart-shaped as viewed from above, with the "apex of the heart" pointed anteriorly. The bodies of all vertebrae, including the thoracic vertebrae, are rimmed superiorly and inferiorly by epiphyseal remnants of bone denser than the rest of the cancellous bone of the vertebral body. When the ossification of these epiphyses in the thoracic spine is disordered during midadolescence, a form of thoracic vertebral wedging occurs called adolescent kyphosis (Scheuermann's disease).

The pedicles of the thoracic vertebrae emerge posteriorly from the upper border of the lateral posterior angle of the vertebral bodies, creating a deep inferior vertebral notch. Each pedicle expands into four processes: the superior articular process, the inferior articular process, the transverse process, and the lamina. On the posterolateral aspect of the body of each thoracic vertebra, at its superior and inferior ends, are joint surfaces called costal foveae. The superior fovea of one vertebra and the inferior fovea of the next superior vertebra form the vertebral articulation for the head of the rib, which takes the numerical designation of the inferior vertebra. Every rib articulates in this fashion with the bodies of two thoracic vertebrae. These articulations are called costovertebral joints.

The planes of the thoracic articular surfaces or facet joints are oriented 10° to 15° from the true frontal plane. The superior facets face slightly superiorly and laterally, and the inferior facets face slightly inferiorly and medially. The articulations of the superior with the inferior facets create the facet joints, which—like all of the facet joints of the spine—are true synovial joints. Normal thoracic facet joints allow for most of the rotation of the trunk, but the orientation of the facets and the attachments to the ribs prevent the thoracic spine from contributing substantially to flexion, extension, or lateral bending. Disorders of these joints can result in thoracic, posterior flank, and abdominal pain, usually worsened by prolonged activity or prolonged inactivity, and abruptly sharpened by straining or by twisting movements.

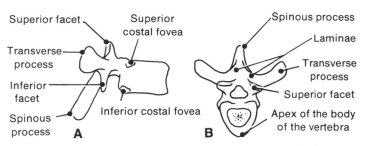

Figure 5.1. *A* and *B*, a thoracic vertebra. Lateral and superior views.

The transverse processes project postero-laterally at an angle of about 45° from the frontal plane and slightly superiorly. At the tip of each transverse process is an articular surface, the costal fovea, which articulates with the tubercle on the dorsal surface of the first 10 ribs. These articulations between the ribs and the transverse processes are called costotransverse joints. The costovertebral and costotransverse joints are true synovial joints. Disorders of the costovertebral and costotransverse joints may result in pleuritic pain.

The laminae of each vertebra fuse at the midline to form the long spinous process, which overlaps the spinous process of the vertebra next inferior. The thoracic nerve root passes through the intervertebral foramen, which is a space bounded by the pedicles superiorly and inferiorly, the facet joints posteriorly, and the superior vertebral body and intervertebral disc anteriorly. The nerve root of each functional unit is designated by the same number as the superior vertebra of that unit. While degenerative arthritis and rheumatoid spondylitis can provoke soft tissue and bony encroachments on these foramina, symptomatic thoracic nerve root compression is uncommon.

Lumbar Vertebrae and Sacrum (Fig. 5.2)

The lumbosacral lordosis is one of the evolutionary adaptations that facilitates standing and erect movement. When standing erect the full weight of the upper body is transferred to the L-4/L-5 and L-5/S-1 functional units, and the lordotic lumbosacral curve so inclines the weight-bearing surfaces of those units that the weight of the upper body applies shearing stress across them. During trunk movements, the entire moment arm of the upper body acts on the L-4/L-5 and L-5/S-1 functional units. These static and dynamic stresses cause the lower lumbar spine to be vulnerable to injury and wear, and to the consequent pain syndromes described later in this chapter.

The bodies of the lumbar vertebrae are elliptically shaped as viewed from above, with the short axis in the sagittal plane. Commensurate with the greater weight they bear, they are four to five times more massive than midcervical vertebrae, and about two times more massive than middorsal vertebrae. The body of the fifth lumbar vertebra is wedge-shaped, with its anterior surface taller than its posterior.

The pedicles of the lumbar vertebrae emerge posteriorly from the upper half of the lateral posterior angles of the vertebral bodies. Their superior borders are near to, but not flush with, the superior border of the vertebral bodies. Each pedicle expands into four processes: the superior facet, inferior facet, transverse process, and lamina.

The planes of the facets between the first through the fourth lumbar vertebrae are very close to the true sagittal plane, allowing for most of the flexion, extension, and lateral bending of the spine but for nearly no rotation. However, the planes of the inferior facets of the fourth lumbar vertebra and the

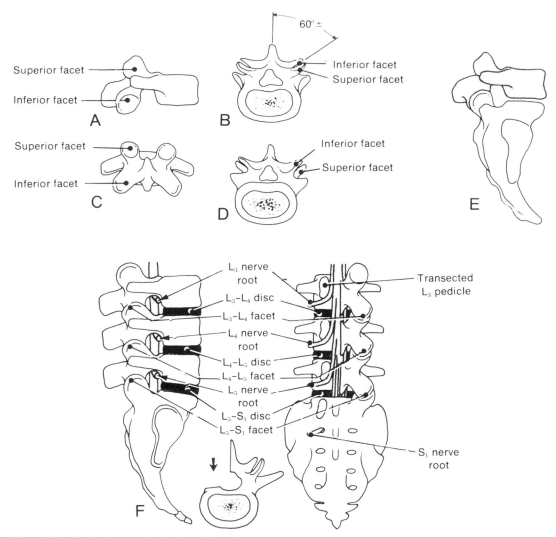

Figure 5.2. The lumbosacral spine. *A* and *B*, the fifth lumbar vertebra. Lateral and superior views. *C* and *D*, the fifth lumbar vertebra. Posterior and inferior views. *E*, the fifth lumbar vertebra, in articulation with the sacrum. *F*, the relationship of nerve roots to discs and the facet joints.

facets of the fifth lumbar and first sacral vertebrae are oriented closer to the frontal plane and allow for some rotation. Disorders of the lumbar and lumbosacral facets can result in posterior flank, inguinal, lumbosacral, buttock, and referred leg pain.

The transverse processes of the lumbar spine project more laterally than posteriorly, and very slightly superiorly. Deep ventral muscles that help effect lumbosacral flexion

and hip flexion take origin from these transverse processes. They can be fractured by blunt trauma to the posterior flanks. Forces that can fracture these processes can also contuse or lacerate the kidney, spleen, or other viscera.

The laminae fuse in the midline to become the spinous process. The spinous process and the laminae project distal to the corresponding vertebral body. This orientation protects the spinal cord from trauma from the posterior direction. The opening between successive laminae can be increased by flexion of the lumbar spine. This maneuver is helpful during lumbar puncture.

The intervertebral foramen is on each side of a functional unit, bounded by the pedicle superiorly and inferiorly, the facet joints posteriorly, and the bodies of the vertebrae and the intervertebral disc anteriorly. A lumbar nerve root passes through the foramen. As each nerve root enters its foramen, it clings to the superior pedicle and is not commonly vulnerable to protrusion of the disc at this site. The nerve root is commonly compressed before it reaches its foramen by protrusion of the disc above the foramen: the L-4 root by the L-3/L-4 disc, the L-5 root by the L-4/L-5 disc, and the S-1 root by the L-5/S-1 disc. Degenerative arthritis can also provoke soft tissue and bony encroachments at these foramina or in the path of the root before it reaches the foramen. These encroachments are more likely to cause irritations of the lumbar nerve roots than are similar encroachments in the thoracic spine. The condition of encroachment on the neural elements by degenerative hypertrophy of the facet joints is termed spinal stenosis. Figure 5.2F illustrates the relationship of nerve roots to disc and facet joints.

LIGAMENTS AND DISCS OF THE THORACIC (DORSAL) AND LUMBOSACRAL SPINE

The supraspinous and interspinous ligaments exist as distinct entities in the dorsal and lumbosacral spines (Fig. 5.3), while they are lost in the ligamentum nuchae of the cervical spine. They are relatively weak ligaments, vulnerable to sprain, that give little support to the spine. The other important ligaments of the dorsal and lumbosacral spine are the ligamentum flavum, a strong segmental ligament chiefly responsible for maintaining the posterior facet joints; the capsular ligaments of the facet joints, rela-

tively lax ligaments that allow for the play of the facet joints necessary for normal range of motion; the posterior longitudinal ligament, a strong multisegmental ligament that limits flexion of the spine; the anterior longitudinal ligament, a strong multisegmental ligament that limits extension of the spine. All of these ligaments are innervated and consequently can be a source of back pain and referred leg pain.

The posterior longitudinal ligament in the cervical spine is a broad ligament across all functional units. In the dorsal and lumbosacral spines, it is wide over the intervertebral discs and narrow over the vertebral bodies (Fig. 5.3). As it crosses the disc, its central portion is strong and its lateral portion is weak. It is at this lateral portion that disc herniation occurs.

The structure of the discs of the dorsal and lumbosacral spines is essentially the same as the structure of the discs in the neck. A central gel, the nucleus pulposus, is surrounded by a concentrically laminated fibrocartilage, the anulus fibrosus, each layer of which passes obliquely between two hyaline cartilage plates that are firmly bound to the bodies of the articulating vertebrae. The nucleus pulposus is eccentrically situated nearer the posterior margin of the disc. Hence, the anulus fibrosus is thinnest, and thus weakest, posteriorly. It is strongly reinforced centrally by the central band of the posterior longitudinal ligament, but is weakly reinforced posterolaterally. Hence, most disc herniations occur posterolaterally.

MUSCLES OF THE BACK (FIG. 5.4)

There are four spinal muscle groups: the splenius, erector spinae, interspinales, and abdominal groups.

The splenius capitis and cervicis originate from the lower cervical and upper thoracic spines. These muscles extend, laterally bend, and rotate the neck. Cervical, upper thoracic, and inner scapular pain can be caused by strain or irritation of these muscles.

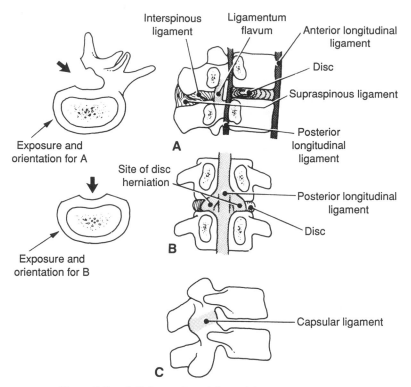

Figure 5.3.   *A–C,* ligaments and discs of the dorsolumbar spine.

The erector spinae are the prominent paraspinal muscles. Over the dorsal back they separate into three divisions, which cannot be distinguished as such through the overlying latissimus dorsi and trapezius. These muscles are the chief extensors of the back.

The interspinales are four pairs of muscles that extend between the five spinous processes of the lumbar spine. They are members of the segmental group and contribute to lumbar extension. Low back pain and referred pain to the buttock and thigh can be caused by strain or irritation of any of these muscle groups.

The abdominal musculature is also important to the function of the spine. The paired rectus abdominis, which span from the rib cage to the pelvis, are the primary flexors of the pelvis and help to prevent excessive lumbar lordosis. The recti, in con-

junction with the external oblique, internal oblique, and transversus, are capable of generating intraabdominal pressure to lessen compressive loads on the axial spine. This action is analogous to fluid pressure within a solid cylinder, i.e., the abdominal wall musculature surrounding the abdominal viscera.

DISTRIBUTION OF NERVE ROOTS L-3 THROUGH S-1 (FIG. 5.5)

The cutaneous dermatomal pattern is variable. Generally the L-3 root innervates the anterior surface of the knee and inner aspect of the thigh, the L-4 root innervates the inner aspect of the lower leg and ankle, the L-5 root innervates the dorsum of the foot, and the S-1 root innervates the lateral plantar aspect of the entire foot.

All leg muscles are innervated by several segments, but L-3 and L-4 dominate control of the quadriceps and the patellar tendon re-

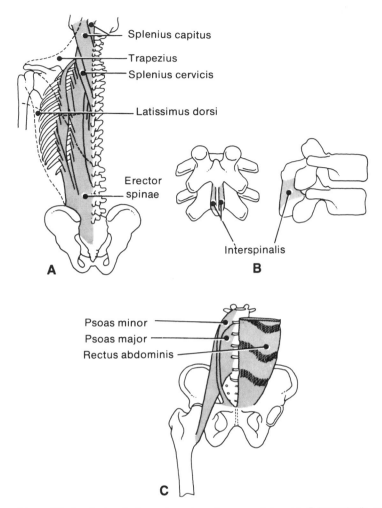

Figure 5.4. Musculature of the back. *A*, splenius and erector spinae muscle groups. *B*, interspinalis, posterior and lateral views. *C*, flexors of the lumbosacral spine.

flexes, L-5 dominates control of dorsiflexion of the ankle and extension of the great toe, and S-1 dominates control of plantar flexion of the ankle and the Achilles deep tendon reflex.

X-RAY ANATOMY

The radiographic evaluation of the spine is an essential part of the evaluation of a patient with a disease process associated with the spine. Panoramic 3-foot anteroposterior (AP) and lateral radiographs of the spine are used in the evaluation of scoliosis. These films, however, do not allow for specific examination of the spinal functional units. Therefore, it is more appropriate to request specific regional radiographs, i.e., thoracic or lumbar spine, when dealing with problems in these areas.

The initial radiographic evaluation of a spinal condition should include an AP radiograph of the spine (Fig. 5.6). On the AP view of the normal spine, the anterior-situated vertebral bodies are aligned in a vertical column. Each vertebral body appears to be a rectangular shape with cancellous bone out-

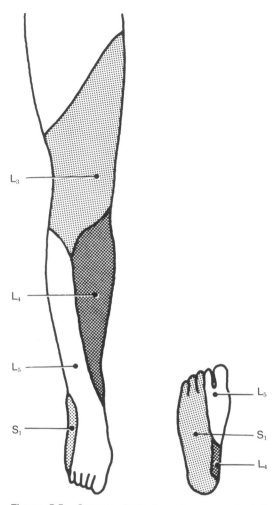

Figure 5.5. Sensory distribution of nerve roots, L-3 through S-1.

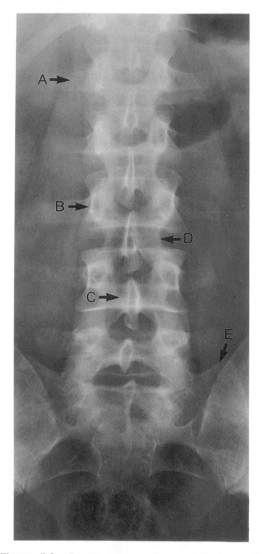

Figure 5.6. Roentgenogram of normal lumbosacral spine. *A*, transverse process. *B*, pedicle. *C*, posterior spinous process. *D*, lamina. *E*, sacrum.

lined by thicker cortical bone. The height of the vertebral bodies in this frontal plane increases from the thoracic to the lumbar spine. Superimposed over the vertebral body are the posterior elements of each vertebra. The pedicles lie at the superolateral corner of the vertebral body. They appear as symmetric oval densities. Lateral to each pedicle, the transverse process projects laterally and slightly superiorly. The posterior spinous process lies in the midline slightly caudal to the vertebral body. The facet joints are difficult to delineate at all levels due to

the overlying bony structures; however, they may be seen at one or two levels. The facet joints lie in line with the pedicles at approximately the level of the intervertebral disc.

On the lateral view of the spine, the normal lordosis of the lumbar region can be well delineated. The height of each vertebral body and intervertebral disc is clearly seen as there are no overlying bony structures on the lateral view. The pedicle extends in a posterior direction from the body near the superior endplate. The pedicle is the superior roof of the neural foramen. The laminae extend from the pedicle in an inferior and posterior direction so that a thin cortical outline of the posterior spinous process can be seen extending from the lamina.

Certain structural anomalies of the lumbosacral spine are common but have not been shown to be significantly associated with symptoms. These include sacralization of the fifth lumbar vertebra, lumbarization of the sacral vertebrae, and spina bifida occulta.

Evaluation of the Patient with Back Symptoms

HISTORY

Back pain is exceedingly common in industrialized society; up to 80% of the population will report an episode of back pain. The severity of this pain can vary from an occasional ache during activities to incapacitating pain. In children, back pain is a less frequent symptom and a complaint of back pain in the skeletally immature person necessitates a thorough search for its etiology. The presence of pain during periods of rest or pain that awakens the child from sleep are ominous symptoms. Patients with infection, bony tumors, and spinal cord tumors may present with pain as a chief complaint with few or no abnormal findings on the subsequent physical examination. Furthermore, pain is not associated with common childhood skeletal deformities, such as scoliosis or leg-length discrepancies. Early referral to an orthopaedic specialist is recommended for the child who complains of back pain.

Because of its prevalence, the presence of back pain in the adult population is less helpful in identifying serious skeletal disease. Also, location of the pain is not usually a specific enough characteristic to allow identification of its underlying etiology.

With the exception of the nucleus pulposus, almost any element of the motion segment could be the source of back pain. In addition, this pain can be referred into the buttock, thigh, and lower leg in a nonradicular fashion. It is important to make this distinction between referred and radicular pain. Radicular pain is secondary to true nerve root irritation or compression and will follow a dermatomal pattern. It is often associated with root tension signs, objective sensory loss, and muscle weakness.

It is important to obtain a detailed history, recognizing that the characteristics of the patient's pain complaints are only marginally helpful. Radicular versus referred pain can usually be suspected on the basis of history. Pain that is present at night or at rest raises concern regarding irritative lesions, such as tumors or infection. The relationship of activity to pain can be significant. For example, activities that cause extension of the back increase the load on the facet joints. Consequently, facet joint pain may be worse with hyperextension activities. Extension of the spine will also reduce the volume of the spinal canal. In these circumstances patients will frequently present with symptoms of stenosis, i.e., back and leg pain with possible associated weakness and sensory alteration. The radicular pain caused by a herniated disc is worse with activities that increase intraabdominal pressure. Consequently, these patients will complain of increased pain with coughing, sneezing, or performing any Valsalva maneuver.

While there is often a traumatic origin to back pain, just as often the initiating event may not be remembered or may seem trivial. Patients may report pain after twisting to see an object behind them or bending forward to pick up something from the floor. These patients often have some degenerative disease of the spine that renders the spine more vulnerable to the stresses of normal activities. Also, it must be remembered that these "normal activities" can dramatically increase the stresses on the lumbar spine. This has been measured as it reflects on the pressure within the intervertebral disc. It has been shown that simple sitting without a spinal support increases the pressure on the disc approximately 40% over the normal standing posture. Sitting with the spine flexed doubles intradiscal pressure. Bending forward to 20° can increase the pressure 120%, and lifting a 20-kg weight can produce a 240% rise in the pressure.

In circumstances where fracture or dislocation of the spine is suspected, there is usually a history of major injury. This may not be the case when there is pathologic fracture because of underlying osteoporosis or tumor. When complaints involve neurologic symptoms, careful description of the pattern is important to help identify the level based on the dermatomal pattern.

Finally, the history is important to exclude many nonorthopaedic conditions that may appear in patients who present with back pain, including abdominal aneurysm, diverticulitis, inflammatory disease, intraabdominal cancer, renal problems, or various forms of intestinal disease.

PHYSICAL EXAMINATION

The patient should be dressed in a loose-fitting gown that opens to allow for visual inspection and palpation of the spine and paravertebral muscles. The visual assessment includes a notation of the height of the right and left hemipelvis, the shape of the spine, the balance of the thorax over the pelvis, and the alignment of the shoulders. In the sagittal plane, the contour of the lumbar and thoracic spines should be noted. Palpation over the paravertebral muscles may reveal localized muscle spasm or tenderness. Palpation directly in the midline will allow for direct percussion of the posterior spinous processes. This will aid in the determination of the presence or absence of scoliosis in an obese patient. Hypersensitivity to light touch with an exaggerated pain response is frequently seen when psychologic overlay is a significant part of the patient's pain symptoms.

Next, the patient is asked to bend forward at the waist. In the normal patient, the lumbar lordosis will be reversed to a gentle kyphosis, which will have a smooth transition through the lumbar spine and into the thoracic spine. Muscle spasm or pain may prevent reversal of the lordosis found in the erect spine. It is helpful to note the degree of forward bend at the waist, as measured in degrees of forward bend or by description of the distal extent of the fingertips, i.e., to the level of the knees, midcalf, ankles, or toes. The forward bend test will also emphasize any rib cage asymmetries that may be present with scoliosis. Palpation at the lumbosacral junction may reveal a step-off, which is seen with spondylolisthesis. Next, the patient is asked to hyperextend the back. Similarly, lateral bending to the right and left are performed. Any pain, muscle spasm, or restriction of motion brought out by these maneuvers is noted.

The patient then assumes a sitting position on the examining table. In this position, straight leg raising is tested by passively extending in sequence the right and left leg. The amount of extension that is possible should be compared with straight leg raising in the supine position, which is performed later in the physical examination. A discrepancy between the amount of straight leg raising in the sitting position compared with the supine position cannot be explained in physiologic terms and consequently serves as a check for "nonorganic" complaints. Deep tendon reflexes are examined at the patellar tendon and the Achilles tendon bilaterally. A segmental innervation of the patellar stretch reflex is L-3 and L-4, while the Achilles tendon stretch reflex is primarily S-1. Individual motor testing of the muscles in the lower extremities is then performed, along with sensory examination. Any abnormalities are checked against the normal patterns of innervation to determine the level of nerve root involvement.

Nontraumatic Conditions of Childhood

SCOLIOSIS

Scoliosis is an abnormal lateral curvature of the spine. When viewed from the front or back, the spine should be straight, centering the head over the sacrum. There are a number of conditions that can produce an apparent scoliosis without a true, intrinsic spinal deformity. These include a leg-length discrepancy, muscular spasm, poor posture, or hysteria. We use the term "scoliosis" to describe a true, intrinsic spinal deformity. Scoliosis may be secondary to congenital bone dysplasia, or metabolic or paralytic conditions. If no primary cause is obvious, it is designated as idiopathic scoliosis. Curvatures under 10°, as measured radiographically, that are not progressive do not require treatment or referral to an orthopaedist. Because scoliosis is often progressive, even the child with a mild degree of curvature greater than 10° should be referred to an orthopaedic surgeon for initial evaluation and possible treatment.

Idiopathic scoliosis is the most common type of childhood scoliosis. This condition occurs in approximately 1% of the adolescent population, and predominantly affects girls. With the advent of mandatory school screening programs, a large number of children with spinal asymmetries that do not represent true scoliosis are seen by the primary care physician. In this setting the evaluation should define the exact nature of the condition. Abnormal posture, leg-length discrepancy, or some painful condition producing an apparent spinal asymmetry must be ruled out. The presence of developmental, traumatic, or paralytic etiology must be evaluated. In the absence of these causes, the diagnosis of idiopathic scoliosis is confirmed. This is an inherited disorder characterized by a sex-linked dominant genetic pattern with a variable expressivity and incomplete penetrance.

Clinical Characteristics

Idiopathic scoliosis is generally a painless disorder in the adolescent. A complaint of back pain warrants thorough investigation to rule out other etiologies, and should not be attributed to the underlying scoliosis. On physical examination the patient presents with asymmetry in the levels of the shoulders, asymmetry in the waist crease, prominence of one iliac crest, and a posterior rib hump prominence most obvious on forward bending. Leg-length measurements will not show significant discrepancy and neurologic examination is usually normal. If there is evidence of neuromuscular disease or metabolic abnormality, or if x-rays reveal a congenital basis, the scoliosis is not classified as idiopathic.

X-ray of the spine is essential for the diagnosis and treatment of scoliosis. To diminish the radiation exposure of the breasts in adolescent girls, it is recommended that the frontal radiograph be performed in a posterior to anterior projection and breast shields be used. The radiograph will establish the extent and the severity of the curvature. The amount of curvature is determined by the Cobb method (Fig. 5.7). Any number of combinations of curves may be encountered (Fig. 5.8). Lateral curvature is always accompanied by rotation of the vertebrae. The rotational component is an important determinant of clinical deformity and is most noticeable when the child bends forward and the examiner sites down the axis of the spine (Fig. 5.9).

Treatment

The treatment of idiopathic scoliosis is based on data obtained from long-term longitudinal studies of the natural history of scoliosis. Curvature of less than 30° at skeletal maturity appears to cause no prolonged

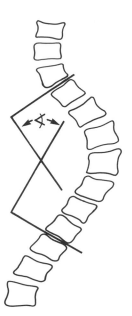

Figure 5.7.   The Cobb method of measuring spinal curvature. (Copyright 1989 CIBA-GEIGY Corporation. Modified with permission from Clinical Symposia by Frank H. Netter, M.D. All rights reserved.)

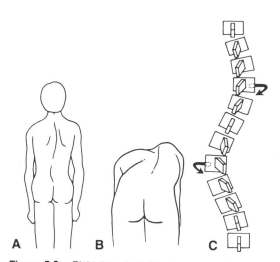

Figure 5.9.   Right thoracic, left lumbar curve. *A*, patient standing upright. *B*, patient bending forward. *C*, the rotation accompanying lateral curvature. (Vertebral bodies rotate toward the convexity, hence clockwise rotation accompanies right thoracic curve, and counterclockwise rotation accompanies left lumbar curve, as viewed from overhead.)

disability as a person matures in later life. Curves that have reached 50° at the time of skeletal maturity, however, tend to progress later in life and may cause restrictive pulmonary disease, cor pulmonale, and severe back pain. Therefore, the treatment of idiopathic scoliosis in adolescents attempts to prevent the curve from progressing to 50°, where later progression in adulthood is inevitable. A curvature of greater than 10° in a

skeletally immature patient needs to be followed by periodic clinical and radiographic examinations until skeletal maturity has been reached. An interval of 6 months between each visit is an acceptable follow-up program. After initial orthopaedic consultation, the primary care physician may follow children in this early stage. However, if while under observation the curve progresses more than 5° or if on presentation the curve is greater than 25°, referral to an orthopaedic surgeon for follow-up and

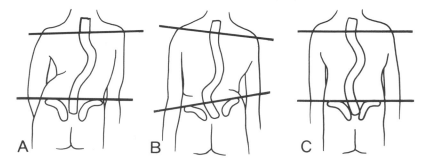

Figure 5.8.   Examples of body contour with scoliosis. *A*, right thoracic curve. *B*, left lumbar curve. *C*, double major curve.

treatment is recommended. It is at this level that brace therapy is initiated.

The spinal orthosis or brace consists of a polypropylene shell that is contoured to provide a corrective force to the spine while the child grows. It is necessary that the child wear the brace for at least 16 hours a day until skeletal maturity is reached. This usually involves treatment for approximately 3 to 4 years. This is difficult for the adolescent patient to accept and the primary care physician can be very helpful in providing guidance, direction, and emotional support to the patient and family. A scoliosis clinic where other similarly affected adolescents are treated can provide a most supportive treatment environment.

If the curvature progresses to a point of 45° to 50°, the patient is at high risk for further progression in adulthood. Therefore, surgical stabilization of the spine with corrective instrumentation is performed to correct the curvature and prevent the inevitable progression.

ADOLESCENT KYPHOSIS (SCHEUERMANN'S DISEASE)

Adolescent kyphosis, also known as Scheuermann's disease, is thought to be secondary to repetitive trauma and stress fractures of the anterior aspect of the vertebral endplates in the growing adolescent. Untreated, the disease leads to permanent kyphosis of a variable degree, which will be established at the end of the adolescent growth period. Nonoperative treatment is effective only when applied prior to the cessation of skeletal growth.

Clinical Characteristics

The patient presents in early adolescence with thoracic or lumbar back pain and/or a kyphotic postural deformity. The child is often taller and heavier than other children of his or her age. Girls are affected as often as boys. When the disease process is in the thoracic area, there is an increased thoracic kyphosis; however, in a few children, the disease affects the lumbar region, in which case that portion of the spine looks abnormally flat. The pain is usually aggravated by prolonged activity or standing for long periods of time, and is relieved by rest. There may be local tenderness. The sensory and motor examinations are normal. The diagnosis is confirmed by a lateral radiograph of the spine, which should be obtained while the patient is standing. The normal thoracic kyphosis measured from T-4 to T-12 by the Cobb method is between 20° and 40°. An increase in the amount of kyphosis associated with anterior wedging of the vertebral body of at least 5° in three or more consecutive vertebral bodies, establishes the diagnosis. Concave osteolytic defects at the endplates, known as Schmorl's nodes, may be noted. These represent herniation of disc material into the weakly ossified vertebral endplate (Fig. 5.10).

Treatment

The primary care physician should refer children to the orthopaedist if the radiographic findings of Scheuermann's disease are present. The treatment of Scheuermann's disease in a skeletally immature patient incorporates the use of a thoracolumbar brace and active physical therapy programs. Such treatment may decrease the amount of inevitable deformity. For severe deformity, however, surgical treatment may be necessary. Corrective spinal fusion with instrumentation can be performed in cases resistant to the above-mentioned modalities. In the absence of radiographic findings of Scheuermann's disease, the "round-back" deformity simply represents a postural habit. In these children, physical therapy is helpful in strengthening the thoracic extensor muscles and flattening the accentuated lumbar lordosis, which is commonly present. The therapy regimen should emphasize antilordotic lumbar exercises and thoracic extension exercises.

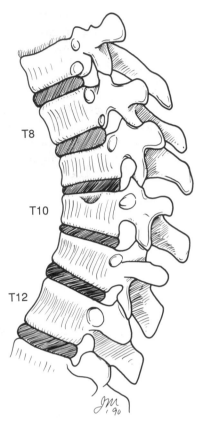

Figure 5.10. Juvenile kyphosis. Anterior vertebral body wedging on three or more consecutive vertebrae.

SPONDYLOLYSIS AND SPONDYLOLISTHESIS

The term spondylolysis refers to a bony defect in the pars interarticularis of the posterior elements of the vertebral body (Fig. 5.11*B*). It is thought to be the result of nonunion of a stress fracture in the posterior elements. The condition most commonly occurs at the L-5 lamina, but has been seen throughout the spine. There is a high incidence in athletes who undergo constant hyperextension activity of the lumbar spine, such as gymnasts and football linemen. Spondylolisthesis refers to an anterior displacement of the vertebral column on a lower vertebra, most commonly an anterior slippage of L-5 on S-1 (Fig. 5.11*A*). This may be due to spondylolysis, articular process malformation, or elongation of the pars interarticularis. Moderate or severe degrees of spondylolisthesis may cause nerve root impingement, and patients with this defect may consequently present with signs and symptoms of nerve root irritation.

Clinical Characteristics

Spondylolysis typically occurs in preadolescent and adolescent children. The initial symptom is an aching pain in the lumbar region, which is associated with activity. It may radiate into the buttock and thigh on the affected side. The pain is typically relieved by rest or limiting the aggravating activity. It is often associated with a feeling of stiffness. This is particularly true for gymnasts or ballerinas, who complain that they are unable to perform their usual routine. This may be difficult to detect on clinical examination because these children are so flexible that even with a decrease in their flexibility they still appear to be within normal standards.

The physical examination reveals that there is spasm in the paravertebral muscles, and there may be a flattening of the normal lumbar lordosis in patients who present with acute back pain. The child with long-standing and severe spondylolisthesis may have a kyphotic deformity at the lumbosacral junction with a compensatory hyperlordosis in the lumbar region. Hamstring tightness is common. This is seen with diminished straight leg raising, increased popliteal angle, and diminished stride length on walking or running. The neurologic examination is usually normal except in those infrequent cases where there is nerve root irritation. The diagnosis is confirmed by radiographs of the lumbar spine (Fig. 5.11*B*). A lumbosacral series should consist of standing lateral and AP views, as well as 45° oblique views of the lumbar spine. Occasionally, a child will present with back pain before the plain film radiographs show the bony defect. In these cases, a bone scan will be helpful.

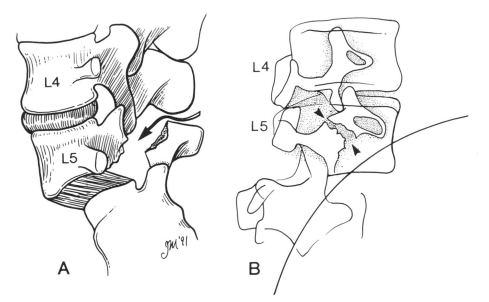

Figure 5.11. *A*, lateral view of spondylolytic spondylolisthesis. *B*, spondylolysis. A 45° oblique view of the lumbar space will show a defect in the pars interarticularis.

Treatment

The goals of treatment in a child with spondylolisthesis or spondylolysis are (*a*) pain relief, (*b*) return to activity, and (*c*) prevention of deformity. It is necessary to follow children with spondylolysis until they reach skeletal maturity. A child with spondylolysis may be treated by the primary care physician with a conservative program consisting of the use of nonsteroidal anti-inflammatory medications, limiting activity below the pain threshold, and a physical therapy regimen. The physical therapy regimen emphasizes antilordotic exercises for the lumbar spine, such as pelvic tilts and modified situps, with stretching exercises for the hamstrings. Patients who do not respond to this therapy should be referred to an orthopaedic surgeon. Any patient who has pain associated with spondylolisthesis should be referred to an orthopaedic surgeon for evaluation. In the adolescent years, a spondylolysis may progress to spondylolisthesis, or a spondylolisthesis may increase in severity; however, this is unlikely to be true for the adult population. For children who do not respond to conservative treatment, a brace may be helpful to control their pain level and allow them to participate in activities. Surgical repair of the spondylolysis or posterolateral fusion of the involved vertebrae are indicated when the patient is unresponsive to conservative treatment, shows progression of a spondylolisthesis, or presents with a severe degree of spondylolisthesis. Surgical fusion is effective in controlling the pain and progression of the disease under these circumstances.

Nontraumatic Conditions in Adulthood

Thoracic and lumbar back pain is a common complaint in the adult population. Back pain accounts for a large number of work-related disabilities with tremendous economic costs. Furthermore, back pain often limits recreational activities. As with any nonspecific complaint, the etiologic cause for an episode of back pain can be taken from a long list of spinal and nonspinal conditions. In this section common degenerative and/or traumatic mechanical causes of low back pain will be discussed. As pointed out earlier in this chapter ("Evaluation of the Patient with Back Symptoms"), the primary care physician must rule out nonmechanical causes of spinal disease, including infection, tumor, and spondyloarthropathy, as well as intraabdominal disease that may accompany back pain. While this section will discuss the diagnosis and treatment of specific etiologies of back pain, it must be recognized that in many patients it will be impossible to determine the exact etiology of back pain because the localization of pain and the physical findings are frequently nonspecific. With a systematic approach, however, the primary care physician should be able to diagnose and treat most cases of back pain and identify the small number that require orthopaedic or other specialty referral. Fortunately for those patients who fall into the "idiopathic back pain" category, symptomatic treatment is often successful and is similar to the initial therapy for many of the specific conditions that will be discussed. It must be remembered that 80% of all patients with acute low back pain will improve within 2 months of the onset of symptoms.

DEGENERATIVE DISEASE

A theoretical scheme of spinal degeneration has been proposed. While there is still debate regarding this theory and how to fit a specific patient into the scheme, it provides a useful perspective for the primary care physician. This theory proposes that facet joint synovitis, hypermobility, and progressive degeneration are "natural" consequences of aging and the repetitive trauma of "normal" activity. These facet joint changes occur concurrently with the degenerative changes in the intervertebral disc, which begin with circumferential tears of the anulus and progress to radial tears and disc herniation. Subluxation of the facet joints with enlargement of the articular processes occurs in parallel

with disc resorption and spinal osteophyte formation. In the early phases of this degenerative process, patients may be identified as having "facet joint syndrome," or after relatively minor trauma the patient may develop an "acute disc herniation." It is important to recognize that the facet joint or the disc is just one part of the motion segment, and it is unlikely that there is isolated trauma or inflammation in one part of the spinal unit (composed of disc, facet joint, ligaments, and bony elements) without associated abnormalities in the complementary parts.

Acute Disc Herniation

Degeneration of the intervertebral disc can lead to both acute and chronic pain conditions. The L-5/S-1 and L-4/L-5 discs are the regions most commonly involved in the degenerative processes. Degeneration of the intervertebral disc is associated with loss of its water content, weakening of the anulus fibrosis, and loss in height of the disc. This weakening of the anulus fibrosis is associated with radial tears in the posterior part of the anulus. In the younger patient, where degeneration is usually not so advanced, actual herniation of the nucleus pulposus through the weakened area of the anulus can occur. This is most common at the posterolateral zone where reinforcement from the posterior longitudinal ligament is weakest. These younger patients present with the syndrome of acute disc herniation. In the older population, the degenerative process continues with degeneration of other parts of the motion segment, including the facet joints. The motion segment may lose its competence to resist shearing stress, which is substantial at the lower lumbar spine. In this circumstance the older patient can develop degenerative spondylolisthesis without a bony defect in the pars interarticularis. In the more chronic form without disc herniation, the patient with degenerative disc disease will have recurrent episodes of pain. These episodes are secondary to inflammation that develops subsequent to tissue injury, which occurs more easily in the face of the degenerative process. Consequently, even normal physiologic stresses can cause injury, as well as excessive stresses of awkward or heavy lifting or exertion.

Clinical Characteristics. While an acute disc herniation can occur in all age groups, it is most typical in patients between 30 and 50 years. This condition is often precipitated by activity, which at times may appear to be physiologic activity without excessive stress. As stated previously, however, the normal physiologic stresses within the disc can be quite high with certain activities. In other instances there is obvious traumatic origin, such as a heavy lifting episode or a fall. The classic presentation is one of acute back pain with radiation into one lower extremity in a dermatomal pattern. Radiation into both lower extremities is much less common but can be seen with more central or massive disc herniations. The clinical presentation will help identify the level of disc herniation. With herniation of the L-4/L-5 disc, it is usually the L-5 nerve root that is affected. Inflammation of this root produces pain in the posterior aspect of the thigh, posterolateral calf, and dorsum of the foot. There is weakness of the extensor hallucis longus and gluteus medius muscles. Weakness of toe flexion and ankle dorsiflexion may also be present because of contribution of the L-5 root to the innervation of these muscles. An alteration in sensation may be present along the posterolateral aspect of the calf and the dorsum of the foot. The Achilles and patellar tendon reflexes are usually normal.

Disc herniation at the L-5/S-1 level produces an S-1 radiculopathy. Back pain radiates into the buttock, posterior and lateral thigh and calf, and plantar lateral aspect of the foot. Weakness of plantar flexion of the ankle is noted along with sensory loss on the lateral and plantar surface of the foot. The Achilles reflex is depressed.

With an acute disc herniation, straight leg raising is limited in the affected leg. This test is considered positive when straight leg raising is abnormally limited by back and leg pain similar to the presenting radicular pain. A strong indicator of an acute radiculopathy is the same response with straight leg raising in the contralateral extremity.

In the differential diagnosis of sciatica, it is important to remember that radiculitis or radiculopathy may be caused by compressive or inflammatory lesions distal to the spinal canal. Lesions that affect the lumbosacral plexus or the sciatic nerve itself can mimic a disc herniation. Although rare, these conditions must be remembered before the patient's pain is attributed to a discogenic cause.

The presence of a disc herniation is confirmed by computerized tomography (CT) or magnetic resonance imaging of the spine. These techniques have essentially replaced myelography in the diagnosis of disc rupture. Electromyograms can be helpful in defining the precise nerve root involved.

Treatment. Except for the patient who presents with significant neurologic loss, the initial treatment of acute disc herniation is conservative. Most patients will have resolution of their symptoms within 8 weeks. An initial period of bed rest for 5 to 7 days is appropriate. Pain relief is often found to be optimal in the supine or side-lying position with the hips and knees flexed. A nonsteroidal anti-inflammatory medication is beneficial in reducing the inflammation about the nerve root, and also has an analgesic effect. A narcotic analgesic may be required in the initial phase when pain may be severe. During the bed rest period, the patient should perform isometric exercises of the abdominal muscles as well as hip and leg muscles as tolerated. Once the acute phase has subsided, a mobilization program begins with a progressive decrease in the amount of time at rest and an increase in the amount of physical activity. Sitting for prolonged periods of time is avoided as the sitting posture increases the pressure in the disc. Walking is a good means of achieving progressive activity and cardiovascular conditioning. A swimming program can be added as tolerated. Supervised physical therapy can help the patient with spinal mobilization and isometric strengthening exercises for the abdominal and paravertebral muscles. Those patients with nonstrenuous occupations can return to work in 3 to 4 weeks. Functional activity should be encouraged during recovery as the likelihood of return to full preinjury function decreases as the length of the patient's disability period increases. Prolonged disability often leads to a chronic pain condition characterized by persistent pain, muscular atrophy, reduced spinal mobility, and failure to function. If a patient is not showing improvement with conservative measures after 2 to 3 weeks, orthopaedic referral should be made. In addition, the patient who presents with significant sensory or motor impairment, or bowel or bladder dysfunction should be referred immediately. Prompt referral is also indicated for the patient who presented initially with minor sensory and motor dysfunction but who has evidence of deteriorating function. The likelihood of recovery from a motor loss is related to the length of time the loss persists before definitive treatment.

Chronic Degenerative Disc Syndrome

A constellation of symptoms grouped under the heading of chronic degenerative disc syndrome occurs in an older population, most commonly over 50 years of age.

Clinical Characteristics. This condition is characterized by recurrent episodes of back pain with referred or radicular symptoms that resolve over a short period of time. After resolution of a painful episode, patients are able to return to their previous level of activity but they are often aware of their propensity for a recurrent back injury. Therefore, they gradually learn to cope with their limitations. Localized back pain is the predominant complaint in this condition. However, on physical examination and often in the history, there are signs and symptoms of a radiculopathy. This may be manifest by radicular pain, motor weakness, or sensory loss in a dermatomal distribution. Minor trauma may often aggravate this condition causing the recurrent symptom complex.

Treatment. The mainstay of the treatment of chronic degenerative disc syndrome is education. The patient must learn the principles of lumbar spine body mechanics and avoid activities that aggravate the condition. This is often presented to the patient in the setting of a "back school." In this setting, protective maneuvers are emphasized as well as weight loss and cardiovascular conditioning. Patients are taught how to cope with their condition so that they maximize the number of pain-free days. For patients who had been employed in occupations requiring manual labor, a change in occupation may be required.

Facet Syndrome

As in all synovial joints of the body, traumatic, degenerative, and inflammatory conditions of the spinal articular joints may cause pain and limited motion. The joint capsules are highly innervated structures that may be stretched from joint subluxation or distention of the joint with fluid. Protective posturing and spasm of the paravertebral muscles lead to diminished spinal mobility and secondary muscle fatigue. As noted above, the facet joints are involved in the scheme of degenerative disease that affects the spinal motion segment. The facet syndrome is commonly seen early in the degenerative process in the young or middle-aged patient. Symptoms frequently develop after an injury or strain, though this injury may not be remembered, with the damage occurring secondary to the "normal stresses" of general activity.

Clinical Characteristics. The pain associated with a facet syndrome is variable. It may be described as a steady ache present after long periods of inactivity. With resumption of activity the pain initially increases but as activity continues, the patient may feel temporarily better. The pain usually intensifies, however, once activity is complete. Patients may complain of intense, sharp pain with abrupt movements and often state that they note a "catching" sensation in the lumbar spine. The pain is often referred to the buttock and thigh, but rarely below the knee, in a true radicular pattern. On physical examination muscle spasm may be noted. There may be loss of the normal lumbar lordosis and inability to flatten the lordosis on forward bending. Motion is restricted in all planes, especially extension. Straight leg raising is often mildly limited as the maneuver invariably causes some motion of the lumbar spine as the legs are elevated, and this in turn causes pain. Neurologic examination is normal.

Radiographic evaluation should include AP, lateral, and oblique views of the spine. The oblique views will allow the best evaluation of the facet joints, where changes typical of degenerative joint disease may be found. The changes consist of hypertrophy and osteophyte formation of the superior and inferior articular processes, loss of joint space, cyst formation, and subchondral sclerosis. In the early phases of the facet syndrome, x-rays may not be remarkable.

Treatment. The acute episodes are best treated by a brief period of bed rest followed by mobilization once the pain subsides. Anti-inflammatory agents are helpful in allowing a quick resolution of this initial exacerbation. Occasionally, an oral narcotic is necessary. Muscle spasm may be relieved by the use of heat. Patients who are resistant to this therapy may benefit from a short course of a muscle relaxant.

Recurrent episodes of acute pain lead to atrophy of the paravertebral and abdominal muscles and a general deterioration in the physical state of the patient. After an acute episode has subsided, a physical therapy program should be initiated, emphasizing abdominal strengthening exercises and spinal mobilization. A corset or lightweight spinal orthosis may be beneficial in allowing the patient to return to a functional state soon after an acute episode of pain; however, the spinal orthosis may lead to further muscular atrophy and it is essential that the patient enter a routine strengthening regimen to maintain the muscular tone of the paravertebral and abdominal muscles. The program must be designed to allow the patient to strengthen these muscles without causing recurrence of the pain. This must be tailored to the individual patient, but in general it is wise to avoid activities that cause axial loading, such as running and jumping. Swimming is an excellent exercise program to increase muscle tone without causing further disability of the spine. Patients who are recalcitrant to the above-mentioned treatment may benefit from injection of the facet joint with a corticosteroid agent. This procedure is performed with radiologic guidance and requires referral to an orthopaedic surgeon or other physician skilled in this technique.

Spinal Stenosis

Spinal stenosis is a term used to describe a reduction in the size of the central spinal canal, the nerve root canal, or intervertebral foramen (Fig. 5.12). Stenosis may occur on a congenital or developmental basis. This can be idiopathic, associated with dysplasia of the bony elements, or seen in achondroplasia. More often, spinal stenosis is an acquired disease secondary to progressive degenerative changes of the facet joints and intervertebral disc. This condition is part of the same scheme of degenerative disease previously outlined. Spinal stenosis develops when this condition becomes severe or is superimposed on a congenitally narrow spinal canal.

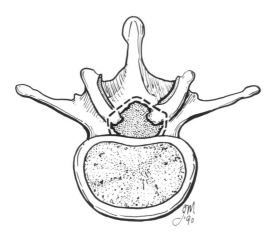

Figure 5.12. Spinal stenosis. Facet joint hypertrophy with thickening of the capsule and ligamentum flavum diminishes available space of the cauda equina. The dotted line marks the normal shape of the canal.

With facet joint degeneration, there is osteophyte formation and hypertrophy with thickening of the capsular ligaments and of the ligamentum flavum of the spine. This produces encroachment on the nerve root canal. The disc at the same level has usually undergone some degenerative changes as well, with narrowing and bulging of the disc and occasionally frank herniation. With severe degenerative disease in the facets and disc, there may be a degenerative spondylolisthesis, which can contribute to the local stenosis. Stenosis may also be seen after a laminectomy, fusion, or fracture. Paget's disease and fluorosis may also be associated with stenosis. The actual cause of the pain and neurologic changes in spinal stenosis is not clear. Various etiologies have been postulated. Many authors believe that the symptoms are produced by transient ischemia of the nerve roots. Because the extended position of the lumbar spine reduces the canal dimension, symptoms are almost always worse when the spine is in relative extension.

Clinical Characteristics. Paresthesia and weakness of spinal stenosis are typically provoked by lumbosacral extension and relieved by lumbosacral flexion. Since most people walk with their lumbar spine somewhat extended, they experience the onset of symptoms with walking. When this condition was originally described it was commonly referred to as "pseudoclaudication" because of the development of leg pain, numbness, and tingling with walking that mimicked the symptoms of patients with true vascular claudication. However, it must be remembered that the classic signs of pseudoclaudication are not present in all patients. The pain is usually worse walking downhill than uphill. Since sitting increases lumbosacral flexion, most patients with symptoms of spinal stenosis experience relief while sitting. The pain is often described as burning, with radiation to the buttocks and thighs. It often has a radicular quality and may be bilateral. Findings consistent with a chronic radiculopathy may be present. Straight leg raising is usually normal. Various sensory and motor deficits may be noted, particularly if the patient is examined once symptoms have been produced by a period of walking. A vascular examination must be meticulously performed to evaluate the aorta and the peripheral vessels to rule out true claudication.

Radiographic evaluation initially begins with plain x-rays of the lumbar spine. This may show degenerative disease of the facet joints and disc, degenerative spondylolisthesis, reduced disc height, and features of congenital stenosis. The diagnosis of spinal stenosis is confirmed by a CT scan of the involved area. The stenosis may involve several vertebral segments in the lumbar spine. Use of a contrast agent may be warranted to also allow evaluation of the nerve root as it exits the spine. An electromyogram may be helpful.

Treatment. The conservative treatment of spinal stenosis should include measures to relieve pain, enhance lumbar flexion, and improve the patient's functional capacity. Reduction of lumbar extension can be accomplished by the use of a lumbar orthosis. The optimal amount of flexion of the orthosis can be determined by a period of trial use of the orthosis in different degrees of flexion. Exercises to improve abdominal strength and reduce lumbar lordosis are also helpful. Cardiovascular conditioning can be accomplished in patients whose walking ability is limited by a program of stationary bicycling.

If this treatment modality fails, referral to an orthopaedic surgeon is warranted. A course of epidural steroid injection may be beneficial. Persistent pain and disability may require surgical decompression of the stenosis by laminectomy with or without fusion.

Traumatic Disorders of the Spine

The functional units of the normal spine articulate with one another to create two lordotic and two kyphotic segments. The lordotic segments, the cervical and lumbar spine, are the most mobile: the cervical spine moves quite freely in all three planes of motion (flexion-extension, lateral bending, and rotation), and the lumbar spine moves quite freely in the sagittal and frontal planes of motion (flexion-extension and lateral bending). The kyphotic segments, the dorsal spine and the sacrum, are the least mobile: the dorsal spine moves predominantly in the transverse plane (rotation), and the sacrum does not move at all except at its articulations with the pelvis. The junctions between the most mobile and the least mobile segments of the spine are the points at which angulating-twisting forces are the greatest. Hence, the most disrupting dorsolumbar injuries tend to involve the functional units T-12/L-1 and L-1/L-2. Though, by this rule, the lower cervical units should be the most vulnerable, the great mobility of all of the cervical units and the angular forces generated by the mass of the head subject all cervical units to a nearly equal vulnerability: the

chances of the moment determine the point at which maximum force will apply.

The spinal cord ends variably at the first or second lumbar vertebra, and the cauda equina, composed of all lumbar and sacral nerve roots, ends near the end of the spinal canal, in the sacrum. Thus, the fractures and dislocations that can injure the cord itself are all those at the L-2 level or higher. Below this level, neural injury involves the nerve roots and consequently carries a better prognosis for recovery.

It is important to recognize that fractures and dislocations of the lower thoracic and lumbar spines are often associated with very troublesome paralytic ileus.

PRESUMPTION OF UNSTABLE INJURY AND METHODS OF TRANSPORTATION

In the conscious patient, neck and back pain following injury should be suspected to represent an unstable fracture or dislocation with a potential for damage to the cord. This suspicion should become a presumption when the individual is reluctant to move, complains of dysesthesia, or demonstrates weakness or paralysis of any extremity, or when deep palpation over and on either side of the spine demonstrates distinct tenderness. In the unconscious patient, spinal column injury should be presumed until ruled out by x-ray evaluation.

Once the presumption is made, the patient must be moved without further spinal injury. The spine can be well-stabilized during transport by immobilization of the patient on a fracture board. For suspected cervical spine injury, any space between the back of the neck and the fracture board should be filled with some folded material (for example, a sweater or towel), and supports to prevent rotation and lateral bending should be placed on both sides of the head and neck (preferably sandbags or some equally stable makeshift equivalent). If a spinal board or narrow stretcher is available, the head position can be maintained by taping. If available, a sternal-occipital-mandibular orthosis, such as a Philadelphia collar, will provide adequate stabilization during transport. For thoracic and lumbar injury, an adequate fracture board must be wide enough to accommodate the patient's shoulders and long enough to support the length of the spine, including the occiput and pelvis. An ideal fracture board extends the length of the patient. The patient should be firmly strapped onto the board.

ESSENTIALS OF ASSESSMENT AND DIAGNOSIS

Vital functions should be assessed and all necessary support provided. When a patient suspected of an unstable neck injury appears to need ventilatory support, introduce an oropharyngeal airway and try to effect adequate ventilation through a mask. If possible, the neck should be stabilized before attempting to introduce any endotracheal airway. When an endotracheal airway must be introduced before the neck can be stabilized, avoid hyperextension of the neck.

Neurologic function should be assessed without moving the spine. If the patient is conscious and able to communicate, test light touch and pinprick sensation in all fingers and over both surfaces of the feet. Test vibratory sensation in both ankles. Ask the patient to move fingers and toes and test the plantar cutaneous reflexes. When paralysis is evident, the level of paralysis should be determined as accurately as can be done without moving the spine. The unconscious accident victim must be presumed to have an unstable spinal injury until disproved by complete spinal x-rays.

The level of neural injury can be quickly approximated by assessing gross regional sensory and motor function in the conscious patient. The patient who is ventilating actively and employing diaphragmatic respirations and has sharp/dull sensory discrimination of the skin over the clavicles demonstrates intact C-4 function. Voluntary contraction of the deltoid and biceps along with intact sensation over the lateral deltoid area of the upper arm demonstrates intact C-5 function. Contraction of the extensor carpi radialis longus or brevis along with intact sensation over the radial forearm, thumb, and index finger indicates C-6 function. Voluntary contraction of the flexor carpi radialis or triceps along with intact sensation over the ring and little finger indicates C-7 function. Flexion of the fingers and intact sensation over the ulnar border of the hand and forearm indicates C-8 function. Intrinsic function in the hand and sensation on the ulnar side of the forearm and elbow indicate T-1 function. The intercostal ventilatory movements are mediated through segments T-2 through T-10. The quadrantal abdominal cutaneous reflexes are mediated through segments T-7 through L-1. Extension of the knee by contraction of the quadriceps muscle is mediated through segments L-3 and L-4. Extension and flexion of the great toe are mediated through segments L-5 and S-1, respectively.

Cutaneous sensation according to dermatomal distribution is indicated in Figure 5.5. Pinprick (anterior cord) and vibratory (posterior cord) sensation can be tested at the various levels to assess anterior and posterior cord function.

It is important to remember when evaluating any spinal column injury that spinal cord segments correspond exactly to the vertebral segments only in the cervical spine. The thoracic segment of the cord extends between C-7 and T-10 vertebrae, the entire lumbar segment between T-10 and T-12 vertebrae, and the sacral and coccygeal segments between T-12 and L-2 vertebrae. Thus, unstable injuries across the T-12 through L-2 vertebrae will produce injury to the sacrococcygeal elements of the cord.

The assessment of the patient who is suspected of having a traumatic spine injury includes a thorough radiographic examination. The initial evaluation should include supine AP and lateral radiographs of the thoracic, lumbar, and sacral spine. These views will reveal the presence or absence of a major spinal fracture or dislocation. If the initial x-rays are normal, further radiographic evaluation to include oblique radiographs can be obtained and the patient can be safely moved. If the initial x-rays are diagnostic of a suspected spinal injury, further evaluation is often necessary. Depending on the clinical situation, this may include a CT scan, plane tomograms, or a myelogram in conjunction with either of the other two modalities. The CT scan is an excellent method of evaluation for subtle fractures or malalignments. Injury to the spinal cord often may require evaluation with a myelogram or magnetic resonance imaging. The need for these further studies should be determined by the orthopaedic surgeon or neurosurgical consultant.

If a fracture or dislocation of the spine is found or a neural deficit noted, immediate orthopaedic consultation should be obtained. The surgeon's therapeutic choices will be strongly determined by the history of paralysis. A clearly recorded, accurate initial examination is critical. The nature of further treatment may depend on whether the paralysis has progressed, remained stable, or regressed since the first examination.

WEDGE COMPRESSION AND BURST FRACTURES OF THE BODIES OF THE VERTEBRAE

Flexion forces and axial compression forces, depending on their magnitude and the resilience of the bony architecture, can produce wedge compression or bursting fractures of the vertebral body (Fig. 5.13). The wedge compression fracture is secondary to flexion force and the injury is confined to the anterior aspect of the vertebral body. A burst fracture occurs when there is more axial compressive force. This results in fracture of the posterior aspects of the vertebral body and posterior body wall. Because in-

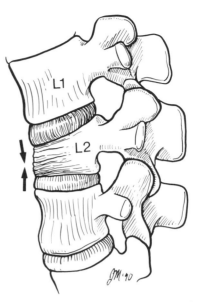

Figure 5.13. Vertebral wedge compression fracture. Loss of anterior body height with normal posterior wall of body.

jury in a wedge compression fracture is confined to the anterior aspect of the body, there is rarely any injury to the spinal cord or nerve roots. The axial compression fracture, however, produces a burst of the vertebral body and fragments of the posterior wall displace posteriorly, where they can contuse or lacerate the spinal cord or nerve roots or interfere with the blood supply to the neural elements.

A burst fracture must be distinguished from a compression fracture. On radiographs, the characteristics that distinguish a burst fracture from a compression fracture are widening of the interpedicular distance noted on the AP view, and loss of height in both the anterior and posterior aspects of the vertebral body as seen on the lateral view. A CT scan may be required in some cases to differentiate a wedge compression fracture from a burst fracture (Fig. 5.14).

Compression or burst fractures of the body of vertebrae can occur at any level or at multiple levels. They can be seen in the cer-

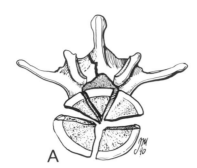

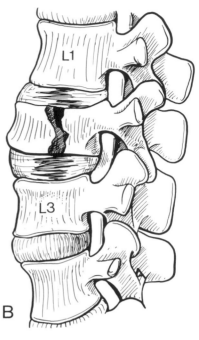

Figure 5.14. Lumbar burst fracture. *A*, axial view showing comminuted vertebral body fracture, including posterior wall of body. *B*, lateral view of lumbar spine burst fracture. Loss of height at the anterior and posterior aspects of vertebral body.

vical, thoracic, or lumbar spine, and are most common in the T-12 through L-2 region.

Wedge Compression Fractures

Clinical Characteristics. Wedge compression fractures usually occur after a fall from a height or a motor vehicle accident in which the victim is thrown from the vehicle. In older adults, especially those who suffer from osteoporosis, minor trauma may result in wedge compression fractures. The patients are generally able to localize their pain to the region of the spine that has been injured. Localized pain is the main symptom, and it is quite rare to have radicular pain associated with a wedge compression fracture. The physical examination will be remarkable for tenderness directly over the involved segment, and loss of the normal sagittal contours of the spine. The neurologic examination will be normal, although motor testing may be difficult in the proximal muscles of the lower extremities as this may ex-

acerbate the pain caused by the spinal fracture.

Treatment. Most wedge compression fractures require supportive and rehabilitative treatment only. However, a wedge compression fracture that causes a 20° kyphosis deformity or is associated with greater than 50% loss of the height of the vertebral body may cause severe progressive deformity. Surgical treatment must be considered under these circumstances. Those injuries that are associated with less than 10° of kyphosis or 25% loss of anterior height of the vertebral body may be treated by a primary care physician; however, the treating physician must be certain that the posterior wall of the vertebral body is intact. If there is any concern about the involvement of this area, an orthopaedist should be consulted. A pathologic basis for the fracture should be ruled out (Chapter 14).

The initial treatment of a mild wedge compression fracture involves hospitalization and a period of rest until symptoms allow resumption of sitting and standing. Initially, narcotic analgesics are provided as necessary until severe pain has passed. Intravenous hydration is provided, as paralytic ileus often develops in association with these injuries. Ileus and the patient's reluctance to strain may result in a rectal impaction and eventually intestinal colic. Liberal use of stimulant laxatives from the onset will eliminate this problem. Initially the patient is kept at strict bed rest on a firm mattress. The head of the bed may be raised to 30° for comfort and meals. As pain permits, more mobility is allowed in bed. As pain improves, active extension exercises are begun in the supine position (Fig. 5.15). In patients who show minor anatomic deformity, reinforced thoracolumbar corsets can be fitted to improve comfort and provide a sense of security as the patient is mobilized. For patients with more significant deformity, a hyperextension orthosis such as Jewett brace or polypropylene jacket is placed for more substantial support. Once the patient is upright, more vigorous extension exercises can be performed, initially while standing against a wall and eventually from the prone position. Most patients are able to get out of bed after

5 to 7 days, and bracing is recommended for 3 months. Extension exercises must be continued until normal movement is possible without pain. Exercises should be done to the point of fatigue, but short of worsening of pain. This should be repeated at least 4 times a day. While the exercises may be easy to describe, instruction and encouragement by a physical therapist will greatly increase the patient's compliance and speed the rehabilitation. Eventual recovery of full painless activity is usual, but can take many months, particularly in the presence of osteoarthritis. Approximately 80% of patients will have mild or no significant residual symptoms after a stable thoracolumbar fracture.

Burst Fractures

The mechanism of injury to a patient who suffers a burst fracture is similar to that which causes wedge compression fractures. Therefore, it is important to critically analyze all radiographs of patients with compressive spinal fractures. The likelihood of a burst fracture increases as the amount of compressive load applied to the spine increases.

Clinical Characteristics. Bursting injuries may occur in the polytrauma patient,

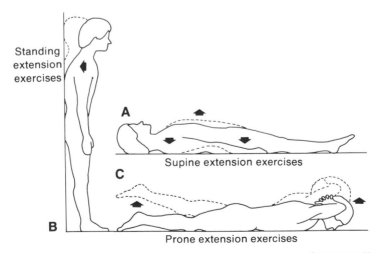

Figure 5.15. Extension exercises. *A*, supine position. *B*, standing. *C*, prone position.

and may be unrecognized as attention is initially paid to more life-threatening concerns. Patients who are conscious will complain of localized pain in the involved spinal segment. They also may have referred pain in a radicular pattern if there is nerve root irritation from the burst fracture. The neurologic picture may vary from a completely normal examination to complete paraplegia, as well as incomplete paraplegia. Under these circumstances, it is important to perform a thorough neurologic examination, including sensory examination of the perianal area.

Treatment.   Burst injuries are unstable spinal injuries that require provisional stabilization and emergency referral to an orthopaedist or neurosurgeon. Definitive surgical stabilization of the unstable spine injury is usually recommended, but in some cases bony healing can be obtained by prolonged bed rest. Early surgical intervention usually provides the best opportunity for anatomic restoration of the spine. It is particularly encouraged when there is spinal cord injury, as it allows a more rapid entry into the rehabilitation process. Throughout the rehabilitation period, the primary care physician helps to coordinate the care of the patient with the consultants in orthopaedics, neurosurgery, physical therapy, and rehabilitation medicine.

FRACTURES AND DISLOCATIONS OF THE VERTEBRAL UNITS

These injuries are a result of flexion, distraction, and/or rotational forces. In the cervical spine, these occur most commonly at the C-5/C-6 segment, though as pointed out previously, they are almost as common at other levels. In the thoracolumbar spine, the injuries are most common at the T-12 through L-2 segments (Fig. 5.16).

Clinical Characteristics

These injuries are the result of severe trauma to the body, as may occur in a fall from an excessive height or a severe motor

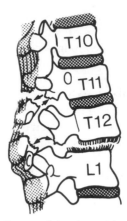

Figure 5.16.   Fracture-dislocations of the spine. This is a very unstable injury due to loss of stability in the anterior, medial, and posterior columns of the spine.

vehicle accident. Again, the patient often has multiple injuries. In this situation, the history is obtained primarily from accident scene witnesses. Patients who are conscious will complain of severe pain in their neck or their back at the area of the fracture or dislocation. Spinal dislocations are usually associated with paraplegia below the level of the injury, although sparing of certain tracts may be found.

Treatment

Stabilization of the spine on a spinal board should be maintained. Immediate consultation with an orthopaedist or neurosurgeon is required. Surgical spinal reduction and stabilization are required to prevent deformity and to allow immediate stabilization of the spine. Surgical stabilization of the spine allows for a rapid entry into the rehabilitation setting. The timing of surgery depends on the status of the patient in terms of other life-threatening injuries. Until the spine can be stabilized, it must be protected from further injury by the use of a spinal turning frame.

TRANSVERSE PROCESS FRACTURES

Fractures of the lumbar transverse processes occur with twisting injuries to the lumbar spine. The transverse processes act as the points of origin for muscles in the retroperitoneum as well as paravertebral muscles and ligaments. The transverse process of L-5 is the site of insertion of the broad lumbosacral ligaments. This transverse process may be avulsed from the L-5 vertebra with pelvic trauma. This may indicate significant soft tissue injury and should alert the physician to other associated injuries, such as splenic or renal contusions (Fig. 5.17).

Clinical Characteristics

The patient may have been involved in a motor vehicle accident or other type of trauma of a significant degree. The physical examination may be relatively benign except for a muscle spasm in the paravertebral muscles. Neurologic examination will be normal. The pain will be localized to the area of concern.

Treatment

The treatment involves symptomatic relief of pain. This will usually require narcotic analgesics for several days until the pain subsides. A lumbosacral corset may be helpful in splinting the injured area for the first 2 weeks after injury. The recovery will subsequently be aided by rehabilitation of the muscles in the back as well as the abdominal musculature. A physical therapist will be

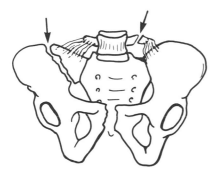

Figure 5.17. Transverse process fracture of L-5 indicates disruption of the lumbar-pelvic unit and signifies severe traumatic injury.

helpful in coordinating the rehabilitation, which should emphasize lumbar strengthening exercises. Functional recovery can be expected in 6 to 8 weeks.

SPINOUS PROCESS FRACTURES

An isolated spinous process fracture in the cervical region may occasionally occur. These are usually the result of an avulsion force. These isolated injuries may be treated symptomatically with a soft collar and analgesics. It is important to note that it is probably more common that spinous process fractures in the thoracic and lumbar regions occur in conjunction with another major spinal injury. Consequently, the radiographs must be carefully scrutinized to look for these injuries. In particular, a flexion distraction injury to the spine may not be apparent on x-ray because the film was taken with the patient supine and the injury has spontaneously "reduced." The evidence of the fracture on the radiograph may be the presence of a posterior spinous process fracture with a subtle widening of the disc space. Separation of two adjacent spinal processes will also be noted. Strong clinical suspicion of this type of injury should be maintained in patients who have sustained "lap-belt" injury. This type of injury occurs when a passenger in a motor vehicle is wearing a lap-type seatbelt and comes to a sudden halt. The momentum of the body causes a distraction flexion force to occur on the spine. This force may be transmitted through the disc space and the posterior elements. This fracture is unstable in a flexed position.

The physical examination may reveal ecchymosis transversely across the anterior abdominal wall. This injury is also associated with severe intraabdominal injuries such as ruptured viscus or spleen. Orthopaedic consultation is mandatory for treatment.

LUMBOSACRAL SPRAINS

Many patients have a history of significant injury to the low back area, with corresponding clinical signs and symptoms and without discernible deformity on radiographic studies. This condition is diagnosed as lumbosacral sprain.

Clinical Characteristics

This symptom complex is one of pain and limited mobility. Stiffness occurs with rest and tends to improve somewhat on activity, but a full functional range of motion is not achieved. Physical examination will reveal spasm of the paravertebral muscles, limited spinal mobility, diffuse tenderness, and a normal neurologic examination. It is often impossible to delineate the exact structure that has been injured because of the complexity of the ligamentous structures at the lumbosacral junction. However, similar to a ligamentous injury at a peripheral joint such as the knee, the healing process predictably will require 4 to 6 weeks before the patient can return to functional activities.

Treatment

Initially, the lumbosacral sprain is best treated by limiting activities with a brief period of bed rest and then slowly increasing activity to the tolerance of pain level. In the situation of a severe lumbosacral sprain in a manual laborer, it can be anticipated that the patient will require at least 3 months of restricted or limited activities before returning to preinjury status. Identifying the expected time course may help to guide the patient and employer in developing a back-to-work program for the injured laborer.

SUGGESTED READINGS

Bradford DS, Lonstein LE, Moe JH, et al. Moe's textbook of scoliosis and other spinal deformities. 2nd ed. Philadelphia: WB Saunders Co, 1987.

Errico GJ, Bauer RD, Waugh T. Spinal trauma. Philadelphia: JB Lippincott Co, 1990.

Floman Y, ed. Disorders of the lumbar spine. Rockville, MD: Aspen Publishers, 1990.

Frymoyer JW. Back pain in sciatica. N Engl J Med 1988;318:291–300.

CHAPTER 6

Pelvis, Hip, and Proximal Thigh

Gerald G. Steinberg, M.D.

Essential Anatomy

Like the shoulder, the hip is a ball-and-socket joint that attaches to the body axis through a bony girdle. There are major differences, however, that are important for understanding the normal function of the pelvis and hip, as well as manifestations of disease.

In contrast to the shoulder girdle, the pelvic girdle is relatively fixed to the body axis. It is capable of significant movement with the body axis only through its joint at the lumbosacral spine. The pelvis is attached to the body axis by the abdominal and spinal muscles and by the stout ligaments of the relatively immobile sacroiliac joints. Because of this immobility, a primary abnormality of the hip or pelvis may create a secondary abnormality in the lumbar spine or at the knee. For example, a patient with a severe flexion contracture of the hip will not ambulate bent forward. The patient will develop a compensatory increase in lumbar lordosis and/or flexed posture at the knee. Also, a primary abnormality in the lumbar spine or knee may create a secondary abnormality in the hip. These must be distinguished when examining a patient with an apparent hip problem.

While the shoulder and hip joints are ball-and-socket types, the shoulder socket is small and flat, providing little inherent stability to the joint. The articular surface of the hip, however, is large and deep, providing substantial mechanical stability. Because of this, the muscles about the hip are more re-

sponsible for postural than for articular stability. The ligaments of the joint are responsible for limiting motion of the hip at the extremes.

Unlike the shoulder, the articular surface of each hip is a weight-bearing surface constantly subjected to high loads. This makes the hip more vulnerable to developing clinical symptoms.

Several areas of functional and anatomic detail are important for evaluating and treating disorders of the hip. These include (*a*) x-ray anatomy, (*b*) bony and ligamentous structure of the pelvis and hip, (*c*) muscular control of the hip joint, (*d*) innervation and blood supply, and (*e*) relationship of the hip to major nerves and vessels of the extremity.

X-RAY ANATOMY

Figure 6.1 shows an anteroposterior (AP) projection of the pelvis and hips with important elements labeled.

BONE AND LIGAMENT STRUCTURE OF THE PELVIS AND HIP

Each hemipelvis is formed by the fusion of the pubis, ischium, and ilium. These bones emerge from separate centers of ossification and fuse into a single bone by early adolescence. Prior to maturity, x-rays show a normal lucency traversing the acetabulum. This is the triradiate cartilage, which is the site of fusion of the three bones of the hemipelvis. Several cartilaginous epiphyses or apophyses are clinically important in the

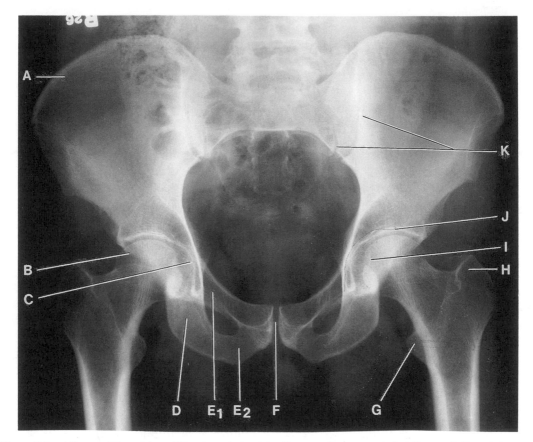

Figure 6.1. AP x-ray of the pelvis and hips. Important points of bony anatomy are noted: *A*, iliac crest. *B*, posterior acetabular margin. *C*, medial acetabular wall. *D*, ischium. *E*, pubis; *E₁*, superior ramus; *E₂*, inferior ramus. *F*, symphysis pubis. *G*, lesser trochanter. *H*, greater trochanter. *I*, fovea of femoral head. *J*, acetabular dome. *K*, sacroiliac joint.

immature individual: the iliac crest, anterior superior and anterior inferior iliac spines, and ischial tuberosity (Fig. 6.2). These begin to ossify by midadolescence but do not fuse to the underlying bone until the mid-to-late 20s. Recognition of these apophyses are important in evaluating certain traction injuries about the pelvis, and in evaluating x-rays of individuals prior to full ossification.

The major pelvic ring is formed by the junction of each ilium at the sacrum posteriorly, and the junction of each pubis at the symphysis pubis anteriorly. The pelvic ring is stable because of the tremendously strong ligaments of the sacroiliac joints and the symphysis pubis, and the locking orienta-

tion of the sacroiliac joint facets. Many ligaments stabilize each sacroiliac joint. The most important of these are the short interosseous sacroiliac ligaments and dorsal sacroiliac ligaments (Fig. 6.3). The short interosseous ligament is a strong structure that forms the fibrous portion of the sacroiliac joint. Only the inferior portion of the sacroiliac joint is a true synovial joint. Above this is a fibrous ankylosis, and the short interosseous ligament forms the fibrous structure. The dorsal sacroiliac ligament passes from the lower third of the sacrum vertically and obliquely upward across the joint to the ilium (Fig. 6.3).

Anteriorly, the pelvic ring is closed by the

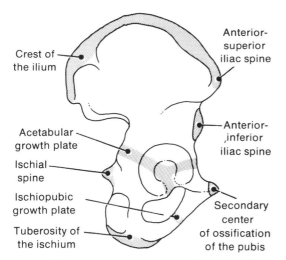

Crest of the ilium

Anterior-superior iliac spine

Acetabular growth plate

Anterior-inferior iliac spine

Ischial spine

Ischiopubic growth plate

Secondary center of ossification of the pubis

Tuberosity of the ischium

Figure 6.2. Growth plates and secondary centers of ossification of the hip.

joint at the pubic symphysis, which is stabilized by a fibrocartilaginous disc and by two ligaments that merge into it (Fig. 6.3A). While the ligaments of the symphysis are strong, the stability of the joint is helped by the structure of the pelvis, which is designed to transmit compressive force across this joint. This reduces the tendency for any distraction or displacement of the joint and helps maintain pelvic stability.

By virtue of its stability, the pelvic ring can withstand the routine forces of bearing weight, effectively transferring body weight across the hip joints to the lower extremities. Because of its inherent stability, an injury of tremendous force is required to produce a dislocation or displaced fracture of the pelvis. A lesser force can cause injury in the pregnant patient because changes in hormonal balance impart increased elasticity to the pelvic ligaments. This increased elasticity accommodates the process of childbirth, but weakens the ligaments and makes them more vulnerable to sprain.

Hip Joint

Each part of the hemipelvis participates in the formation of the acetabulum (Fig. 6.4).

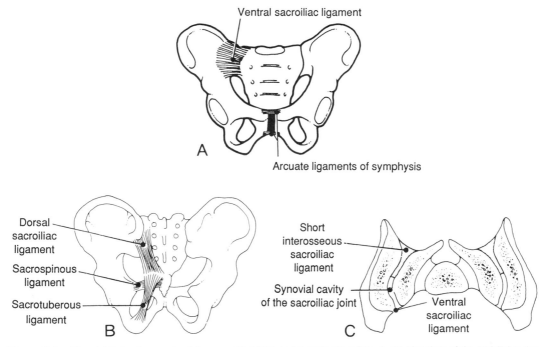

Ventral sacroiliac ligament

Arcuate ligaments of symphysis

A

Dorsal sacroiliac ligament

Sacrospinous ligament

Sacrotuberous ligament

B

Short interosseous sacroiliac ligament

Synovial cavity of the sacroiliac joint

Ventral sacroiliac ligament

C

Figure 6.3. The stabilizing ligaments of the sacroiliac joint and symphysis pubis. *A*, anterior view of the stabilizing ligaments. *B*, posterior view of the stabilizing ligaments. *C*, coronal section of the sacroiliac joint.

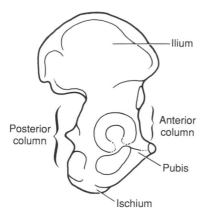

Figure 6.4. The right hemipelvis showing the convergence of the ilium, ischium, and pubis in the formation of the acetabulum. The posterior and anterior columns are marked.

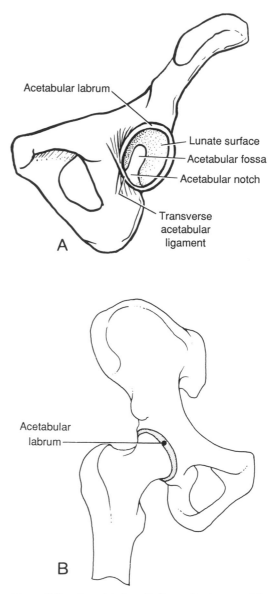

Figure 6.5. *A*, acetabulum. *B*, fibrocartilaginous acetabular labrum containing the femoral head.

The superior ramus of the pubis and the body of the ischium form its anterior and posterior walls, respectively. The body of the ilium forms the superior acetabular wall. The posterior ilioischial column connects with the anterior iliopubic column to form the strong arch of bone making up the superior acetabulum. The anterior columns form a bridge between the two posterior columns, and function as a compression-resisting strut for the medially directed forces generated at the hips. As the anterior and posterior acetabular walls converge inferiorly, an inferior medial deficiency forms the acetabular notch (Fig 6.5).

The surface of the acetabulum is composed of an incomplete ring of hyaline cartilage that surrounds the central acetabular fossa, which in turn merges with the acetabular notch inferiorly. The fossa contains the ligamentum teres and does not have a hyaline cartilage covering. The walls of the acetabulum are expanded by a fibrocartilaginous extension called the acetabular labrum. Inferiorly, the labrum continues across the acetabular notch as the transverse acetabular ligament (Fig. 6.5). The labrum and transverse acetabular ligament extend beyond the hemisphere of the femoral head, deepening the acetabulum and increasing its coverage to about two-thirds of the head.

The capsule of the hip joint extends from the femur to the acetabulum, overlying the acetabular labrum proximally. The capsule inserts on the femur along the intertrochanteric line anteriorly, and on the distal aspect of the femoral neck posteriorly. The capsule is composed of four recognizable ligaments. The strongest, the iliofemoral ligament (Fig.

6.6), is the main capsular restraint to extension and internal rotation.

The synovial membrane of the capsule completely lines its surface, and reflects back along the neck of the femur where the capsule makes its femoral attachment. The synovium completely covers the femoral neck, ending at the peripheral border of the cartilage of the head of the femur. The entire femoral head and most of the neck are intrasynovial (Fig. 6.7). This anatomic circumstance allows a septic arthritis to develop

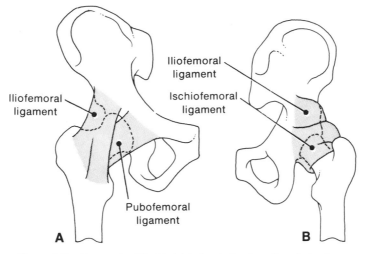

Figure 6.6.   Ligaments of the hip joint. *A*, anterior view. *B*, posterior view.

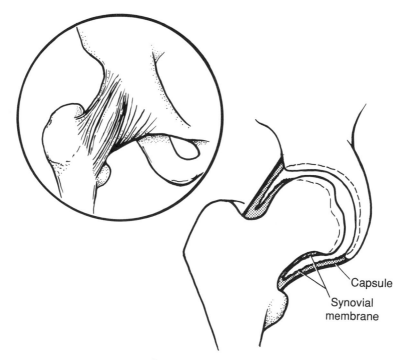

Figure 6.7.   The synovial covering of the hip joint renders the entire femoral head and most of the femoral neck intrasynovial.

from a focus of metaphyseal osteomyelitis of the femoral neck.

Proximal Femur

The neck of the femur forms an angle of approximately 135° with the femoral shaft in the coronal plane (Fig. 6.8). In the sagittal plane, the average angle of anteversion (apex posterior) is approximately 15° in the adult. The angulation of the proximal femur provides improved range of motion as it brings the femur away from the acetabulum, providing better clearance. This angulation, however, causes weight-bearing forces to generate substantial bending moments in the proximal femur that dictate the pattern of bony architecture. The trabecular architecture of the upper end of the femur is oriented to bear these forces of tension and compression most efficiently (Fig. 6.8). This is a demonstration of Wolff's fundamental law of bony architecture, that bony form accommodates function and applied force.

The lateral placement of the hip joints provides increased stability when an individual stands stationary in double-limb stance. During single-limb stance, however, such as while walking or running, the lateral placement of the hip joints necessitates strong abductor muscle force to maintain stable erect posture. Figure 6.9 shows dia-

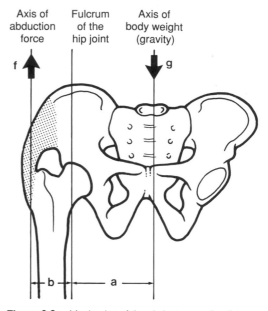

Figure 6.9.   Mechanics of the abductors: *a*, the distance or moment arm along which gravity or body weight acts with one extremity weightbearing; *b*, the abductor moment arm; *g*, the force of gravity or body weight; *f*, the abductor force. At equilibrium (when an individual stands stationary on one leg) $f \times b = g \times a$. Consequently, $f = g \times a/b$. In this individual, the ratio of a to b is approximately 3. Consequently, $f = 3g$. (When $g = 70$ kg, $f = 210$ kg)

grammatically the abductor muscle group mechanics across the hip. Assuming an equilibrium, that is, someone standing on one leg maintaining an erect posture, the forces of the abductor muscles exerted on the greater trochanter must balance the forces of body weight exerted on the pelvis. To maintain a stable, erect posture, abductor muscle forces are very high and are the dominant force across the hip joint. Abductor muscles are consequently subject to considerable wear and tear. Deficiencies in these muscles lead to abnormalities of hip function that are manifest during many activities of daily living, such as walking, running, and stair climbing. This will be addressed in more detail later in this chapter.

The abductor muscles have a broad attachment to the proximal femur at the greater trochanter, which forms the upper

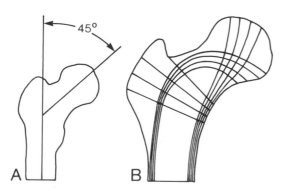

Figure 6.8.   Architecture of the upper end of the femur. *A*, neck of the femur angulates medial to the axis of the femoral shaft. *B*, trabecular architecture parallels the lines of tension and compression within the bone.

pole of the body of the femur. The greater trochanter also provides the site of attachment for the external rotators. The lesser trochanter arises posteromedially at the junction of the neck and shaft of the femur and provides attachment for the major hip flexor, the iliopsoas. The bony ridge on the posterior surface of the proximal femur, just distal to the greater trochanter, is the site of attachment of the direct tendon of the gluteus maximus, the major hip extensor (Fig. 6.10). The head and trochanters of the femur develop as epiphyses that begin to ossify in childhood: the capital femoral epiphysis begins to ossify during the 1st year of life, the greater trochanter at 5 years, and the lesser trochanter at 9 years. These all fuse with the metaphysis in adolescence, with the capital epiphysis fusing last. Like any epiphysis, they are vulnerable to traumatic separation, but the capital femoral epiphysis is most vulnerable to slippage. This will be discussed later in this chapter.

The femoral head is approximately two-thirds of a sphere. It is covered by articular cartilage except at the insertion of the ligamentum teres. The femoral neck is smaller than the femoral head, providing improved range of motion so that the neck does not impinge on the margins of the acetabulum.

MUSCLES CONTROLLING THE HIP JOINT

Numerous short and long muscles control the hip joint. The main function of the musculature is to meet the requirements of efficient walking: to maintain stability of the weight-bearing leg despite continued change in limb and body position, and to move the body forward. Stability is gained by muscle action to resist the force of gravity that acts to pull the body downward. Because the human frame is top-heavy, with much of its mass above the pelvis, large muscular forces are required to maintain stability. Also, because the center of gravity must move from behind the supporting stance phase foot to ahead of the stance phase foot to move the body forward, the demands on the muscles are constantly changing. The force to propel the body forward is derived from accelerating the swing phase limb during the gait cycle and posi-

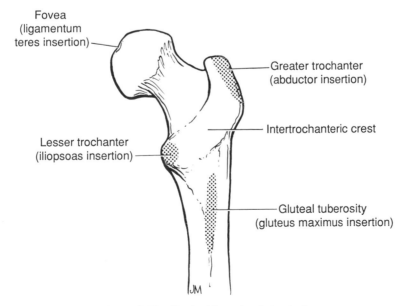

Figure 6.10. Proximal femur (posterior view).

tioning the stance phase limb to allow the body to fall forward. Hip muscles participate in both these functions. The gait cycle presents complex and progressively changing demands to the hip musculature, and abnormalities of these muscles causing weakness or pain distort the gait cycle, producing a limp. It is convenient to think of the muscles in functional groups when describing muscular control; however, an individual muscle may contribute to more than one functional movement. These groups are described as the abductors, flexors, adductors, extensors, and rotators. The innervation of these muscles will be noted so that the physician can interpret the effect of neurologic disorder on hip function.

Abductor Group

The origins and insertions of the gluteus medius, gluteus minimus, and tensor fascia lata are demonstrated in Figure 6.11. The tensor fascia lata extends its tendinous fibers with the fibers of gluteus maximus to form the iliotibial tract on the lateral aspect of the thigh. The muscles of this group are innervated by the superior gluteal nerve, which is composed mainly of fibers from the fourth and fifth lumbar nerve roots. The muscles of this group are required to maintain pelvic stability during the stance phase of gait. During stance phase, body weight forces the bearing hip into adduction. Unless the abductors contract with normal strength, there is an excessive pelvic tilt. With deficient abductor function, the individual will compensate by leaning the trunk over the stance phase limb. This compensatory gait pattern is called an abductor lurch (Figs. 6.12 and 6.13) and reduces forces across the hip.

Hip Flexors

The primary flexors of the hip are the iliopsoas, rectus femoris, and sartorius. The pectineus and tensor fascia lata also function as flexors. The strongest flexor is the double-bellied iliopsoas muscle (Fig. 6.14). The iliopsoas is innervated by the femoral nerve,

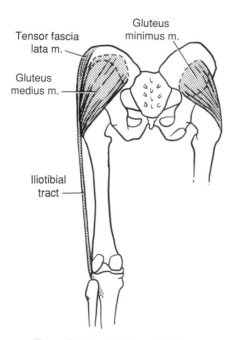

Figure 6.11.   Abductors of the hip.

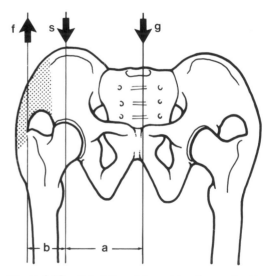

Figure 6.12.   Calculation of force (s) acting on the hip joint during normal gait; a = gravity or body weight moment arm with right extremity weight bearing; b = abductor moment arm; g = force of gravity (body weight); f = abductor force. At equilibrium $f \times b = g \times a$, $f = g \times a/b$. If a/b = 3/1, then $f = g \times 3$. When g = 70 kg, f = 210 kg. The force across the hip is $s = g + f = 70 + 210 = 280$ kg.

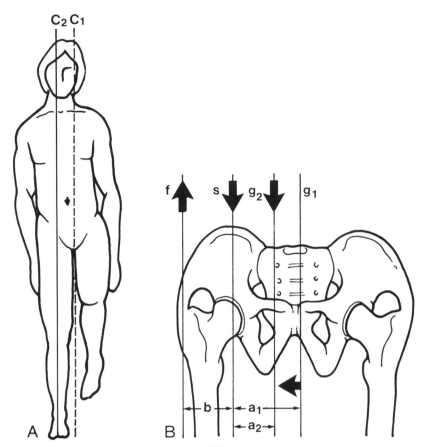

Figure 6.13.   Leaning gait (abductor lurch). *A*, illustrates shift in center of gravity during single limb stance with individual leaning toward the stance phase side; c_1, normal axis; c_2, axis with leaning. *B*, calculation of hip joint force; a_1, gravity moment arm in normal gait; a_2, gravity moment arm during leaning gait. $f \times b = g_2 \times a_2$. If $a_2/b = 2$, then $f = 2g_2$. When $g_2 = 70$ kg, $f = 140$ kg. $s = f + g_2 = 210$ kg.

composed of fibers originating from the second through fourth lumbar segments. The sartorius and rectus femoris muscles are less powerful flexors and are innervated by the femoral nerve. During gait, hip flexors are important as swing phase is initiated. These muscles contract to accelerate the leg forward. The patient with weak hip flexors circumducts the leg and compensates further by pivoting the body about the opposite stance phase foot, giving the characteristic circumduction limp. The hip flexors are also important in elevating the limb during stair climbing and in such activities as kicking. The rectus femoris contracts strongly with

kicking, and its origin through an apophysis at the anterior inferior iliac spine may be avulsed in adolescence.

Adductor Group

The adductor group is comprised of five muscles: the adductor longus, brevis, magnus, the gracilis (Fig. 6.15), and the pectineus (Fig. 6.14). The adductor longus and brevis, the gracilis, and much of the adductor magnus are innervated by the obturator nerve. The posterior portion of the adductor magnus, which is predominantly an extensor of the hip, is innervated by the sciatic nerve. The pectineus is innervated mainly by the

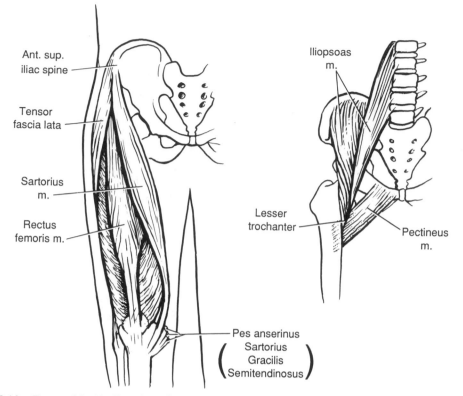

Figure 6.14. Flexors of the hip. The primary flexors are the iliopsoas (most powerful), and the rectus femoris and sartorius (less powerful).

femoral nerve. Like the hip flexors, these muscles are largely controlled by the second through fourth lumbar segments.

The adductor group has a varied role during gait. At the beginning of stance phase, the adductor magnus is important in assisting the hip extensors to resist flexion of the hip. The adductor longus acts as a hip flexor at the end of the stance phase and as an extensor at the end of the swing phase.

Extensor Group

The extensors consist of the gluteus maximus and hamstring muscles, including the long head of the biceps femoris, the semitendinosus, and the semimembranosus. The posterior portion of the adductor magnus is also an extensor (Fig. 6.16). The gluteus maximus is innervated by the inferior gluteal nerve, which is predominantly composed of fibers from the fifth lumbar and first sacral segments. The hamstrings are all innervated by the sciatic nerve, with fibers originating from the eighth lumbar through second sacral segments.

The hip extensors are responsible primarily for preventing hip and trunk flexion during gait, especially during the early stance phase of gait. The extensors are also responsible for slowing down the accelerating swing phase leg at the end of swing phase. If these muscles fail to function properly, gait becomes unsteady. The gluteus maximus, along with the adductor magnus, is also responsible for climbing and rising from a sitting posture.

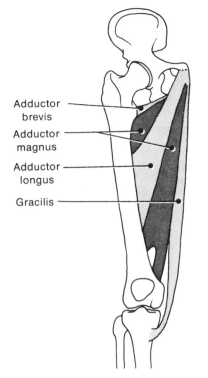

Figure 6.15. Adductors of the hip (anterior view).

Adductor brevis
Adductor magnus
Adductor longus
Gracilis

External Rotators

Extending across the posterior surface of the hip joint are the short external rotators, including the piriformis, superior and inferior gemelli, obturator externus and internus, and the quadratus femoris (Fig. 6.17). Except for the obturator externus, which is innervated by the obturator nerve, the short rotators are innervated by branches of the sacral plexus.

Internal Rotators

There are no pure internal rotators of the hip. A number of muscles provide internal rotation as well as other functions. For example, the anterior fibers of the gluteus minimus may internally rotate the hip.

INNERVATION AND BLOOD SUPPLY
Innervation

Branches of the lumbar and sacral plexus innervate the hip joint. These nerves derive from the second through fifth lumbar segments. Several of the branches originate from the obturator nerve. That other branches from the obturator nerve innervate the anterior portion of the knee joint fits with the characteristics of pain referral from the hip: patients with hip pathology may have anterior knee pain in the absence of significant complaints about the hip. Occasionally, knee pain may be referred to the hip.

Blood Supply

Blood supply to the hip joint in general is profuse, but the blood supply to the femoral head itself is more tenuous. The femoral head blood supply is carried by a retinacular arterial system that runs along the neck of the femur. There are two major retinacular vascular systems, posterosuperior and posteroinferior. These vessels are supplied by perforating capsular branches that derive from an extracapsular arterial ring, formed predominantly by the medial femoral circumflex artery with contributions from the lateral circumflex vessel. When the epiphyseal growth plate is well-formed, no metaphyseal vessels traverse the plate to help supply the femoral head. This renders the femoral head particularly susceptible to vascular interruption. Consequently, avascular necrosis is commonly seen in the child with a femoral neck fracture. It may also explain the development of avascular necrosis in the pediatric patient with pyogenic arthritis. The tense pressure in the joint shuts down the retinacular arterial system, and the epiphyseal plate blocks any communication between the femoral neck metaphyseal vessels and the femoral head epiphyseal vessels.

In the adult, following closure of the epiphyseal plate, anastomosis occurs between the metaphyseal and epiphyseal vascular systems. Therefore, the femoral head is at a reduced risk, but blood supply still remains tenuous. For example, in the adult with a displaced intracapsular fracture of the neck, the metaphyseal vessels traveling into

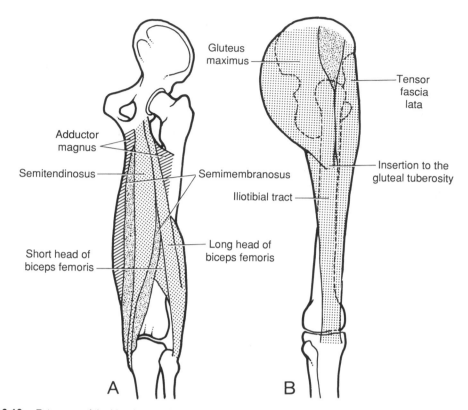

Figure 6.16. Extensors of the hip. *A*, posterior view of the hamstring muscles. *B*, lateral view of the gluteus maximus and its relationship to the tensor fascia lata and the iliotibial tract.

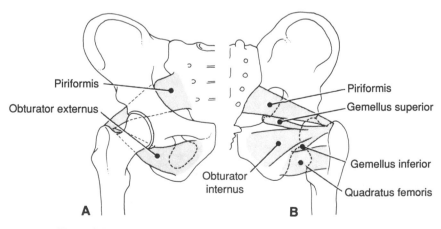

Figure 6.17. Pure external rotators. *A*, anterior view. *B*, posterior view.

the head and the subsynovial retinacular vessels may be disrupted. This can result in aseptic necrosis of the head of the femur. In most individuals, the artery carried in the ligamentum teres does not supply adequate circulation to prevent avascular necrosis. Avascular necrosis can also be seen in patients who have sustained a dislocation of the hip, tearing and stretching the arterial system. Because of this potential for avascular necrosis, a dislocation of the hip must be treated as an orthopaedic emergency.

RELATIONSHIP OF THE HIP JOINT TO THE GREAT VESSELS AND NERVES

The sciatic nerve emerges from the sacral plexus through the greater sciatic notch between the piriformis and the obturator internus (Fig. 6.18). In the sciatic notch, it is vulnerable to injury from pelvic fractures, and distal to the notch, vulnerable to injury from posterior dislocation of the femoral head. The femoral artery, vein, and nerve enter the thigh lying on the iliopsoas and pectineus muscle. They are cushioned by these muscles and are not likely to be injured by hip dislocation or pelvic fractures.

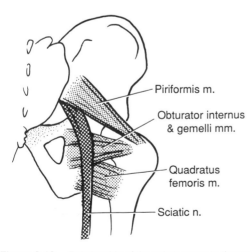

Figure 6.18. Relationship of the sciatic nerve to the posterior aspect of the hip joint and the external rotators.

Piriformis m.

Obturator internus & gemelli mm.

Quadratus femoris m.

Sciatic n.

Evaluation of the Patient with Hip Symptoms
HISTORY

Pain is usually the chief complaint of patients with hip problems. These patients may present with pain over the anterior or lateral aspect of the hip, in the groin, or more medially in the region of the adductors (corresponding to the obturator nerve distribution). Pain may radiate distally to the knee. Pain referred to the hip may be secondary to spinal problems, and this must be considered in the differential diagnosis of patients with "hip" pain.

Most patients with hip pain have increased pain with activity. Those who complain of pain at rest usually have some inflammatory component to their disease. An infectious or neoplastic process may be present. Many patients will report increased pain as they begin activity. Pain is increased when the patient loads a joint that has been at rest. As the joint accommodates the new level of activity, pain subsides.

Patients with chronic progressive disease such as osteoarthritis report progressively severe pain. They often report prior problems like injury or childhood disease, including congenital dysplasia, avascular necrosis, or slipped capital femoral epiphysis. Adults with avascular necrosis may describe the onset of pain months or years after cortisone use. Excessive alcohol ingestion may be a contributing problem.

Patients will complain of stiffness. This may be worst in the morning, or may be a more constant problem affecting many activities of daily living. To obtain an accurate analysis, patients should be questioned to determine their impairment in the activities of walking, dressing, stair climbing, and foot hygiene.

PHYSICAL EXAMINATION

The patient must be adequately undressed for proper examination. Inspection normally reveals a level pelvis. Pelvic obliquity suggests leg-length discrepancy or scoliosis, which may or may not be associated with hip disease. Range of motion of the spine will help demonstrate any true spinal abnormality. Contracture of the hip may cause a compensatory obliquity of the pelvis. If inspection of the pelvis is difficult because of the patient's size, palpation should be performed at the bony prominences to determine position and symmetry.

Observe the resting posture of the hip. The ligaments of the hip are so oriented that pressure in the joint space is least when the hip is slightly flexed, abducted, and externally rotated. Therefore, patients with an acute synovitis or effusion tend to maintain the hip in this position.

The Trendelenburg's test is performed following inspection. The patient is asked to stand on one leg and lift the other leg with hip and knee flexed. Normal patients will lift the pelvis contralateral to the stance limb. Patients with deficient abductor muscles or hip pathology that causes pain on contraction of the muscles have an impairment of this normal mechanism. Consequently, these patients will allow the pelvis to drop contralateral to the stance phase side, or may shift the upper body over the stance phase leg to reduce muscular demand (Fig. 6.13).

The patient's gait should be observed. Many limps are secondary to abnormality of the hip. The antalgic limp results from decreased time in the stance phase on the painful side, producing an abnormality in the normal rhythm. The short-leg limp is secondary to leg-length inequality, which may be associated with hip disease. There is an obvious increase in the up and down movement of the head and shoulders. This occurs when the body falls onto the shortened stance phase leg and then rises up on the long contralateral leg when stance phase begins on that side. The abductor sway is characterized by increased sway of the head and upper body over the stance phase limb. As noted above, this may be associated with a painful hip or with chronic weakness of the hip abductor muscles.

Following observation of gait, the hip is palpated to elicit areas of tenderness. There may be tenderness over the greater trochanteric bursa or ischial bursa. Palpation over the posterior superior iliac spine often reveals tenderness that may be a trigger zone for spinal pain, or there may be pain in this area from sacroiliac disease. There can be tenderness in various muscles, such as the tensor fascia lata or gluteus maximus.

Leg lengths are measured following palpation. Reliable measurement of true leg length can be obtained by noting the distance from the anterior superior iliac spine to the medial malleolus. Range of motion should be determined. Flexion contracture of the hip is often noted with serious hip disease. This is detected with the patient supine, as demonstrated in Figure 6.19. When checking abduction and adduction of the hip, it is also important to isolate hip motion from pelvic motion on the lumbosacral spine. Following range of motion, strength of muscle groups can be determined.

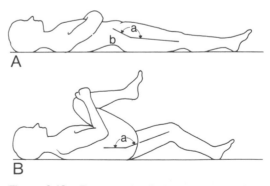

Figure 6.19. Demonstrating flexion contracture of the hip. *A*, with the patient lying supine and both hips extended, there is an increased lumbar lordosis (*b*) compensating for the true flexion contracture (*a*) of the hip. *B*, with the right hip flexed to flatten the lordosis, the true flexion contracture of the left hip becomes apparent.

Nontraumatic Conditions of Childhood

CONGENITAL DYSPLASIA OF THE HIP

Congenital hip dysplasia is the most common disorder of the hip in patients during the first 3 years of life. The term congenital dislocation is commonly applied to the full spectrum of congenital hip disease, which includes dysplasia without subluxation, the subluxatable hip, and the dislocated hip. The incidence of true congenital dislocation of the hip is approximately 1.2 in 1000 live births. Congenital dysplasia of the hip is more commonly associated with low birth weight infants, breech deliveries, and ligamentous laxity. It is much more common in female patients, is most often unilateral with predilection for the left hip, and there is a familial pattern. Because the development of the acetabulum and femoral head are dependent on normal physiologic stress, untreated congenital dysplasia or dislocation may lead to secondary developmental changes of both the acetabulum and femoral head, further compounding the initial deformity.

The pathology of congenital dysplasia of the hip is variable depending on the severity of the condition. Infants may be born with minimal dysplasia, in which there is some deformity of the acetabulum but the hip is not actually dislocated. In other infants, the hip may be dislocatable or dislocated, and in the most severe form, there is obvious teratologic deformity of the joint and soft tissue with complete dislocation.

The diagnosis of congenital hip instability or dislocation is a clinical one requiring careful examination of the newborn and infant during the "well baby visits."

Clinical Characteristics

The clinical presentation of congenital dysplasia varies according to the age of presentation and the pathologic state of the joint. In most infants and children, abduction will be limited. However, in the newborn and infant, while abduction may be limited, there may actually be more extension of the involved hip and knee with absence of the normal mild flexion contracture seen in these joints in the newborn. The affected extremity may appear short in comparison with the normal side. There may be asymmetry of the gluteal, inguinal, and thigh skin folds. The hip may be dislocatable and relocatable with alternating abduction and adduction of the flexed hip (Fig. 6.20).

In the newborn, the Barlow test is performed to demonstrate dislocatability of the hip. Direct pressure is applied along the lon-

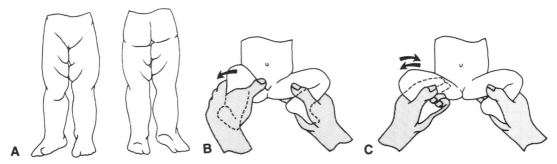

Figure 6.20.   Physical characteristics of congenital hip dislocation (the right hip is dislocated). *A*, asymmetry of skin folds, anterior and posterior views. *B* and *C*, manipulation: with the hip flexed to 90°, range of abduction may be restricted (*B*), or recurrent dislocation and relocation may be produced by alternate abduction and adduction (*C*). This movement in and out of the joint will be detected as a click.

gitudinal axis of the femur while adducting the hip to demonstrate dislocation. This is associated with a dislocation click. With traction/abduction, there may be a soft relocation click. It should be noted that a child may be born with dysplasia of the acetabulum without dislocation or dislocatability, and this may present at a later age.

When an infant presents at age 3 to 6 months and the femoral head has been dislocated for several months, it may not be possible to relocate the hip during examination. The hip appears more adducted. This is secondary to contracture of the adductor musculature, and palpation of the adductor tendon at the pubic tubercle will demonstrate this. Significant asymmetry of skin folds is more common at this stage. It is also possible to observe slight proximal migration of the hip. Palpation of the greater trochanter will indicate that the involved hip is higher than the opposite hip and leg-length measurement will confirm this.

When a child presents after walking has begun, the chief complaint may be that of a limp. This is in fact a "Trendelenburg" gait pattern with drooping of the contralateral side of the pelvis during stance phase on the involved limb, or an abductor sway may be noted.

When congenital dysplasia of the hip is suspected, x-rays should be obtained (Fig. 6.21). When the hip is subluxated or dislocated, Shenton's line (the continuous curve of the inner margin of the femoral neck and the superior margin of the obturator foramen) is broken. There is often delay in ossification of the capital femoral epiphysis so the bony portion of the epiphysis appears smaller in the dysplastic hip. When the femur is laterally subluxated, its malposition may be demonstrated relative to a vertical line (Perkins' line) dropped from the superior lip of the acetabulum perpendicular to a line drawn through the center of both acetabula. The beak of the neck of the normally articulating femur lies well medial to this line, while the beak of the neck of the dislocated femur lies closer to or lateral to this line. When the acetabulum is dysplastic, the slope of the superior margin is increased.

In the newborn or infant, in whom the femoral head is largely cartilaginous, ultrasound, when well done, can give a more sensitive and accurate representation of the hip joint. The cartilaginous structure is not seen

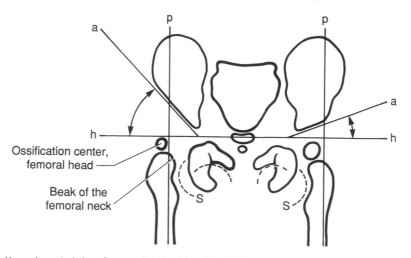

Figure 6.21. X-ray characteristics of congenital hip dislocation. (1) The arc of Shenton's line (*S*) is discontinuous on the dislocated side. (2) The beak of the femoral neck and the ossification center of the femoral head are displaced laterally and upward toward or beyond Perkins' line (*p*) and Hilgenreiner's line (*h*). (3) The angle between the acetabular line (*a*) and Hilgenreiner's line (*h*) is increased.

on x-ray but is seen on ultrasound. This is an important adjunct to the clinical diagnosis.

Treatment

Once the diagnosis of congenital dislocation or dysplasia of the hip is made, referral to the orthopaedist is indicated. It is the orthopaedist's responsibility to further define the nature of the abnormality and then recommend and monitor progress and treatment. The principle in treatment of the dislocated hip is to reduce the hip and maintain reduction to allow for normal development. In general, for patients who present from birth to 6 months, successful treatment can be instituted with a spica cast or dynamic harness (Pavlik harness). If treatment with this is unsuccessful, further measures are considered, including traction, closed reduction, and possible surgical intervention. In a child presenting between the ages of 6 to 18 months, treatment is more difficult. Success of dynamic strapping is less predictable and the need for closed reduction or surgical treatment is more likely.

NONSPECIFIC OR TRANSIENT SYNOVITIS OF THE HIP

This is a self-limited synovitis of the hip joint most commonly seen in children between the ages of 3 and 5 years. Its etiology is unclear, but unrecognized injuries and viral infections have been considered. This condition must be differentiated from pyogenic arthritis and from avascular necrosis of the hip (Legg-Calvé-Perthes disease). When suspicion of pyogenic arthritis exists, the joint must be aspirated. The distinction from aseptic necrosis is made by clinical follow-up and x-ray.

Clinical Characteristics

The child presents with complaints of pain in the groin, anteromedial thigh, or knee. There is an associated limp. Duration of pain is from several days to 2 weeks. Low-grade fever may be present with slight leukocytosis and slight increase in the sedimentation rate. The affected hip is maintained in a flexed and externally rotated position. The child resists efforts to move the hip rapidly or to the extremes of motion. The child does not appear seriously ill and the onset of disease is not as dramatic as pyogenic arthritis. X-rays are unremarkable except for evidence of soft tissue swelling, which may be subtle.

Treatment

Initial treatment should consist of bed rest. Crutches should be used with nonweight-bearing gait. Acetaminophen may be given on a symptomatic basis. If simple bed rest is not adequate, a few days of Buck's traction (Chapter 10) will almost always produce symptomatic relief. This can be done at home with orthopaedic consultation. Patients may begin full weight bearing when they have regained full painless range of motion and can ambulate without pain and without a limp. They may then return to normal activity as tolerated. If there is persistent or recurrent pain, or suspicion of pyogenic arthritis or aseptic necrosis, orthopaedic consultation should be obtained promptly. Even if the child becomes asymptomatic and returns to normal activity without restriction, a follow-up visit at 8 to 12 weeks is recommended. At that time, repeat x-ray should be obtained to rule out aseptic necrosis.

AVASCULAR NECROSIS OF THE FEMORAL HEAD (LEGG-CALVÉ-PERTHES DISEASE)

This condition affects children between the ages of 2 and 11. The cause of the interruption of the blood supply to the femoral head is not known. After infarction, reparative tissue grows into the necrosed head, and healing occurs by a process of creeping substitution with resorption of dead bone and deposition of new bone. The process of necrosis and reconstitution can take 2 to 3 years. There may be deformity of the femoral head and subsequently the acetabulum if the disease is extensive and exceeds the remodeling and healing capacity of the developing epiphysis. Younger children have a better prognosis, as do those children with smaller areas of involvement of the femoral head.

Clinical Characteristics

Pain is usually in the groin, anterior thigh, and sometimes the knee. The onset is usually insidious. The patient has usually been symptomatic for several months prior to presentation. Some children present without pain but almost all limp, some intermittently. Limping increases with activity. While the disease may occur in children between the ages of 2 and 11, the incidence is highest in children between ages 5 and 9. Children with this condition frequently present with synovitis, which is associated with muscle spasm and restricted motion. X-ray changes are variable depending on the stage of the disease. The first bony change noted may be increased density of the femoral epiphysis, and later an irregular mottled appearance and subchondral fracture.

Treatment

Orthopaedic referral should be made. Treatment is based on the principle that containment of the femoral head within the acetabulum will lead to the best healing and remodeling of the infarcted femoral head. Patients who are young, 4 years or under, with involvement of less than 50% of the head, and who lack certain x-ray changes, may be simply observed with symptomatic treatment. For most other patients, containment of the femoral head within the acetabulum can be achieved with an external brace or cast. For some patients, osteotomy of the femur or pelvis is necessary.

One of the problems for the primary care practitioner is distinguishing the child presenting with aseptic necrosis from the child presenting with nonspecific synovitis of the hip. X-rays are most important in making this distinction. Orthopaedic consultation is indicated if there is suspicion of avascular necrosis. Also, it is important to reexamine patients who present with "nonspecific synovitis" to make certain they do not continue to be symptomatic or have restricted motion, suggesting avascular necrosis.

SLIPPED CAPITAL FEMORAL EPIPHYSIS

During the period of rapid growth during adolescence, there is relative weakness at the capital femoral epiphyseal plate. The exact cause of this condition remains unknown. Various etiologies have been suggested, including hormonal dysfunction. Whatever the cause, it appears that the stresses of normal activity exceed the strength of the epiphyseal plate through the zone of cartilage hypertrophy. This results in slowly progressive slippage of the capital femoral epiphysis, in a posterior and medial direction. In some patients, the condition has an insidious onset; however, in many there is an acute presentation associated with injury. Many patients report some preinjury pain and have an acute slip superimposed on a chronic condition.

Clinical Characteristics

A child between the ages of 11 and 16 presents with a history of insidious hip, thigh, or knee pain associated with limp. The patient may also present with a history of acute hip pain following an injury, with or without prior history of intermittent hip pain and limp. Male patients are more commonly affected, and the patient is often obese with somewhat delayed development of secondary sexual characteristics. The condition may be bilateral and the opposite hip must be examined. In the acute phase there is significant muscle spasm and synovitis with restricted range of motion; internal rotation is usually significantly limited. Because of the limitation in internal rotation when the hip is flexed, the extremity tends to externally ro-

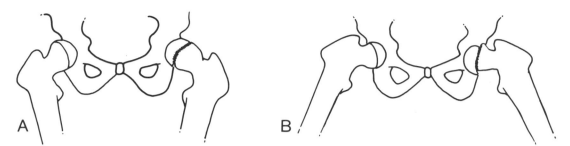

Figure 6.22. X-ray evidence of slipped capital femoral epiphysis. Anteroposterior and frog-leg lateral views of both hips and pelvis are done to provide comparison. *A*, on the AP view, the change is subtle and more difficult to appreciate. It is helpful to draw a line along the lateral neck to demonstrate the medial translation of the epiphysis. *B*, frog-leg view highlights the posterior slippage of the epiphysis.

tate. X-rays demonstrate posterior and medial displacement of the epiphysis (Fig. 6.22). The change may be subtle and often apparent only on the lateral view of the hip.

Treatment

Once this diagnosis is made, orthopaedic referral and treatment should be obtained. The treatment is usually surgical. With small or moderate degrees of slip, fixation of the epiphysis may be performed in situ. This leads to fusion of the epiphysis and long-term stability. Shortening of the extremity is not usually a problem. In slips of greater degree, more extensive surgical reconstruction may be necessary.

Nontraumatic Conditions in Adulthood

DEGENERATIVE ARTHRITIS OF THE HIP

Osteoarthritis of the hip is one of the most common diseases affecting this joint. This condition is often secondary to an underlying abnormality of the hip such as congenital dysplasia, Legg-Calvé-Perthes disease, or slipped capital femoral epiphysis. In some cases, however, there is no identifiable cause, and in those situations the osteoarthritis is considered primary or idiopathic.

The pathophysiology of osteoarthritis is reviewed in Chapter 12. As a result of these changes, motion in the hip becomes progressively restricted first by painful synovitis and muscle spasm, then by secondary soft tissue contracture. In more advanced stages of the disease, there is loss of joint congruity, osteophyte formation, and mechanical block to motion superimposed on the soft tissue contracture.

Pain in osteoarthritis can be from this synovitis, muscle spasm, capsular contracture, and pain fibers in bone and reparative granulation tissue.

Clinical Characteristics

The patient presents with pain, which may be felt in the groin, buttock, anterior thigh, or knee. Pain is usually worse with weight bearing, although there may be pain at rest. Initially, the pain may be intermittent, but with time it becomes more frequent, lasts longer, and becomes progressively severe. The patient may limp. This may be an antalgic limp or an "abductor sway" (Fig. 6.13).

Motion is restricted, and may be demonstrable as a flexion contracture. Abduction and internal rotation are usually more restricted than adduction and external rotation. The leg shortens with advanced disease. X-ray of the hip demonstrates varying changes, including narrowing of the joint space, subchondral bone irregularity with cyst and osteophyte formation, sclerosis of the subchondral and trabecular bone, and lateral or superolateral subluxation of the hip.

Treatment

Conservative measures can be helpful in reducing the symptoms and associated disability of degenerative arthritis of the hip. One of the most important measures of conservative treatment is reducing the stress across the hip. The patient should walk less, avoid running, jumping, climbing stairs, and other impact-type activities. An overweight patient can reduce the stress on the hip by losing weight. In Figure 6.12, if body weight was 90 kg instead of 70 kg, the force across the hip joint would be 360 kg, not 280 kg. This is nearly a 25% difference. A cane is another effective means of reducing stress across the hip. A cane used on the side opposite the affected hip can reduce hip joint force by as much as 30%. The cane should be approximately 1 to 2 inches longer than would be necessary to reach the ground when held in a weight-bearing grip with the elbow fully extended.

While rest reduces symptoms, it also produces atrophic muscular weakness. Consequently, a patient may maintain muscular strength by performing daily exercises that are of fairly low stress. Range of motion exercise will help to preserve motion. Muscle strengthening and range of motion exercises as outlined in Figure 6.23 are recommended if well tolerated. The patient should omit any exercise that produces pain. If these strengthening exercises are painful, the patient may perform isometric exercises. In addition to these exercises, a regular swimming or stationary bicycle program is beneficial. These are excellent general conditioning activities, and will not lead to the type of joint stress and increased wear that impact activity would. It is difficult for a patient to maintain optimum weight without an exercise program.

The use of heat and/or cold may reduce the symptoms of osteoarthritis of the hip. Anti-inflammatory medication (aspirin, nonsteroidals, and corticosteroids) may provide relief from pain of synovitis associated with osteoarthritis. Systemic corticosteroids have serious side effects and should be avoided in routine treatment of osteoarthritis. Intraarticular steroid injection may be beneficial and can be employed on a limited nonrepetitive basis. While nonsteroidal anti-inflammatory drugs can be beneficial, there is some evidence suggesting that prolonged use of these medications may impair the reparative processes about the diseased hip, and there may be more rapid bone deterioration.

Surgical Treatment

When conservative treatment is unsuccessful, surgical treatment is considered and orthopaedic referral is necessary. Three forms of surgical treatment are commonly considered. Arthrodesis of the hip provides pain relief by surgical ankylosis of the joint. The patient trades movement for a stable, painless hip. Osteotomy of the femur or pelvis attempts to improve the weight-bearing condition of the hip by changing the weight-bearing relationship of the femoral head and acetabulum. An attempt is made to increase the weight-bearing area of the hip to decrease the relative force per unit area and to bring the femoral head into a more "congruous" relationship with the acetabulum. This procedure should be done relatively early in the arthritic process when the patient still has a fairly good range of motion. Therefore, early orthopaedic referral is important, particularly for younger patients. The most common therapy for osteoarthritis of the hip is total hip arthroplasty. The technique of this procedure has improved substantially as it has evolved over the last 25 years. It is a highly successful procedure, and prostheses are now designed to be inserted without bone cement. Though experience with these new devices is still limited, there is optimism that they will provide more durable, long-term, pain-free function.

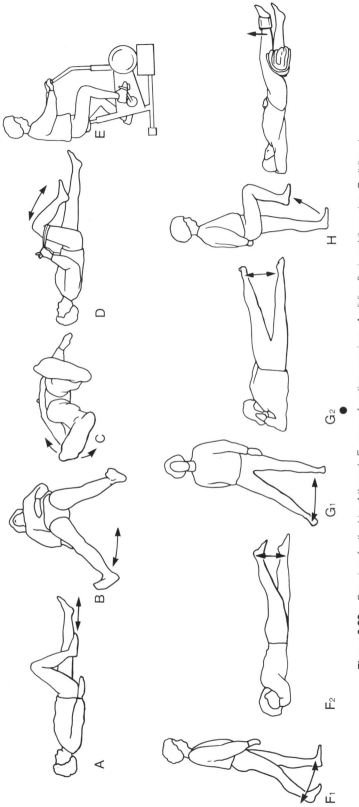

Figure 6.23. Exercises for the hip: A through E, range of motion exercises. A, sliding flexion while supine. B, sliding abduction/adduction while supine. C, internal and external rotation while supine (this can be repeated with the hip flexed). D, active and self-assisted further flexion using hands or exercise strap. E, stationary bicycle with low resistance on pedal. F through I, strengthening exercises. F, hip extensor strengthening, erect (F_1) and prone (F_2) (more advanced). G, hip abductor strengthening, erect (G_1) and side-lying (G_2) (more advanced). H, hip flexor strengthening, supine (see Fig. 6.23A) and erect (more advanced). I, quadriceps strengthening.

179

INFLAMMATORY ARTHRITIS OF THE HIP

Chapter 12 describes the various arthritides. These can affect the hip as any other synovial joint. Any patient who appears to have synovitis of the hip that is refractory to treatment should be referred for orthopaedic or rheumatologic evaluation. A variety of conditions must be considered, including rheumatoid arthritis, spondyloarthropathies, collagen vascular disease, crystalline arthritis, primary and metastatic malignancy, pigmented villonodular synovitis, avascular necrosis (see below), and infection (see below).

INFECTIONS OF THE HIP

Adult patients rarely develop septic arthritis of the hip. Those patients who develop septic arthritis are frequently immunocompromised, i.e., patients with diabetes or renal failure, or those taking corticosteroids or chemotherapeutic agents. The intravenous drug abuser is also at increased risk. The healthy patient who develops septic arthritis presents acutely ill with high fever, exquisite pain, and decreased motion. The immunocompromised patient may present without high fever and may not appear acutely ill. Range of motion may not be as painful.

Tuberculosis can occur in the hip joint as in any other synovial tissue. Pain, limited motion, subcutaneous abscess, or draining sinus may be part of the presentation. In the advanced stages of this 'disease, x-ray changes are significant and demonstrate bone and joint destruction.

A patient suspected of having infectious arthritis of the hip must undergo joint aspiration and should be referred immediately to the orthopaedist.

AVASCULAR (ASEPTIC) NECROSIS OF THE HIP

Avascular necrosis of the femoral head is well recognized in association with fractures of the femoral neck and dislocations of the femoral head in both adults and children. The cause of avascular necrosis of the femoral head following trauma is an interruption of the arterial supply to the femoral head as a direct result of the injury. Aseptic necrosis of the femoral head without recognizable injury is not well understood. When this condition affects children (Legg-Calvé-Perthes disease), there is a good potential for repair and recovery. In adults, however, this condition is more often associated with an unfavorable outcome.

The pathologic change associated with the early phase of this disease is a segmental necrosis of the femoral head. The overlying articular cartilage is unaffected. With time, there is reparative tissue ingrowth with resorption of necrotic bone, accompanied by formation of new bone on necrotic trabeculae. With resorption there is a weakening of the area of segmental necrosis, and there can be a subchondral fracture. Patients often have a marked increase in pain when the fracture occurs.

The precise cause of nontraumatic aseptic necrosis in adults is unknown and may be multifactorial. In patients with sickle cell disease, it is thought to be associated with vascular thrombosis. Aseptic necrosis has been associated most commonly with alcoholism and steroid use. It has also been noted in gout, Gaucher's disease, caisson disease, and in patients with altered hemostasis.

The disease is clinically categorized in stages based on the x-ray appearance of the hip. The condition is frequently bilateral.

Clinical Characteristics

Patients with avascular necrosis may be asymptomatic in the earliest stages. It is not uncommon for patients who present with pain in one hip to already have subtle x-ray changes on the asymptomatic opposite side. Patients who are symptomatic present with pain in the groin and anterolateral hip. There may be pain in the thigh or radiation to the knee. In some patients, an episode of severe pain develops after a period of milder pain; this is frequently at the time of subchondral fracture. The patient may have an antalgic limp or an abductor sway. Motion is restricted by pain in the early stages of the disease, and by mechanical obstruction in the later stages when secondary degenerative arthritis develops.

Treatment

Treatment of this condition is surgical, and orthopaedic referral is necessary. In the early stages, prior to collapse, a "core decompression" of the avascular segment can be performed by drilling into the head from the lateral femoral cortex. This decompression may be followed by healing. Once any collapse occurs, this form of treatment is not predictable and other procedures, including osteotomy, debridement, grafting, and hip arthroplasty, must be considered. Early referral of the patient is important to salvage the femoral head.

BURSITIS

Bursitis about the hip is a common condition secondary to inflammation of one of the three major bursae about the hip: the trochanteric bursa, the iliopsoas bursa, and the ischiogluteal bursa. These bursae facilitate the gliding of musculotendinous or ligamentous structures. Bursitis may be secondary to direct injury or overuse of the adjacent musculotendinous structures, and/or degenerative changes in these structures. Because bursae are lined by true synovial tissue, bursitis can also occur with systemic disease causing synovitis.

Trochanteric Bursitis

The trochanteric bursa is a large bursa that lies between the greater trochanter and the overlying junction of the gluteus maximus and tensor fascia lata, as these merge to form the fascia lata and iliotibial tract (Fig. 6.24).

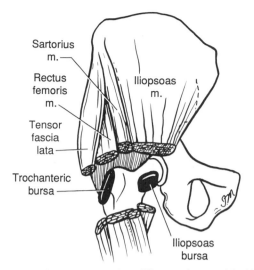

Figure 6.24. Trochanteric and iliopsoas bursae of the hip joint, anterior view.

Clinical Characteristics. Patients complain of pain over the lateral aspect of the hip; there is frequently radiation into the lateral thigh and posterolaterally toward the posterior aspect of the trochanter and into the buttock. Patients complain of pain when they turn onto the affected hip or with hip movement, particularly rotation. The pain may develop abruptly or insidiously, and may be mild or severe. There is tenderness over the trochanter laterally and posterolaterally, but rarely swelling or redness. Rotation of the hip may increase pain, especially if this is combined with compression over the trochanter. X-rays are usually noncontributory, but they should be obtained to rule out other conditions. There may be signs of soft tissue swelling or calcification in the adjacent tendinous structures. Fracture of the greater trochanter in the elderly patient with osteoporosis can mimic trochanteric bursitis.

Treatment. Treatment consists of rest, heat or ice, and the use of nonsteroidal anti-inflammatory medication. Local steroid injection can also be helpful, but one must be careful to inject this in the bursa and avoid intratendinous injection.

Ischiogluteal Bursitis

This is inflammation of the bursa between the ischial tuberosity and the overlying gluteus maximus. It is usually associated with injury or with occupations requiring long periods of sitting.

Clinical Characteristics. The patient complains of pain over the ischial tuberosity aggravated by sitting, and the pain may radiate into the posterior thigh. There is tenderness overlying the ischial bursa. Swelling is rarely noted. X-rays are usually noncontributory.

Treatment. Treatment is the same as for trochanteric bursitis. Resolution usually occurs in 1 to 2 weeks.

Iliopsoas Bursitis

This is inflammation of the iliopsoas bursa, located between the iliopsoas muscle and the pelvis proximally and between the hip capsule and psoas tendon distally (Fig. 6.24). Communication between the hip joint and psoas bursa is common.

Clinical Characteristics. Pain is felt in the groin and may radiate into the anterior aspect of the thigh. The pattern of pain is difficult to distinguish from true hip arthritis. The patient may complain of pain on walking. Local tenderness is difficult to elicit because the structures are deep. There may be some pain with deep palpation over the anterior aspect of the hip. Pain is increased with flexion of the hip against resistance or hyperextension of the hip. X-rays are noncontributory.

Treatment. Treatment consists of rest, heat, ice, and nonsteroidal anti-inflammatory medication.

When treating bursitis in any location, a gentle program of stretching exercise within the limits of pain and active exercise of the involved muscles should be instituted once pain has subsided. Brief, frequent periods of exercise are recommended, as opposed to one long period of exercise, which tends to produce fatigue and may cause reinjury. If symptoms persist after 2 weeks of treatment, orthopaedic referral is indicated.

PERIARTICULAR MYOFASCIAL PAIN SYNDROMES

A variety of myofascial pain syndromes occur about the hip joint. These syndromes usually occur in middle-aged or older patients. The pain site varies in location according to the specific muscular unit that is involved. The pathophysiology is not clear, and some authors argue the existence of these syndromes. Nevertheless, many patients present with localized muscular pain and consistent areas of tenderness (trigger points). These areas of tenderness may be somewhat firm, or the muscle may have a cord-like thickening. The distinction of these syndromes depends on the location of pain and tenderness, and a fairly characteristic pattern of referred pain (as noted below).

Gluteus Medius Syndrome

Pain is felt over the upper and midportion of the gluteus medius. There may be referred pain to the posterior or lateral thigh (Fig. 6.25). Passive stretch or contraction against resistance may aggravate the pain.

Gluteus Maximus Syndrome

Pain is felt more centrally in the buttock. Referred pain may be felt in the posterior thigh (Fig. 6.25).

Tensor Fascia Lata Syndrome

Pain is felt more anteriorly over the tensor fascia lata muscle, with referred pain to the lateral and anterolateral thigh. Pain may go below the knee (Fig. 6.25).

Hamstring Syndrome

Pain is felt over the ischium or proximal thigh posteriorly, associated with tenderness in the region of the hamstring origin and muscles.

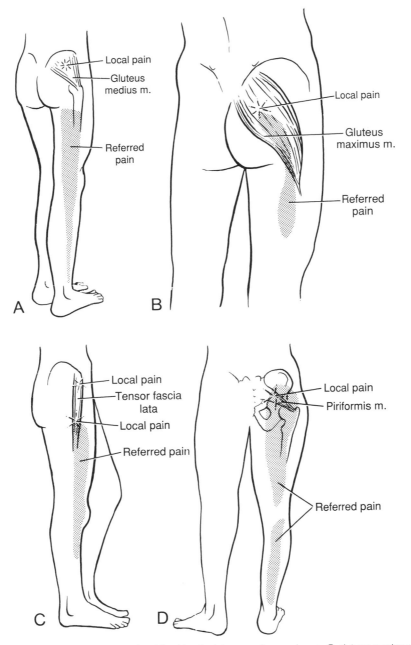

Figure 6.25.   Myofascial pain syndromes about the hip. *A*, gluteus medius syndrome. *B*, gluteus maximus syndrome. *C*, tensor fascia lata syndrome. *D*, piriformis syndrome.

Piriformis Syndrome

Pain is felt in the region of the sciatic notch (Fig. 6.25). There may be referred pain, felt more generally in the buttock, posterior thigh, or lower leg. Because of the proximity of the adjacent sciatic nerve, a patient with "sciatica-type" pain may present with inflammation of the piriformis. There is local tenderness over the piriformis. Pain may be increased with passive forced internal rotation or resisted external rotation. Patients may complain of pain in the rectal or vaginal area, which can be reproduced on rectal or vaginal examination by fingertip pressure just at and medial to the ischial spine.

Treatment

In all of the myofascial pain syndromes, rest, heat or ice, and oral anti-inflammatory medication may be helpful. Injection with a local anesthetic with or without depository steroid may be helpful, but intratendinous injection must be avoided. Success has also been reported with "cold spraying" of the affected muscle, using a fluoromethane spray, followed by manual stretching.

SACROILIAC SYNDROME

Inflammation of the sacroiliac joint can occur with a variety of the spondyloarthropathies. Reiter's syndrome, psoriatic arthritis, ankylosing spondylitis, and inflammatory bowel disease commonly occur with sacroiliitis. In other patients, there may be sacroiliac pain without other signs of spondyloarthropathy. Pain may be from true synovitis of this joint, or from inflammation of the overlying muscles or ligaments.

Clinical Characteristics

There is pain over the sacroiliac joint region with referred pain into the lower buttock and thigh. Pain over the greater trochanter and groin pain may also be present. There is tenderness over the sacroiliac joint and in the region of the posterior superior iliac spine. The Patrick's test may elicit pain in the involved joint. With the patient side-lying, strong compression of the pelvis may cause pain. Hyperextension of the hip may also produce pain. X-rays frequently show no significant change. In the case of spondyloarthropathy, however, there may be irregularity or osteopenia of the subchondral bone leading to a "blurring" of the joint space. These changes are most commonly seen in the lower (synovial) part of the joint. Patchy areas of lucency and sclerosis may develop. With further progression, there is marked narrowing of the joint space, and there can be ankylosis.

Treatment

When sacroiliitis is a manifestation of an underlying spondyloarthropathy, treatment is dictated by the underlying inflammatory disease. In isolated cases of sacroiliac syndrome, symptomatic relief can be achieved by rest, application of local heat or ice, and use of nonsteroidal anti-inflammatory medication. A sacroiliac belt may also be helpful.

Traumatic Disorders of the Pelvis and Hip
PELVIC SPRAINS

Because of their strength, disruption of the sacroiliac joints and pubic symphysis occur as a result of severe injury. Because the pelvis is a stable bony ring (see "Essential Anatomy" section), injuries that involve actual displacement of one of the pelvic joints usually occur in conjunction with a secondary site of injury elsewhere in the bony ring. For example, a disruption of the symphysis may occur in conjunction with a sacroiliac dislocation, sacral fracture, or iliac fracture.

Women in the later stages of pregnancy are more subject to sprains of the pelvic ligaments with lesser degrees of injury. Also, isolated pubic symphysis sprains can occur as a result of a fall directly onto the symphysis or perineum, such as when an individual slips off a bicycle seat onto the frame.

Clinical Characteristics

Sprain of the sacroiliac joint is associated with pain over the region of the joint and posterior superior iliac spine, with referral into the buttock and thigh. Sprains of the pubic symphysis are associated with pain in that region. Pain is referred into the groin and inner thigh, and may be bilateral. There is localized tenderness in the region of the joints. Weight bearing can increase pain, and transfer of weight from one extremity to another may aggravate symptoms. In pregnancy, pain may persist until delivery. X-rays are usually noncontributory except if there has been actual displacement of the joint. Cases with displacement are usually the result of violent trauma, and sacroiliac or symphyseal dislocation is often associated with a fracture of the pelvic ring.

Treatment

In the case of obvious displacement of the sacroiliac joint or pubic symphysis, orthopaedic consultation should be obtained immediately for further evaluation and treatment. Even if there is no obvious x-ray abnormality, orthopaedic consultation should be obtained when there is a history of violent injury and significant pubic symphysis or sacroiliac injury is suspected.

In other circumstances, treatment is rest, heat or ice, and nonsteroidal anti-inflammatory medication. During pregnancy, medication is usually avoided. After a brief period of rest, activity can be increased progressively within the limits of pain as tolerated. Some patients benefit from a sacroiliac-belt.

MUSCULAR STRAINS AND AVULSION INJURIES

Muscular strains are distinguished from the myofascial pain syndromes by the recognition of their immediate onset following an injury. These injuries are secondary to violent stretch or contraction of the muscle against resistance, or less often as a result of blunt impact. Contusion of the muscle can occur anywhere in its substance, and can disrupt the fascial muscular envelope as well as the actual muscle fibers. Bleeding occurs, with associated swelling and ecchymosis. There is local tenderness and pain with passive stretch or active contraction of the muscle. The area of hematoma may become the site of new bone formation, which can cause prolonged pain and swelling, and limited motion secondary to muscular contracture. This is known as myositis ossificans.

Any of the major muscle groups about the hip can be injured. A common injury is the "groin pull." This is an injury of the adductors. It is often secondary to forced abduction of the hip in a fall, twisting injury, or collision. Pain is felt at the adductor tubercle, about the inferior pubic ramus, or within the adductor tendon region.

An abrupt, strongly resisted, sudden hip flexion, which might occur in a kicking injury, produces a strain of the iliopsoas or rectus femoris muscles. Pain is felt over the anterior iliac spine or anterior aspect of the hip. There is tenderness in these regions and pain with passive extension or active flexion.

In adolescence, passive stretch or strong contraction against fixed resistance may produce avulsion injuries of a musculotendinous unit. This occurs because these muscles join the bone at apophyses that are still unfused during adolescence. An abruptly resisted hip flexion, such as might occur when a kick is blocked, may cause avulsion of the rectus femoris at the anterior inferior iliac spine, avulsion of the sartorius at the anterior superior iliac spine, or avulsion of the lesser femoral trochanter by the iliopsoas. Severe stretch of the hamstrings, which can occur doing the splits, may cause avulsion of the hamstrings from the ischial tuberosity. Abruptly opposed hip adduction or hip extension, as may occur during a fall or the splits, can avulse the origins of the adductor group from the inferior pubic ramus and ischial tuberosity.

Clinical Characteristics

Pain and tenderness are localized to the injured muscle or its site of origin or attachment. There may be associated swelling and ecchymosis. Passive stretch or voluntary contraction is painful and may be inhibited. X-rays may show avulsion injuries at the bony apophyses.

Treatment

If gross disruption of the musculotendinous unit is suspected or there is an avulsion injury on x-ray, orthopaedic referral should be obtained. The orthopaedist must then decide whether immobilization is indicated, or whether actual repair of the injury should be considered. It is unusual that these injuries require operative repair.

For the majority of these injuries, the goal of treatment is reduction of symptoms, allowing a comfortable period of rest and restricted activity for healing to occur. The duration of restriction and symptomatic treatment depends upon the severity of injury.

Initially, rest, use of crutches, and application of ice are helpful. When there is injury to a muscle belly, it is helpful to provide support to reduce symptoms and further minimize intramuscular bleeding and swelling. For injuries about the hip, a pelvic elastic bandage spica is effective. Another helpful device is elasticized shorts that provide good muscular support.

If the injury is minor with little swelling, mild tenderness, and no pain with weight bearing, it usually resolves over several days. Stretching and active exercise may progress as soon as symptoms allow. Ice is applied initially, and after the first 24 to 48 hours applications of heat may be helpful.

With more severe injuries, where there is marked swelling and tenderness several hours after injury and significant pain with weight bearing, a more major disruption of the muscle tissue is presumed. Treatment is initiated with rest and ice, and the patient is instructed in crutch use. This must continue for several weeks and then, as pain recedes, stretching and active exercise and increased weight bearing may begin. Pain is used as a guide to initiation and progression of activity. Return to sporting activity is allowed when the patient feels pain-free during activities of daily living and has regained nearly full motion and strength. With a severe hamstring pull, it is not uncommon to have patients restricted for 2 months.

SPRAINS AND DISLOCATIONS OF THE HIP JOINT
Sprains

Sprains of the hip joint are secondary to the same kinds of forces that cause dislocations, but are of a lesser magnitude. Also, it must be remembered that the hip joint is intrinsically stable and, except with violent force, is not subject to sprain or dislocation. Therefore, sprains of the hip are much less common than those of the knee or ankle. When this injury occurs, synovitis may be associated with the stretch or partial tear of the hip capsule and ligaments.

Clinical Characteristics.   Sprain of the hip joint is characterized by pain and limited motion in the hip following acute injury.

Treatment.   Treatment includes rest and ice. For minor sprains, as comfort returns within 24 to 48 hours, weight bearing may be resumed and range of motion and strengthening exercises begun. With more severe injuries, a more prolonged period of rest and restricted weight bearing is recommended.

Dislocations of the Hip Joint

Hip dislocations are most prevalent among young patients whose bones are strong and whose activities carry the risk of violent injury. Elderly patients with more fragile bones are more likely to suffer a fracture of the hip.

The hip can dislocate in three directions: posterior, anterior, and central. The posterior dislocation is the most common. An acetabular fracture often occurs with dislocation of the hip, and the exact nature of the injury depends upon the magnitude and precise direction of the forces applied.

Posterior Dislocation. Posterior dislocations are produced by forces that act along the axis of the femur, driving the femoral head posteriorly into the posterior acetabular wall. The most common mechanism of posterior dislocation is a motor vehicle accident in which the knee of the victim riding in the front seat strikes the dashboard. With the hip flexed and adducted, the head of the femur is driven over the posterior rim of the acetabulum (Fig. 6.26) as it bursts through the posterior capsule and ligament. When the hip is flexed but in less adduction, a fracture through the posterior wall of the acetabulum may occur.

Clinical Characteristics. The patient presents with complaints of hip pain. The hip is usually adducted and internally rotated and shortened (Fig. 6.27). There may be evidence of sciatic dysfunction with numbness, tingling, and muscular weakness or absence of muscular function in the sciatic distribution.

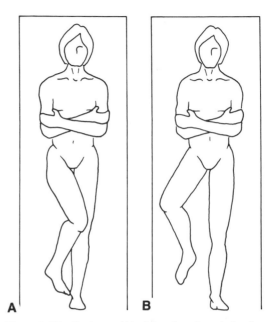

Figure 6.27. Postures of hip dislocation. *A,* posterior dislocation. *B,* anterior dislocation.

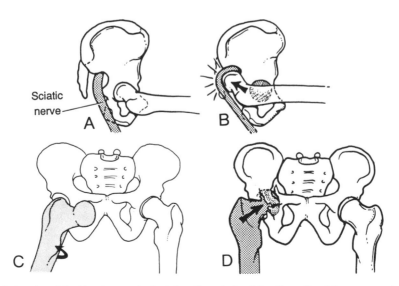

Figure 6.26. Dislocation of the hip. *A,* normal articulation. *B,* posterior dislocation with sciatic nerve on stretch. *C,* anterior dislocation. *D,* central dislocation.

X-ray will demonstrate the dislocation. A true lateral film of the hip is often necessary to confirm the direction of dislocation.

Anterior Dislocation. The anterior dislocation is produced by a violent force that externally rotates the extended hip. The head of the femur disrupts the anterior inferior capsule and may come to rest over the pubis or may lodge in the obturator foramen (Fig. 6.26).

Clinical Characteristics. Pain is felt in the hip and anterior and medial thigh. The hip is usually held in slight abduction, in relative extension, and in external rotation (Fig. 6.27). X-rays demonstrate the dislocation.

Central Dislocation. Central dislocations are produced by violent forces that drive the head of the femur through the medial wall of the acetabulum (Fig. 6.26). This injury can be produced by a variety of combined forces.

Clinical Characteristics. The patient presents with severe pain in the hip, groin, and anterior and medial thigh. The hip may be externally rotated or shortened slightly. X-rays demonstrate the dislocation with medial wall fracture.

Complications of Dislocation. The immediate complication of posterior dislocation of the hip is injury to the sciatic nerve (Fig. 6.26), which may affect its peroneal and/or tibial branches. Peroneal injury is more common, and manifests as decreased sensation of the anterolateral leg and dorsum of the foot, with weakness or inability to dorsiflex the ankle and toes. Posterior tibial nerve dysfunction manifests as decreased sensation on the posterior aspect of the lower leg and plantar aspect of the foot and heel, with weakness or inability to plantar flex the ankle or toes.

The other complication of dislocation of the femoral head is interruption of the blood supply to the head, leading to avascular necrosis. This can be associated with actual tearing of the vessels, or there may be interruption secondary to stretch of these vessels.

The effects of this vascular interruption may not be noted for months or years following the initial injury.

Because of potential sciatic nerve injury and interruption of the blood supply, dislocations of the hip must be reduced as rapidly as possible. The sciatic nerve is put on stretch by the protruding femoral head, and removal of this deforming force is important to reduce the potential for increasing nerve injury. Also, stretching of the vessels supplying the femoral head may cause ischemia, and with reduction those blood vessels that are not actually disrupted can resume circulation and minimize the subsequent development of aseptic necrosis. Finally, dislocation of the hip often causes injury to the articular cartilage, and it is not uncommon for these patients to develop some degree of posttraumatic arthritis.

Treatment. Dislocations of the hip are often associated with other injuries secondary to violent force. Consequently, comprehensive evaluation and support of the patient are necessary prior to treatment of the hip dislocation. It is especially important to check for ipsilateral knee injury. Reduction of the dislocated hip is an orthopaedic emergency, and orthopaedic referral should be made immediately. In those circumstances where this is not possible or may be delayed for several hours, the primary care physician should proceed with reduction of the hip. Such reduction should only be performed with good pain control and muscle relaxation. This can often be achieved in the emergency department in an otherwise stable patient, taking care that full resuscitative facilities are available.

For posterior dislocation, the hip can be reduced with the patient either supine or prone. The more common method is with the patient supine (Fig. 6.28). The hip is flexed. An assistant stabilizes the pelvis, and the operator applies traction to the leg from behind the flexed knee. The hip is often in adduction initially and the operator should

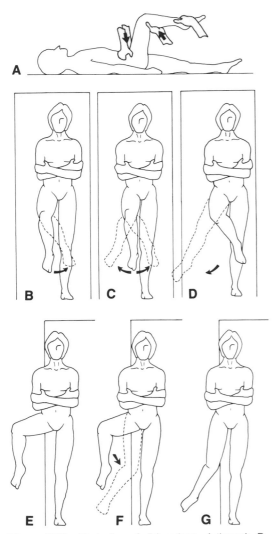

Figure 6.28. Reduction of dislocations: *A* through *D*, posterior dislocation. *A*, upward traction with hip flexed progressively to 90°. *B*, external rotation while continuing traction. *C*, alternate external and internal rotation while continuing traction. *D*, extension and abduction while maintaining traction and external rotation. *E* through *G*, anterior dislocation. (Note the position of the patient at the edge of the examining table.) Maneuver begins with strong traction to the hip through the flexed knee. *E*, hip abducted while maintaining flexion. *F* and *G*, reduction accomplished with continued traction and usually some internal rotation; adduction and extension complete the maneuver.

not attempt to correct this position initially. Traction should be applied along the line of the limb, and maintained as the hip is brought gently into flexion to a position of approximately 90°. With continued traction, the hip can be gently rotated using the lower leg as a lever. Reduction usually occurs with external rotation, but it may be necessary to alternate gentle internal and external rotation.

With reduction of the hip, there is usually a palpable and at times audible click. This is less apparent with posterior rim fractures. Also, certain dislocations are quite unstable, and redislocation will occur if traction is released and the hip allowed to internally rotate in flexion.

An x-ray is obtained following reduction, and inspected to confirm a congruous reduction of the hip and to evaluate the presence of any acetabular or femoral head fractures.

If this supine method is not successful, the patient is placed prone with the hip flexed over the end of the table. In this position, gravity works with the operator to facilitate reduction. Access to the patient is limited, however, so the patient must be breathing in a normal spontaneous way and must be cooperative to do this safely. While considerable traction is necessary, excessively rough or ballistic-type movements should be avoided. If reduction is not possible, the patient must be prepared for general or spinal anesthesia and possible open reduction. This is preferable to traumatic manipulation. In this situation, orthopaedic referral becomes mandatory.

For anterior dislocation, the technique of reduction is strong continuous traction along the line of the femur with the patient supine (Fig. 6.28). The hip is usually externally rotated and abducted, and traction should be applied to the femur in this position. Traction is continued with progressive flexion of the hip. Usually, internal rotation and then extension with adduction will complete the reduction. As with posterior dislocation, repetitive traumatic attempts at reduction should be avoided. If these measures are not successful, the patient must be prepared for general anesthesia and possible open reduction. In this situation, orthopaedic referral becomes mandatory, even if delay is necessary.

Following reduction of the hip, an x-ray is obtained to confirm congruous reduction and to rule out fractures of the acetabulum or femoral head.

The central dislocation of the hip is actually a combination of fracture of the medial and superomedial acetabular dome and medial displacement of the femoral head. Prolonged longitudinal traction is usually necessary to effect reduction. This fracture-dislocation may be unstable and operative methods may be necessary. Definitive treatment of this injury requires orthopaedic referral.

Postreduction Care and Rehabilitation. If the hip is stable after reduction of a simple dislocation, patients are maintained in skin or light skeletal traction for 1 to 2 weeks. When patients are comfortable and have regained good leg control, they may get up with light partial weight bearing using crutches. Limited range of motion exercise can begin. In the case of posterior dislocation, patients are instructed to avoid flexion beyond 90°, and combinations of flexion with internal rotation and/or adduction. Weight bearing may be slowly progressed using the rule of no pain/no limp. Full weight bearing is allowed when patients can ambulate without pain or limp and have regained good strength. This is usually possible by 6 weeks. Follow-up x-rays are obtained at this point. If the patient has been non-weight bearing, a disuse osteopenia of the hip should be present. This is a good sign, indicating that the femoral head blood supply is intact. The femoral head of a patient with avascular necrosis may not show this disuse osteoporosis because the bone resorption that is the basis of disuse osteoporosis requires intact circulation.

FRACTURES OF THE HIP

Fractures of the hip are most prevalent among elderly women, in whom osteoporosis is common. In this group of patients, the forces that produce these fractures are often surprisingly mild. A fall from which a younger person may get up with a sore hip and limp can cause a fracture in the elderly patient. In some circumstances, a twist of the weight-bearing extremity when a patient is trying to avert a fall may result in fracture. The architecture of the upper end of the femur is well suited to resist the forces of weight bearing. In the elderly osteoporotic patient, however, it is not as well suited to resist twisting and shearing forces, and it is often these forces that result in hip fracture.

Hip fractures may be classified into two large groups: fractures of the femoral neck (subcapital or transcervical) and fractures of the intertrochanteric region (Fig. 6.29). The femoral neck fractures are usually intracapsular and the intertrochanteric fractures are extracapsular. The importance of this distinction derives from the vascular anatomy of the head and neck of the femur (as summarized in the "Blood Supply" section). Intracapsular femoral neck fractures may disrupt the blood supply to the femoral head, resulting in avascular necrosis. Because the younger patient with a hip fracture has usually been subject to greater violence than the elderly patient, there is often more tissue injury and as a consequence there is a higher rate of avascular necrosis in the young patient.

Most fractures of this type, whether intracapsular or extracapsular, are unstable and displaced. A minority of these injuries are firmly impacted and may withstand substantial weight-bearing forces. These patients may be able to ambulate on the fracture with only mild or moderate pain.

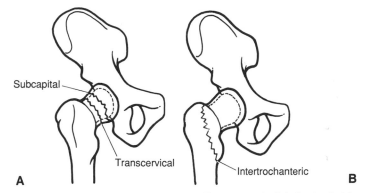

Figure 6.29. Fractures of the hip. *A*, intracapsular. *B*, extracapsular (intertrochanteric).

Clinical Characteristics

The elderly patient has fallen or twisted a hip, while a younger patient has been subject to much more substantial injury. The patient complains of pain in the hip, groin, or thigh, and is unable to bear weight or move the extremity. The uncommon exception is the patient with an impacted femoral neck fracture, in which there is moderate stability and only mild pain. The injured extremity is usually shortened and externally rotated, although minimally displaced and impacted fractures may not show this deformity. Motion is painful and limited. X-rays of the hip and pelvis demonstrate the fracture. In minimally displaced, impacted fractures of the femoral head, the fracture line may be difficult to see.

Treatment

Most of these injuries are treated surgically with reduction and internal fixation. In displaced femoral neck fractures in elderly patients, prosthetic replacement of the femoral head is commonly performed. This is true when displacement is severe, osteoporosis is significant, and definitive treatment is delayed. All of these factors increase the chances of avascular necrosis and problems with healing, even with fixation.

In the elderly patient with a fractured hip, the primary practitioner must first identify the presence and nature of the fracture. Once this is done, orthopaedic referral should be made promptly. It is important to proceed with comprehensive evaluation of the patient's medical status, as these patients require surgical treatment. The primary care practitioner should coordinate the timing of surgery with the treating orthopaedist based on the patient's medical status. It is important to optimize the patient's condition prior to surgery, and this can usually be done within the first 24 to 48 hours.

FRACTURES AND DISLOCATIONS OF THE PELVIS

Because of the stability of the pelvic ring, fractures of the pelvis, unless they involve the osteoporotic bone of the elderly, are usually caused by violent forces. These injuries are commonly the result of a fall from a height, or impact during a motor vehicle accident. Fractures and dislocations of the pelvis can be associated with massive hemorrhage and severe genitourinary and rectal injury. Therefore, evaluation of patients with pelvic fractures must include assessment of hemorrhage and hypotension, and evaluation of the genitourinary and lower gastrointestinal systems.

The pelvis is commonly thought of as a rigid ring. Therefore, for the shape of the pelvic ring to be distorted, it must be disrupted at two points. The example of a "pretzel ring" is helpful. One cannot imagine breaking a crisp pretzel ring in only one location by applying a compressive or shearing force: it will break in two locations. Of course, the pelvis is not a truly rigid ring. There are two rigid half-rings that are connected at the symphysis and sacroiliac joints, and these joints provide yield points during applied stress. These yield points allow isolated fractures of the pelvic ring to occur and to present with a nondisplaced or minimally displaced appearance. When a fracture occurs, the pelvis yields at the sacroiliac joints or symphysis, or there may be some deformation in the bony ring. If the deformation of the symphysis or sacroiliac joint is slight, it may not be readily apparent on x-ray. When there is displacement at one site in the bony pelvic ring, one must anticipate and search for the second site of ring disruption. For example, a widely displaced dislocation of the symphysis pubis anteriorly will be associated with a posterior iliac fracture, sacral fracture, or sacroiliac dislocation posteriorly (Fig. 6.30).

Pelvic injuries can be classified as "closed ring" or "open ring" fractures (Fig. 6.30). The closed ring injuries include the nondisplaced and minimally displaced single rami or two ipsilateral rami fractures, and fracture near or subluxation of the symphysis pubis or sacroiliac joint without significant dislocation. These injuries are stable and can usually be treated symptomatically with rest and then progressive mobilization. Open ring injuries involve double breaks in the pelvic ring and are more commonly unstable to either vertical or lateral plane forces. These injuries require more aggressive treatment, including skeletal traction and internal or external fixation. Fractures of the acetabulum must be considered as a separate category. These are evaluated based on the relative stability of the hip and disruption of the articular surface. They may occur with closed or open ring fractures of the pelvis.

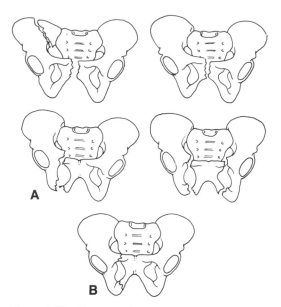

Figure 6.30.   Fractures of the pelvis. *A*, four examples of open ring fractures. *B*, closed ring fracture.

Open ring fractures of the pelvis are more likely to be associated with injury to the genitourinary system and/or rectum. It is important to recognize this during the evaluation and initial treatment of patients with pelvic injuries.

Clinical Characteristics

The patient has been involved in a violent accident and if conscious will complain of pain, which often girdles the hips or localizes unilaterally in the buttock or groin. Attempts to actively or passively move the lower extremities increase the pain. There may be obvious ecchymosis or swelling about the pelvis, groin, scrotum, or perineum.

Manipulation of the pelvis increases the pain. Downward pressure on the anterior superior iliac spine may be associated with posterior displacement or external rotation of the ilium if there has been disruption of the symphysis anteriorly and/or injury of the sacroiliac joint posteriorly. Downward pressure on the pubic symphysis may cause pain if there is injury at this location. Central compression over both trochanters or iliac crests may demonstrate medial-lateral instability of one or the other hemipelvis. Vertically directed force applied to the hemipelvis through the femur may demonstrate vertical displacement of the hemipelvis. These maneuvers help to demonstrate the location of the fracture and degree of stability.

Hematuria or urinary retention may be present. There may be blood in the urethral meatus, rectum, or vagina indicating injury in these locations. X-rays of the pelvis reveal the fracture.

Treatment

The role of the primary care practitioner is in the initial assessment and stabilization of the patient with a pelvic injury. Once the patient is stabilized, physical examination, including genitourinary and rectal examination, should be accomplished. With suspected genitourinary injury, urethrogram and cystogram are considered first, then intravenous pyelogram. Prompt orthopaedic referral is indicated.

Nondisplaced and minimally displaced closed ring fractures are usually stable and can be treated symptomatically with bed rest and progressive mobilization as symptoms allow. Usually, bed-to-chair activity and partial weight bearing are possible within 1 to 2 weeks. After the initial consultation, these patients can be followed by the primary practitioner.

The treatment of open ring fracture of the pelvis must be deferred to the orthopaedic surgeon. Skeletal traction or internal and/or external fixation may be used based on the degree of instability and other characteristics of the fracture.

SUGGESTED READINGS

Bennett JT, MacEwen JD. Congenital dislocation of the hip: recent advances and current problems. Clin Orthop 1989;247:15–21.

Canale ST, Barr JS Jr, eds. Problems and complications of slipped capital femoral epiphysis. Instruct Course Lect 1989;38:281–290.

Canale ST, King RE. Pelvic and hip fractures. In: Rockwood CA Jr, Wilkins K, King RE, eds. Fractures in children. Philadelphia: JB Lippincott Co, 1984:733–844.

Coleman SS. Diagnosis of congenital dysplasia of the hip in the newborn infant. Clin Orthop 1989;247:3–12.

DeLee JC. Fractures and dislocations of the hip. In: Rockwood CA Jr, Greene DP, eds. Fractures in adults. Philadelphia: JB Lippincott Co, 1984:1211–1356.

Fernbach SK. Avulsion injuries of the pelvis and proximal femur. Am J Roentgenol 1981;137:581–584.

Haueisen DC, Weiner TS, Weiner SD, et al. The characterization of transient synovitis of the hip in children. J Pediatr Orthop 1986;6:11–17.

Hely DP, Salvati EA, Pellicci PM. The hip. In: Cruess RL, Rennie WR, eds. Adult orthopaedics. New York: Churchill Livingstone, 1984:1209–1274.

Herring JA, Barr JS Jr, eds. Legg-Calves-Perthes disease. A review of current knowledge. Instruct Course Lect 1989;38:309–315.

Kane WJ. Fractures of the pelvis. In: Rockwood CA Jr, Greene DP, eds. Fractures in adults. Philadelphia: JB Lippincott Co, 1984:1093–1210.

Lovell WW, Winter RB, eds. Pediatric orthopedics. Philadelphia: JB Lippincott Co, 1990.

Ponseti IV. Growth and development of the acetabulum in the normal child: anatomical, histological and roentgenographic studies. J Bone Joint Surg 1978; 60A:575–585.

Tachdjian MO. Pediatric orthopedics. Philadelphia: WB Saunders Co, 1990.

CHAPTER 7

Knee

Dudley A. Ferrari, M.D.

Essential Anatomy

The knee is a weight-bearing, modified-hinge joint. Its motion is controlled and stabilized by muscles and ligaments, as well as the shape of the opposing bone surfaces and their associated meniscal cartilages. It is a highly efficient structure that can provide support for the body and meet the changing demands of multiple locomotor tasks. Because it is subject to high forces exerted along lengthy lever arms (tibia and femur), it is vulnerable to injury during the course of normal daily activities and during sports.

Knee motion is a complex function. Flexion and extension of the knee require rotation as well as some degree of abduction and adduction. The rotation effect can be demonstrated by placing the fingers over the tibial tubercle and noting that the tibia internally rotates as the leg goes into flexion and externally rotates as it goes into extension. This rotation is dependent on the relative size of the medial and lateral femoral condyles, the shape of the tibial condyles, and the effects of the controlling ligaments (Fig. 7.1). As the femoral condyles move through their rotational arc, they both roll and slide on the tibial condyles (Fig. 7.2). If the femoral condyles did not slide, the femur would simply roll off the tibia posteriorly at the extremes of flexion. In fact, the rolling motion is combined with a sliding motion, and it is this combination that allows for the full arc of stable flexion of the knee. Rolling and sliding varies between the medial and lateral sides of the knee. The lateral condyle rolls more and the medial condyle slides more, producing external rotation as the knee goes into full extension. The rolling and sliding mechanism is passively controlled by the anterior cruciate ligament as the knee flexes and by the posterior cruciate ligament as the knee extends.

X-RAY ANATOMY

Figure 7.3 shows radiographs of the knee with important elements labeled.

Skeletal and Articular Structure of the Knee

Femur (Fig. 7.4). The shaft of the femur extends from the trochanters to the condyles. It is triangular in cross-section with its apex, the linea aspera, directed posteriorly. It is slightly bowed with anterior convexity, and inclines from the trochanters to the condyles in slight adduction. Posteriorly, the linea aspera provides insertion for the adductors and extensors of the thigh, while the anterior surface of the midshaft and the trochanteric area provide origin for the extensors of the knee. As the shaft approaches the condyles, it broadens laterally and medially, and the ridges of the linea aspera merge with the supracondylar ridges. These ridges outline a triangle, called the popliteal surface, to which no muscles are attached.

The femoral condyles are the rounded ends of the femurs that articulate with the tibia. Anteriorly, the condyles merge to form

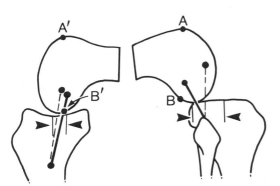

Figure 7.1. Unequal motion of the condyles is due to (*a*) the unequal length of the condyles (A to B is greater than A′ to B′ on the medial condyle); (*b*) the shape of the condyles (the medial tibial condyle is concave, the lateral is convex, allowing more posterior rolling); and (*c*) the direction of the collateral ligament (the medial collateral is stretched faster and the lateral is more posterior, allowing the condyle to move farther back). (Adapted from Kapandji IA. The physiology of the joints, vol 2. 2nd ed. Edinburgh: E & S Livingstone, 1970:195,196.)

the patella articular surface. The medial condyle is larger in surface area than the lateral condyle, which diverges from the medial condyle. While the lateral condyle is smaller in total area, it is longer in length than the medial (Fig. 7.4). The condyles of the tibia are the widened platforms that articulate with the condyles of the femur (Fig. 7.5). The medial side is concave and the lateral side

convex from front to back. The medial and lateral tibial condyles are separated by the intercondylar eminence; its medial and lateral spines articulate with the femur. The cruciate ligaments maintain contact between the spines and the femur. The actual center of rotation may vary but in static systems is considered to be near the medial spine.

The anatomy of the lower extremities is such that the hips are wider apart than the ankles. Consequently, a physiologic valgus alignment is produced at the knee for the joint to remain parallel to the ground, which is biomechanically the most efficient orientation (Fig. 7.6).

Ossification Centers about the Knee

There are three ossification centers about the knee. The femoral condylar epiphysis is evident at birth and completes ossification by age 20. Ossification of the distal aspect of the femoral condyles can sometimes proceed in an irregular pattern. This must not be confused with osteochondritis (see section on "Nontraumatic Conditions of Childhood"). The tibial condylar epiphysis is usually evident at birth and completes ossification by age 20. This epiphysis includes the tibial tubercle as well as the tibial condyles. The patella ossifies from a single center that be-

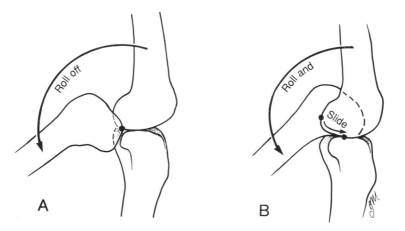

Figure 7.2. *A*, position of femur if only rolling occurred. *B*, normal rolling and sliding motion of the femoral condyles. Initial rolling is followed by sliding to maintain position on the tibial condyle.

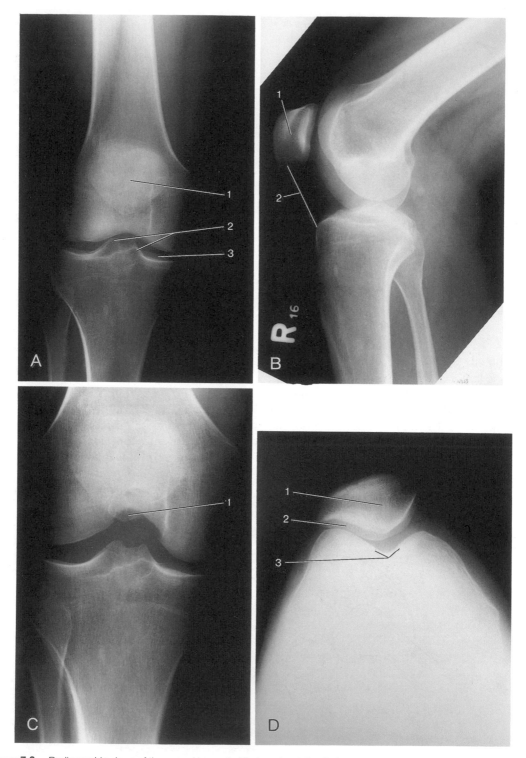

Figure 7.3. Radiographic views of the normal knee. *A*, AP view; *1*, patella; *2*, tibial spines; *3*, medial joint space. *B*, lateral view; *1*, patella; *2*, patellar ligament. *C*, tunnel view; *1*, intercondylar notch. *D*, tangential view; *1*, patella; *2*, lateral patellar facet; *3*, trochlear groove.

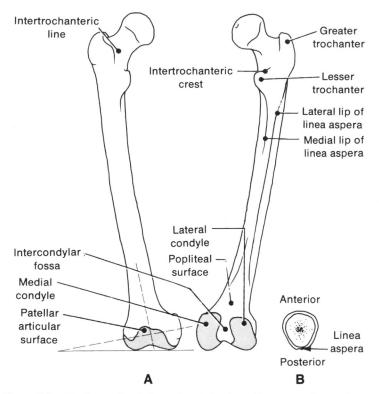

Figure 7.4. The femur. *A*, anterior and posterior views. *B*, cross-section, midfemur.

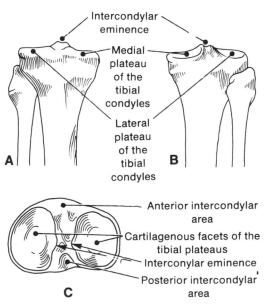

Figure 7.5. The proximal condyles of the tibia. *A*, anterior view. *B*, posterior view. *C*, superior view.

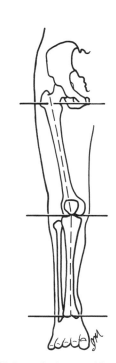

Figure 7.6. To keep the knee, pelvis, and ankle parallel to the ground, an angle is created by the wider pelvis and the knee.

197

comes radiologically evident by age 6. Ossification is completed during puberty.

Synovium of the Tibiofemoral Articulation

Figure 7.7 illustrates the three-dimensional form of the synovial space and the lines of attachment of the synovium to the articular borders of the femur and tibia. The menisci are included within the synovial space but the cruciate ligaments are excluded.

Within the synovium there can be shelves or bands, called plicae. These are remnants of membranes that separated the compartments of the knee during embryonic development. There are three types and they vary in size (Fig. 7.8). The suprapatellar plica divides the suprapatellar pouch from the rest of the knee. The infrapatellar plica separates the medial and lateral compartments anterior to the cruciate ligaments. The medial plica originates from the medial synovium near the suprapatellar plica and extends to the infrapatellar fat pad. The medial plica is the one band that often becomes symptomatic by being caught between the patella and medial femoral condyle or against the medial condyle alone, producing medial patellar pain. This will be discussed further in the section "Injury of the Patellofemoral Articulation."

Menisci

The two menisci are semilunar fibrocartilaginous wedges that rim and cushion each tibiofemoral articulation. The radius and circumference of the medial meniscus are larger than those of the lateral meniscus. The ends of the lateral meniscus attach to the intercondylar eminence, and the ends of the medial meniscus attach to the intercondylar areas. Outer rims attach to the synovial

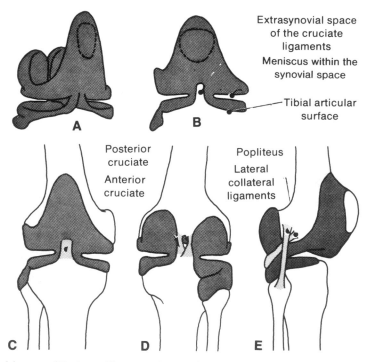

Figure 7.7.   Synovial space of the knee. Diagrammatic cast of the synovial space. *A*, three-quarter anterior view. *B*, full-face anterior view. *C–E*, the cast of synovial space applied to the femur, patella, tibia, and fibula to indicate the margins of attachment of the synovial membrane to those bones.

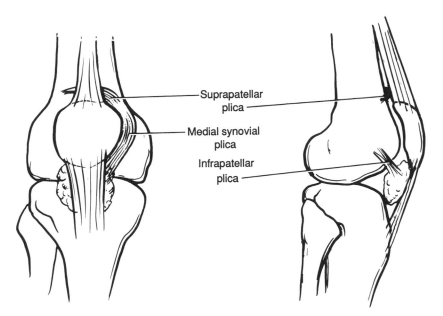

Suprapatellar plica

Medial synovial plica

Infrapatellar plica

Figure 7.8. Suprapatellar plica divides the suprapatellar pouch and knee. Infrapatellar plica extends from the infrapatellar fat pad to the intercondylar notch, and medial plica extends from the fat pad to the suprapatellar plica.

membrane of the articular capsule (Fig. 7.9). The menisci sit on the tibial surfaces and assist in weight distribution through the knee. The medial meniscus shares half the load with the exposed weight-bearing area of the tibial condyle. The lateral meniscus shares more of the weight-bearing load than the exposed area of the lateral tibial condyle.

This weight distribution varies with activities (Fig. 7.10). The weight-bearing area of the tibial condyle is posterior in flexion. The menisci become wedges that act as stabilizers in addition to accepting weight. The menisci are pushed back in flexion and pushed forward in extension. In addition to these passive motions, the ligaments also affect the movement of the menisci. For example, the medial collateral ligament pulls the medial meniscus posteriorly during flexion and internal rotation of the tibia, and anteriorly during extension and external rotation of the tibia. On the lateral side, the popliteus muscle pulls the lateral meniscus posteriorly during flexion or during external rotation of the femur. The movement of the menisci is syn-

chronous and obligatory. Consequently, abnormal stresses to the knee often produce meniscal tear. Because the lateral meniscus is less firmly attached to the capsule and more free to move about, it is injured less frequently than the medial meniscus.

Ligaments (Fig. 7.11)

The ligaments of the knee guide and check the movements of the articular surfaces. The lateral and medial patellar retinacula are continuations of the fascia lata and quadriceps tendon on their respective sides of the patella. They merge with and reinforce the anterolateral and anteromedial aspects of the knee capsule. The retinacula limit the motions of the patella.

The medial collateral ligament extends in two layers from the medial femoral condyle to the medial tibial condyle. The superficial layer is a broad, triangular ligament with its apex extending posteriorly over the posterior aspect of the medial femoral condyle and joint line. The deep layer is a stout structure that blends intimately with the capsule and

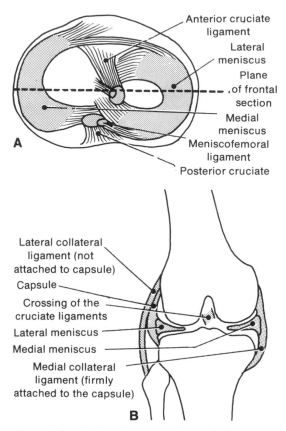

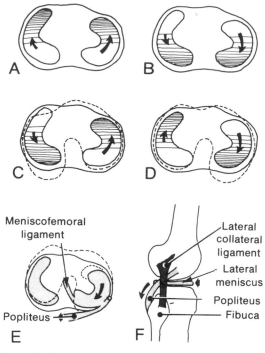

Figure 7.9. Relationship between the menisci, the capsule, and the ligaments of the knee. *A*, superior view of the menisci and cruciate ligaments. *B*, posterior view of a frontal section of the knee through the middle third.

Figure 7.10. *A–D*, shifts in tibial weight-bearing points and passive accommodations of the menisci during flexion-extension and rotation. *Shading* indicates weight distribution. *Arrows* indicate accommodative passive movements of the menisci. *Longer arrows* over the lateral meniscus symbolize its greater mobility. *A*, full extension. *B*, near full flexion. *C*, medial rotation of the femur. *D*, lateral rotation of the femur. *E* and *F*, active accommodations of the menisci during knee movement. During external rotation of the femur, the movement of the meniscofemoral ligament and the contraction of the popliteus muscle pull the lateral meniscus posteriorly and medially.

has an attachment to the medial meniscus. The posterior portion of the tibial collateral ligament or posterior oblique ligament is located on the medial posterior corner.

The lateral collateral ligament is a cord-like structure with its main attachments extending from the lateral femoral condyle to the fibula. It does not blend with the capsule. The popliteus tendon is also part of the lateral stabilizing complex, and this runs beneath and attaches to the femur in front of the lateral collateral ligament. The arcuate ligament and short external collateral ligament are also on the lateral corner.

The anterior cruciate ligament extends from the anterior intercondylar area of the tibia to the medial aspect of the intercondylar area of the lateral femoral condyle. The posterior cruciate ligament extends from the posterior intercondylar area of the tibia anteromedially to the intercondylar surface of the medial femoral condyle.

Function. Because of the orientation of its fibers and the shape of the condyles, some portion of the medial collateral ligament is tight from extension through flexion. The posterior fibers are taut in extension and the anterior fibers are taut in flexion. The medial collateral ligament is the primary stabilizer to valgus stress at the knee. The posteromedial capsule and anterior cruciate ligament

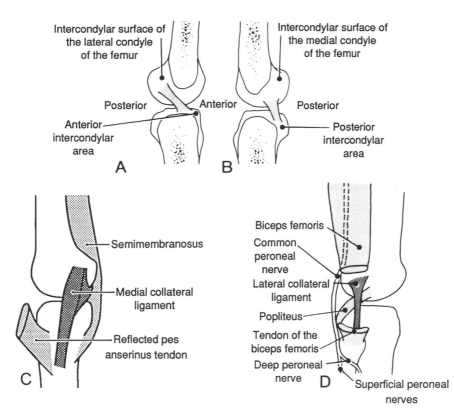

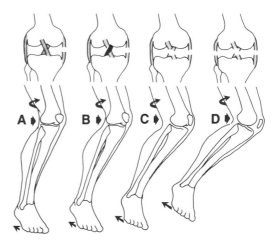

Figure 7.11.   Cruciate and collateral ligaments. *A*, medial view of the anterior cruciate ligament. *B*, lateral view of the posterior cruciate ligament. *C*, medial view of the medial collateral ligament. *D*, lateral view of the lateral collateral ligament.

are secondary stabilizers. Consequently, a valgus force to the knee may first cause injury to the medial collateral ligament, but as this force continues, the anterior cruciate, posterior capsule, and posterior cruciate may be disrupted (Fig. 7.12).

The lateral collateral ligament is taut in extension and relaxed in flexion. The iliotibial tract assists in the range of 5° to 40° of flexion. The lateral collateral ligament is the primary stabilizer to varus stress. Secondary restraint is provided by the posterolateral complex, consisting of the popliteus tendon, short external collateral ligament, and arcuate ligament. A varus force will likely injure the lateral collateral ligament first, the posterolateral complex next, and if large enough, the posterior and anterior cruciate ligaments.

Figure 7.12.   Order of vulnerability of ligaments of the knee to a valgus force. *A*, medial collateral ligament. *B*, medial collateral ligament and anterior cruciate. *C*, medial collateral ligament, anterior cruciate, and posterior cruciate. *D*, medial collateral ligament, anterior cruciate, posterior cruciate, and lateral collateral ligament.

The anterior cruciate ligament consists of two bands, the anteromedial and posterolateral. The anteromedial band tightens in flexion and this tightening, along with a twisting of the entire anterior cruciate ligament about the posterior cruciate ligament, controls anterior displacement of the tibia and compresses the joint surfaces. The posterolateral band of the anterior cruciate tightens in extension, maintaining contact. The anterior cruciate restricts anterior translation and resists internal rotation as well as hyperextension. As a secondary stabilizer to varus and valgus forces, it may be injured, as noted previously.

The posterior cruciate also demonstrates two bands, the anterolateral and posteromedial. The posteromedial band is tight in extension and, as the knee flexes, the entire ligament becomes tight. It is the main restraint to posterior displacement of the tibia.

A force applied to the front of the tibia is resisted mainly by the posterior cruciate with little restraint from the posterior capsule. The posterior cruciate ligament can be injured in hyperflexion.

MUSCLES CONTROLLING THE KNEE
Extensors

The major extensor of the knee is the quadriceps muscle, which forms the anterior bulk of the thigh. It is made up of four parts: the rectus femoris, vastus lateralis, vastus medialis, and vastus intermedius. The origins and insertions are illustrated in Figure 7.13.

The vastus medialis lies deep to the rectus femoris proximally and emerges distally to create the medial curve of the distal thigh. The vastus medialis has a special orientation at its distal end. The direction of its fibers applies a medial- and proximal-directed force

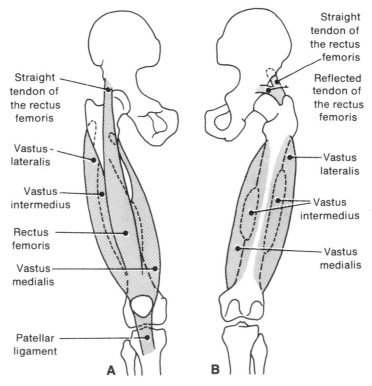

Figure 7.13. The quadriceps muscle. *A,* anterior view. *B,* posterior view.

to the patella during the last 15° of extension. This is important in maintaining patella stability and alignment. Both the vastus lateralis and medialis are in continuity with the knee capsule and can produce knee extension even in the presence of patella fracture as long as there is not complete disruption of the anteromedial and anterolateral capsule (Fig. 7.14A).

All of the extensors are innervated by branches of the femoral nerve, which is derived from the second through fourth lumbar roots.

Flexors

The main flexors of the knee are the gracilis, semitendinosus, semimembranosus, and biceps femoris muscles. The origins and insertions are illustrated in Figure 7.14. The gracilis and semitendinosus along with the sartorius insert into the medial aspect of the shaft of the tibia and anterior to the tibial collateral ligament, just inferior to the attachment of the patellar ligament to the tibial tubercle. This sweep of tendons over the tibial collateral ligament is known as the pes an-

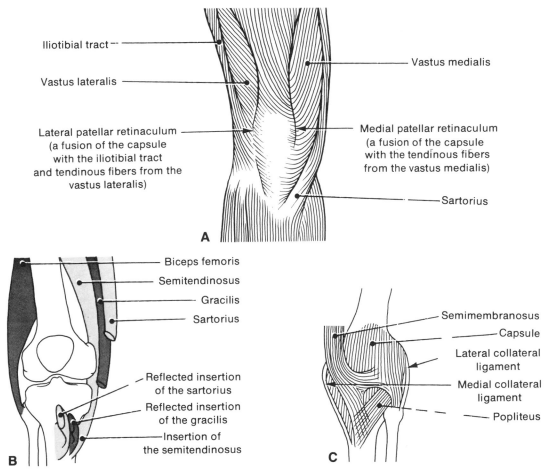

Figure 7.14. Tendinous expansions merging with capsule of the knee joint. *A*, anterior view showing the patellar retinacula. *B*, anterior view showing the tibial insertion of the sartorius, semitendinosus, and gracilis medially, and the fibular insertion of the biceps femoris laterally. *C*, posterior view showing the relationship of the semimembranosus to the capsule medially and posteriorly. The medial head of the gastrocnemius overlies posterior to the semimembranosus tendon (not illustrated).

serinus. There is a bursa related to the pes anserinus that is a common site of bursitis, particularly in patients with osteoarthritis of the knee.

The knee flexors have other actions in addition to flexing the knee. With the knee flexed, they can serve as rotators of the leg: the gracilis, semitendinosus, and semimembranosus internally rotate the leg and the biceps femoris externally rotates the leg. The internal rotators are slightly stronger than the external rotators of the leg.

The popliteus muscle arises on the posterior surface of the tibia. The tendon passes beneath the arcuate ligament and attaches to a depression on the anterior part of the groove of the lateral condyle of the femur. This muscle unlocks the knee, initiating flexion and rotation.

The sartorius, along with all the anterior muscles of the thigh, is innervated by branches of the femoral nerve. The gracilis, with all of the adductors of the hip, is innervated by branches of the obturator nerve, with contribution from the third and fourth lumbar nerve roots. The other three flexors of the knee are innervated by branches of the sciatic nerve.

Fascia Lata

All the muscles of the thigh are enclosed within the fascia, a tough, unyielding covering. The fascia merges medially and laterally with the intermuscular septa. In combination with the fascia, the septa divide the thigh into anterior and posterior compartments. As this fascial covering will not yield, extravasation of enough blood or edema into either of the two compartments of the thigh may produce a compartment syndrome.

INNERVATION AND BLOOD SUPPLY (FIG. 7.15)

The knee joint receives fibers from both the femoral and sciatic distributions. Because the femoral nerve also innervates the hip, patients with hip pathology may present with knee pain.

The femoral artery gives rise to the deep and superficial femoral arteries in the femoral triangle. The deep artery carries the major blood supply to the muscles of the thigh, and the superficial artery carries the major blood supply to the leg and foot. The deep artery penetrates deep to the adductors and eventually comes to lie between these muscles and the posterior surface of the femur. In this location, the artery and its accompanying veins are vulnerable to injury by the fragments of a fractured femoral shaft. In the distal third of the thigh, it passes posteriorly around the femur to lie directly on the popliteal surface of the femur, anterior to the sciatic nerve. In this area it is vulnerable to injury with dislocation of the knee or juxtaarticular fractures.

Evaluation of the Patient with Knee Symptoms
EXAMINING FOR EFFUSION

Ambulatory patients should first be examined with both knees flexed 90°. Inspect the area on either side of the patellar ligament. Moderate effusions cause a bulging in these areas that is not present in the normal knee.

With the knee fully extended and the extensor apparatus relaxed, compress the knee above and on either side of the patella, and attempt to subject the patella to ballottement with a finger. Sufficient effusion forces the patella away from the femur and allows ballottement (Fig. 7.16).

If neither of these observations suggests an effusion, attempt to flex the knee fully, unless a suspected injury to the extensor apparatus contraindicates this. An effusion can interfere with full flexion of the knee.

EXAMINATION OF THE EXTENSOR APPARATUS

Palpate the quadriceps tendon, the body of the patella, and the patellar ligament to look for defects and tenderness. Obtain x-rays if there is evidence of a defect over the

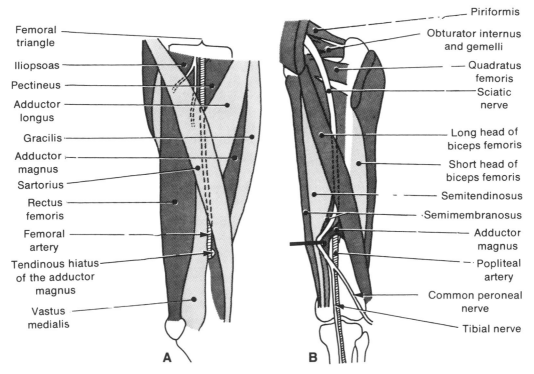

Femoral triangle
Iliopsoas
Pectineus
Adductor longus
Gracilis
Adductor magnus
Sartorius
Rectus femoris
Femoral artery
Tendinous hiatus of the adductor magnus
Vastus medialis

Piriformis
Obturator internus and gemelli
Quadratus femoris
Sciatic nerve
Long head of biceps femoris
Short head of biceps femoris
Semitendinosus
Semimembranosus
Adductor magnus
Popliteal artery
Common peroneal nerve
Tibial nerve

A   B

Figure 7.15. Relationships of the major vessels and nerves in the thigh. *A,* anteromedial view. *B,* posterior view.

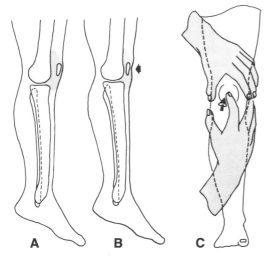

A   B   C

Figure 7.16. Examination for knee joint effusion. *A,* patella forced away from the femur by the effusion. *B,* patella forced downward onto the femur by ballottement maneuver. *C,* illustration of the ballottement maneuver.

quadriceps tendon or the patellar ligament, or if the body of the patella is tender or palpably fractured. A rupture of the extensor apparatus should be presumed if the x-ray reveals a fracture of the body of the patella or avulsion from the superior border or the inferior pole, or if the examination by palpation demonstrates an apparent defect in the quadriceps tendon or patellar ligament. Further examination should be discontinued and orthopaedic referral made.

When there is no evidence of rupture of the extensor apparatus, displace the patella laterally and medially to test for a retinacular tear or strain. Subluxation or dislocation of the patella should be suspected if this type of patella manipulation is associated with apprehension. Displace the patella proximally while forcing it posteriorly into its femoral articulation to test for pain and crepitus associated with chondromalacia patellae.

EXAMINATION OF THE COLLATERAL LIGAMENTS

Test the integrity of the medial and lateral ligaments by applying valgus and varus stress, attempting to open the joint line of the knee with the knee flexed to 30° (Fig. 7.17). If the knee opens in comparison to the opposite knee given the same stress and position, and there is local tenderness and a history of injury, a disruption of the ligament or ligament complex is present. Any opening indicates a complete or third-degree sprain. An opening of 1 to 5 mm is grade I, an opening of 5 to 10 mm is grade II, and an opening greater than 10 mm is a grade III injury. With higher grade injuries, the likelihood of injury to the secondary stabilizing ligaments increases. In addition to testing the ligaments with the knee flexed, stress testing should also be done with varus-valgus force with the knee extended. Instability in extension indicates more global ligamentous disruption.

EXAMINATION OF THE CRUCIATE LIGAMENTS
Anterior Cruciate

Perform the **anterior drawer test**. With the knee flexed to 90° and the hip flexed to

45°, the examiner sits on the foot to keep it stabilized and uses both hands to grasp the tibia from behind. Keeping the hamstring relaxed, the pull is straight forward. If the foot is placed in external rotation, this maneuver tests the anterior cruciate ligament and also the secondary stabilizers in the posterior medial corner (Fig. 7.18). The movement of the injured knee is compared with the uninjured knee, as it is for all ligament stability testing.

Perform the **Lachman test** (Fig. 7.19). Place the patient supine and flex the knee to 20°. Stabilize the distal femur with one hand and the proximal tibia with the other. The tibia is moved forward on the femur and the degree of displacement noted. Compare the

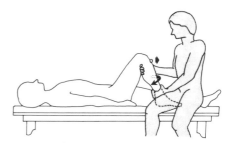

Figure 7.18. Examination for laxity of the anterior cruciate ligament.

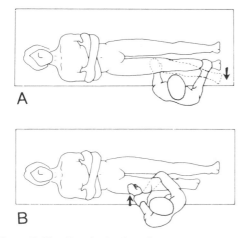

Figure 7.17. Examination for collateral ligament injuries. *A*, applying valgus stress. *B*, applying varus stress.

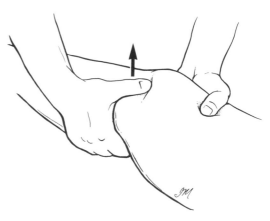

Figure 7.19. Lachman test. The knee is flexed 20°. The proximal tibia is grasped and moved forward while the femur is held with the other hand. (Adapted from Torg JS, Conrad W, Kalen V. Clinical diagnosis of anterior cruciate ligament instability in the athlete. Am J Sports Med 1976;4:84–92.)

degree of displacement with the unaffected side.

Perform the **pivot shift test** (Fig. 7.20). This is pathognomonic of a tear of the anterior cruciate ligament. The test can be performed in many ways, each producing anterior subluxation of the lateral tibial condyle and subsequent relocation, which produces the "pivot shift." One good method is for the examiner to place the patient's ankle beneath the examiner's arm with the hip in abduction. The hands support the proximal tibia, exerting a valgus internal rotation and anterior translation force. With this combination of forces applied in relative extension, the tibia subluxates. As the knee is further flexed from this position, the tibia falls backward to anatomic position, producing a shifting sensation. This sensation reproduces the feeling of "giving way" that the patient experiences functionally.

Posterior Cruciate

Prepare to perform the **posterior drawer test** (Fig. 7.21). The patient's leg is positioned in a fashion similar to the anterior drawer test, with the knee flexed to 90° and the foot on the examining table. In this position, the injured leg should be examined and compared with the opposite leg. There may be a posterior "sag" of the injured tibia relative to the femur. This is an important observation and is pathognomonic of posterior instability. Recognizing this also allows the examiner to avoid misinterpreting "pseudo" anterior laxity of the knee. In this condition, the tibia begins from a posteriorly displaced position and, consequently, there is increased laxity on anterior drawer. In fact, this represents a posteriorly subluxated tibia.

After making the observation for posterior sag, a posterior force is placed against the proximal tibia. The degree of laxity is compared with the opposite side. A positive posterior drawer test or a sag that occurs with the knee flexed indicates posterior cruciate ligament injury. Laxity may be difficult to detect and quantify. In an isolated injury there may not be an effusion and the pain may be manifest posteriorly. Ecchymosis present posteriorly should suggest posterior cruciate injury. The presence of varus or valgus laxity in full extension is also suggestive of posterior cruciate ligament injury.

EXAMINATION FOR MENISCUS INJURY

Palpate the joint lines. Shortly after an acute tear or displacement of a chronic tear, the associated joint line will be tender. Palpate the joint lines while rotating the leg back and forth. A torn meniscus may cause a palpable click during this maneuver (Fig. 7.22).

Perform **McMurray's test** (Fig. 7.23). Flex

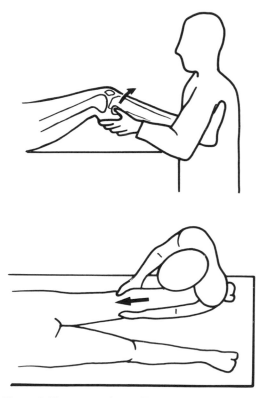

Figure 7.20. Pivot shift test. The ankle and leg are held under the axilla. The leg is abducted and the knee extended. The hands are under the proximal tibia applying gentle anterior and internal rotation force. The tibia will subluxate forward and, as pressure is applied in line with the leg, the tibia will flex and reduce.

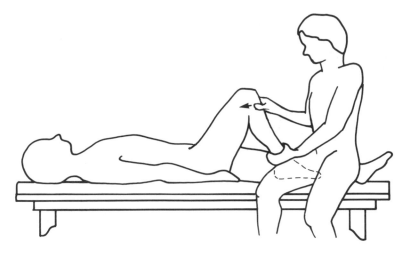

Figure 7.21.   The posterior drawer test. With the knee at 90° of flexion, push back on the tibia to see whether there is increased motion or sag compared with the opposite leg.

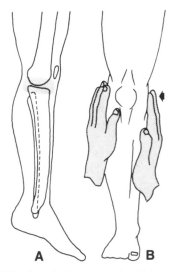

A   **B**

Figure 7.22.   Examination for meniscal injury. *A*, area of tenderness. *B*, palpation for tenderness.

the knee fully, with the leg externally rotated when testing for medial meniscus tear, and internally rotated when testing for lateral meniscus tear. While maintaining rotation, extend the knee with a firm controlled movement. A painful click in early or midextension is suggestive of a meniscus tear.

Perform **Apley's test** (Fig. 7.24). With the patient lying prone, flex the knee to 90°.

While applying upward traction on the leg, rotate the leg internally and externally. Pain during this maneuver is more compatible with ligament injury than with meniscal tear. Repeat the rotation while bearing downward on the leg. Pain during this maneuver is more compatible with meniscal injury.

Nontraumatic Conditions of Childhood

TIBIAL APOPHYSITIS (OSGOOD-SCHLATTER DISEASE)

Apophysitis of the tibial tubercle occurs at the time the apophysis undergoes the transition from cartilage to bone. It commonly occurs between ages 12 and 14. Traction of the patellar ligament on the apophysis may result in microfractures.

Clinical Characteristics

Pain in the region of the tibial tubercle is related to activity, and it may be relieved by rest. Swelling and tenderness are present over the tibial tubercle and along the patellar ligament. A lateral x-ray may or may not show irregular ossification or fragmentation of the tibial tubercle. While this is not evi-

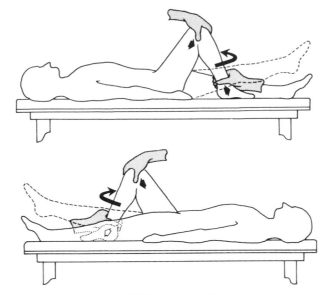

Figure 7.23.   McMurray's test.

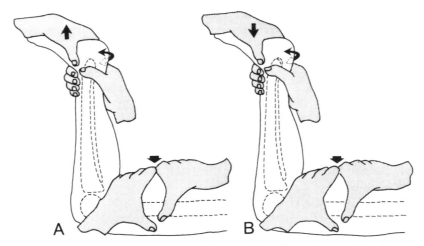

Figure 7.24.   Apley's test. *A,* pain is compatible with ligament injury. *B,* pain is compatible with meniscal injury.

dent early in the disease, it may persist long after the disease has become asymptomatic.

Treatment

Instruct the child to avoid all activity that requires resisted knee extension—for example, climbing, running, kicking—until pain and tenderness have fully remitted. This restriction usually applies for 6 to 8 weeks.

When pain is severe and recurrent, casting in a walking cylinder for 2 to 3 weeks lessens symptoms. When pain persists after skeletal maturation and ossification are complete, the usual cause is the presence of non-united ossicles within the tuberosity or tendon. This will be seen on x-ray. Surgical excision of the loose ossicles relieves symptoms, although it is rarely necessary.

NECROSIS WITHIN THE POLES OF THE PATELLA (LARSEN-JOHANSSON'S DISEASE)

This condition occurs in children aged 8 to 13. The initiating event is unknown. Clinical characteristics include pain that occurs during resisted extension of the knee and during kneeling. Onset is insidious and activity-related. There is also swelling and tenderness over the inferior pole of the patella. X-rays may or may not show fragmentation of bone near the affected pole. Treatment and prognosis are the same as those presented for Osgood-Schlatter disease.

NECROSIS WITHIN THE CONDYLAR EPIPHYSES OF THE FEMUR (OSTEOCHONDRITIS DISSECANS)

Osteochondritis dissecans is the result of avascular necrosis in the area of subchondral bone. The medial femoral condyle is involved in 75% of cases, but the lateral condyle may be affected. These lesions may heal, particularly if the adolescent growth plates are open. The etiology is probably traumatic from impingement of the tibial spine on the femoral condyle.

Clinical Characteristics

Osteochondritis dissecans is characterized by aching pain in the knee at rest that becomes worse with weight bearing, causing the patient to limp. The onset is insidious. Physical examination may demonstrate a restriction in range of motion, but usually range of motion is normal. Rarely, an effusion will be evident. If the fragment detaches it may produce locking or symptoms of a loose body. AP, lateral, and tunnel x-rays of the knee will usually demonstrate a characteristic lesion that appears as a half-moon defect or irregularity of the subchondral bone.

Treatment

As the prognosis is unpredictable, the patient should be referred at the outset to an orthopaedist. A decrease or elimination of weight bearing with immobilization may be prescribed until the lesion heals. A loose body may be removed and the defect drilled. The fragment may be drilled to promote revascularization and healing, or fixed by screws.

Nontraumatic Conditions in Adulthood

OSTEONECROSIS

As in the hip, avascular necrosis can occur in the knee. It most commonly involves the medial compartment, with the femoral condyle more frequently involved than the tibial condyle. In some patients, an associated systemic factor will be noted, such as previous history of alcoholism, steroid therapy, or bone marrow disease. In most patients osteonecrosis of the knee is idiopathic.

Clinical Characteristics

The patient usually presents with an acute onset of pain in the knee, most often on the medial side. Patients are usually over 50 years of age and women are more commonly affected. A minority of patients have a more subacute onset of pain. The pain initially may be severe, but subsequently is more moderate. Patients often complain of stiffness and swelling, and an effusion is commonly noted.

X-rays taken early in the disease are often negative and the lesion can only be found by bone scan or magnetic resonance imaging. Later in the disease, x-rays become abnormal, usually showing a lucent region of the subchondral bone with surrounding sclerosis. There may be secondary degenerative changes.

Treatment

The initial treatment of osteonecrosis should be conservative with restricted weight bearing, anti-inflammatory medication, and analgesics. Many patients will improve with conservative management. For those who continue to have significant symptoms, orthopaedic referral is indicated for possible surgical intervention. Successful treatment usually requires osteotomy or knee replacement.

BURSITIS

Thirteen bursae have been described about the knee (Fig. 7.25). Of these, five are of particular importance to the primary care clinician. They are the prepatellar bursa that lies between the patella and the skin, the superficial infrapatellar bursa that lies between the lower end of the patellar ligament and the skin, the deep infrapatellar bursa that lies between the lower end of the patellar ligament and the tibia, the anserine bursa that lies between the medial collateral ligament and the pes anserine tendons; and the bursa of the semimembranosus that lies between the semimembranosus tendon and the medial head of the gastrocnemius. This bursa can communicate with the synovial cavity of the knee joint.

Prepatellar and Superficial Infrapatellar Bursitis

The prepatellar and superficial infrapatellar bursae are to the knee what the olecranon bursa is to the elbow. As such, they are ex-posed and vulnerable to trauma. The chronic form of prepatellar bursitis is classically referred to as "housemaid's knee." Thickening of the bursa is seen in patients whose occupations require kneeling, for example, carpet layers. The thickened bursa may not be symptomatic, but on occasion is sensitive. The bursal thickenings may be small, firm, and mobile, giving the feeling of nodules or bone chips. Bursal swelling is usually localized to the prepatellar area and not to the surrounding tissue. Often bursal swelling is initiated by trauma, sometimes trivial. When trauma causes a laceration or abrasion over the bursa it is difficult to differentiate between traumatic or septic bursitis.

Clinical Characteristics. The patient usually presents with localized pain and swelling in the bursa. There is no effusion of the knee itself. There may be tenderness. Patients with chronic bursitis may have mild swelling but little tenderness, and rarely experience extreme pain. A patient with an infected bursa presents with more severe pain, tenderness, and surrounding cellulitis.

Treatment. Chronic forms of bursitis are treated with anti-inflammatory medication. The patient should use padding to avoid repeated trauma. Chronic, recurrent, or persistent bursitis may require excision of the bursa. Acute bursitis is treated with rest,

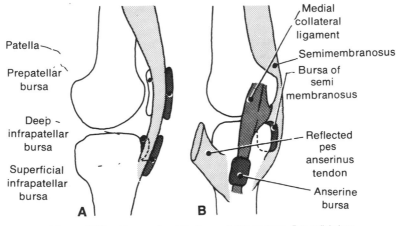

Patella
Prepatellar bursa
Deep infrapatellar bursa
Superficial infrapatellar bursa
A

Medial collateral ligament
Semimembranosus
Bursa of semi membranosus
Reflected pes anserinus tendon
Anserine bursa
B

Figure 7.25. Bursae about the knee. *A*, lateral view. *B*, medial view.

ice, and anti-inflammatory medication. If fluid is present, it can be aspirated. A purulent aspirate indicates a septic bursitis. Both acute and chronic bursitis may respond to cortisone injection, but infection must first be ruled out. Septic bursitis should be treated by incision, drainage, and antibiotics.

Anserine Bursitis

Individuals who are unaccustomed to lengthy, vigorous, weight-bearing exercises may occasionally experience acute inflammation of the anserine bursa.

Clinical Characteristics. Patients usually complain of knee pain that begins following some traumatic episode or unaccustomed weight-bearing exercise. They experience an intense aching pain at rest that becomes worse when resisting extension or flexion. Swelling may be evident, and tenderness is elicited over the pes anserine tendon or just superficial to its tibial attachment.

Pain and tenderness over the anserine bursa must be distinguished from several other conditions, including medial joint line tenderness associated with meniscal derangement or degenerative arthritis of the medial compartment. In the latter conditions, tenderness is localized to the joint line, whereas anserine bursitis causes tenderness below the joint line in the region of the bursa. Osteonecrosis of the tibial plateau or stress fracture of the tibia may be more difficult to distinguish because pain may be in the area of the anserine bursa. X-ray and bone scan are helpful in distinguishing these conditions. Stress fracture usually occurs in association with a history of recent increase in activity. Finally, patients with fibromyalgia may have pain in this area.

Treatment. Instruct the patient to minimize weight-bearing activities and avoid resisted extension (i.e., no climbing, jumping, running, squatting). The patient should apply ice packs over the inflamed bursa four times daily. Quadriceps-setting exercises can begin as soon as pain subsides. When pain

and tenderness are fully remitted, range of motion and full quadriceps exercise can begin. Injecting a depository corticosteroid into the inflamed bursa can result in a dramatic remission. Oral anti-inflammatory agents may be prescribed, but these are less effective than local corticosteroid injection (Chapters 11 and 14).

Baker's Cyst

"Baker's cyst" is a term that is commonly applied to the formation of a swollen bursa posterior to the knee joint. This is most often caused by fluid distention of the bursa between the semimembranosus and medial gastrocnemius, but there are other posterior bursae that can be associated with a Baker's cyst. Because these bursae can communicate with the synovial cavity of the knee joint, they often form because of inflammation and effusion in the knee secondary to intraarticular derangement. Because of this, the physician must rule out medial meniscal tear, degenerative joint disease, and rheumatoid or other arthritides.

Clinical Characteristics. Patients complain of a mass behind the knee that may or may not be slightly tender. If there is an underlying meniscal tear or arthritis, additional symptoms will be present. A fluctuant mass is palpable on the medial side of the popliteal fossa when the patient lies prone with the knee extended. Clear serous fluid is readily aspirated from the cyst, causing the cyst to collapse. X-rays may show evidence of degenerative arthritis.

Treatment. Aspiration not only confirms diagnosis, it removes the mass and usually relieves the patient's symptoms. Patients are often fearful that these masses are malignant tumors. To search for the cause of a chronic knee joint effusion, the examiner must obtain more detail about knee symptoms. Take note of range of motion, test patellar and tibiofemoral stability, examine for meniscus tear, and obtain x-rays for evidence of degenerative arthritis. The physician should perform a review of systems and a general orthopaedic examination, and obtain an erythrocyte sedimentation rate if any points of the history suggest an inflammatory arthritic disorder.

When the underlying disorder is obvious and its treatment is within the limits of primary practice, proceed appropriately. When no underlying disorder can be found or conservative treatment is ineffective, orthopaedic referral should be made.

TENDINITIS

Tendinitis is tendon degeneration without inflammation or with peritendinous inflammation, usually at the area of insertion or at the musculotendinous junction. This condition is probably related to microscopic tears that lead to pain. Repeated tearing results in tendon degeneration and scarring, and the scarred tendon is weaker and subject to rupture. Tendinitis is a common overuse syndrome in athletes.

Patellar Tendinitis

Patellar tendinitis, or "jumper's knee," is a common problem for athletes involved in sports that require jumping. There is pain during activity but often not enough to curtail the activity. There is also pain after activity, usually after sitting for a long period of time. Tenderness is noted at the inferior pole of the patella.

Quadriceps Tendinitis

Quadriceps tendinitis involves the superior pole of the patella at the tendon junction. This type of tendinitis is common for athletes involved in sports that require running, jumping, and acceleration-deceleration activities. Pain and tenderness are noted over the superior pole of the patella.

Iliotibial Tract Tendinitis

The iliotibial tract is a condensation of some of the fibers of the fascia lata. It attaches to Gerdy's tubercle and overlies the lateral epicondyle and fibular collateral ligament. Pain develops from friction between the underlying structures and the iliotibial tract. This is most commonly seen in runners and in patients with an abnormally tight iliotibial tract. The examination reveals tenderness in the lateral epicondylar area that is amplified by pressure over the area as the knee goes through a range of motion.

Popliteus Tendinitis

The popliteus tendon attaches to the lateral aspect of the lateral femoral condyle and runs beneath the fibular collateral ligament. Tendinitis often develops with excessive downhill running, but it can also occur with excessive squatting activities. Tenderness in this area must be differentiated from lateral joint line tenderness associated with lateral meniscus injury.

Treatment

Treatment of tendinitis is nonoperative and should begin with a period of rest. Ice after activity is helpful since it reduces inflammation, and anti-inflammatory medication is also helpful. After pain is relieved by the above methods, the patient should begin to gently stretch the scar tissue, then follow a graduated strengthening program. Cortisone injection into tendon sheaths to reduce inflammation is acceptable, but cortisone injection into the tendon leads to tendon weakness and subsequent rupture.

Traumatic Disorders of the Knee

INJURIES TO THE EXTENSOR APPARATUS (FIG. 7.26)

The quadriceps muscle and tendon, patella, patellar ligament, and patellar retinacula constitute the extensor apparatus. Direct and indirect forces can disrupt the extensor apparatus at the knee.

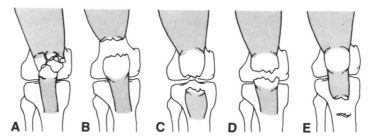

Figure 7.26. Injuries of the extensor apparatus. *A*, comminuted fracture of the patella. *B*, avulsion of the quadriceps tendon. *C*, avulsion of the patellar attachment of the patellar ligament. *D*, transverse fracture of the patella. *E*, avulsion of the tibial attachment of the patellar ligament.

Direct Impact Forces

These forces are typically generated in injuries that occur when an individual falls onto the knee or the knee is otherwise struck.

Direct blows to the quadriceps muscle result in varying degrees of injury. There is always some hemorrhage within the muscle. Tenderness and ecchymosis develop and there may be an associated knee effusion. Tenderness is localized to the area of impact. Contusions of the quadriceps tendon at its insertion on the patella or at the site where it merges with the patellar retinacula are fairly uncommon because the area is not as exposed to impact. These injuries present with an indistinctly circumscribed swelling above the patella that may be associated with fluctuance if bleeding into the suprapatellar bursa has occurred. Pain may inhibit active extension.

Direct blows to the patella can contuse the patellar cartilage or fracture the patella. Such fractures are usually comminuted and may or may not be displaced. The prepatellar bursa is always contused when these injuries occur, causing a hemorrhage into the bursa. Therefore, patients with impact injuries to the patella present with circumscribed swelling over the patella and variable pain on lateral compression and manipulation of the patella. Pain may inhibit active extension.

Direct blows to the insertion of the patellar ligament contuse the superficial infrapatellar bursa and the patellar ligament at its attachment to the tibial tubercle. Patients with these injuries present with an indistinctly circumscribed swelling and tenderness over and just above the tibial tubercle. Pain may inhibit active extension.

Indirect Distracting Forces

When extension is applied with abrupt violence, as can occur when kicking or jumping, the resultant force may strain or rupture the extensor apparatus. Strain is suggested when there is tenderness over the quadriceps tendon or patellar ligament and the anatomy is palpably intact. Rupture is indicated by one of the following clinical pictures.

The quadriceps tendon may be avulsed from its patellar insertion and from its merger with the patellar retinacula. Such an injury is rare and patients having it present with a depression just above the patella, a fluctuant mass about the depression reflecting hemorrhage into the suprapatellar bursa, and an inability to actively extend the knee without a significant extensor lag.

More commonly, the patella may be fractured. The inferior pole may be avulsed with the patellar ligament, or the patella may fracture into two fairly equal pieces. Patients with the injury present with a fluctuant swelling, a palpable disruption of the patella, and an inability to actively extend the knee fully.

The patellar ligament may be avulsed from the inferior pole of the patella. Patients with this injury present with a distinctly circumscribed swelling about the patellar ligament, an elevated patella, a palpable tendon defect when the knee is flexed to 90°, fluctuance above the tibial tubercle when hemorrhage has occurred into the deep infrapatellar bursa, and an inability to actively extend the knee fully.

Any complete disruption of the extensor mechanism, whether patella, ligament, or tendon, prevents full active extension of the knee. However, the patient may be able to lift the leg or have limited extension to *minus* 30° even with the rupture.

As soon as injury to the extensor apparatus is suspected, an x-ray of the knee should be obtained to rule out fracture. This will prevent the examiner from converting an undisplaced fracture to a displaced fracture that may require operative treatment. A tangential view of the patella may show a vertical fracture line, often missed by standard AP and lateral views. However, a tangential view should not be requested if the injury is suspected to have occurred from distraction forces. This view requires that the knee be markedly flexed, which may complete the displacement partially produced by distraction forces.

Treatment

A simple contusion or strain may be treated symptomatically with rest, immobilization, and ice packs until active extension and range of motion are nearly painless. Quadriceps exercises (Fig. 7.27) and weight bearing to the point of tolerable pain can then begin and progress as pain recedes. When the prepatellar bursa is swollen and fluctuant, the bursa should be aspirated.

An undisplaced fracture of the patella with injury to the patellar cartilage should be immobilized in a cylinder cast for 4 to 6 weeks. Weight bearing as tolerated is allowed while the extremity is immobilized.

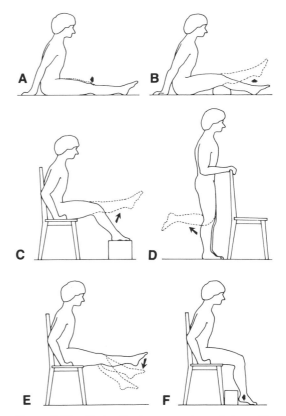

Figure 7.27. Restorative knee exercises. *A*, isometric quadriceps exercise. *B* and *C*, isotonic quadriceps exercises. *D*, gravity-resisted isotonic flexion exercise. *E*, gravity-assisted isotonic flexion exercise. *F*, isometric flexion exercise.

When the immobilization is removed, only partial weight bearing is allowed. The patient should be instructed in active quadriceps exercises, and active range of motion exercises are begun. Progressive weight bearing is allowed as range of motion and quadriceps strength are restored. Full weight bearing is permitted when the patient can walk without pain or limp.

When the extensor apparatus has been ruptured, either through the quadriceps tendon, through the patella, or by an avulsion of a patellar ligament from the inferior pole of the patella, the knee should be splinted in extension and the patient should be referred to an orthopaedist for definitive treatment. Operative repair is usually required.

MENISCAL INJURY

Meniscal injury occurs when rotation of the femur on the tibia exceeds the normal physiologic range, when the normal synchronous internal rotation with flexion or external rotation with extension does not occur, or when excessive axial compressive loads exceed the meniscus strength. For example, consider the fall that occurs with the foot fixed in external rotation. As the individual falls, the knee flexes. Physiologically, this requires internal rotation, but the tibia is held in external rotation. The femoral condyle pushes the meniscus backward. The meniscus is held forward, however, by the medial collateral ligament. The meniscus is subjected to excessive stress and may be torn.

The medial meniscus is injured more frequently than the lateral meniscus because of its anatomy. The medial meniscus is trapped within the concavity of the medial tibial plateau and has more ligamentous tethers. The lateral meniscus is more mobile and can slide posteriorly more easily, thus avoiding the weight bearing of the condyle. The pattern of injury is also different for the medial and lateral menisci, with the medial more likely to sustain longitudinal tears and the lateral more likely to sustain radial tears (Fig. 7.28).

After age 40, a different type of injury occurs to the meniscus. A horizontal splitting occurs as a result of a lifetime of bending, squatting, turning, and twisting. The horizontal lesion is seen in a large percentage of people over the age of 55 and is not necessarily symptomatic. This injury is more common in the medial meniscus and usually occurs at the junction of the middle and posterior one-third.

Clinical Characteristics

Patients complain of pain at the time of injury that usually persists and interferes with weight-bearing activity. Symptoms may subside initially but recurrent episodes with minor stress are common. The pain is usually medial and often posteromedial, in the case of the medial meniscus tear. Lateral meniscal pain is usually along the lateral joint line but may be referred anteriorly or medially.

Effusion may develop, which may be minimal and noted as a feeling of tightness in the knee. If the joint communicates with one of several posterior bursae, swelling may be present in the back of the knee (see "Baker's Cyst"). Cystic swelling at the joint line with meniscal tear is more likely to develop on the lateral side because of the opening of the popliteus recess. Cystic swelling on the medial joint line is rare.

The patient often describes pain or inability to extend the knee fully. This is sometimes termed "locking." It is not true locking in the sense of not being able to move the knee at all, but it is the lack of full extension. Because of the interposition of the meniscus or the interference of the torn meniscus with normal rotation, there is no external rotation in extension. Therefore, the leg does not come into full extension and is considered to be "locked."

Many patients report a feeling of giving way, describing a sense that the knee is going to collapse. While this may occur as a result of a torn meniscus with interposition of meniscal tissue preventing normal rotation, it is a nonspecific symptom. It can also result from pain or from various instabilities of the knee if the femorotibial or patellofemoral surfaces are moving abnormally.

In long-standing meniscal derangement, quadriceps atrophy is common because the

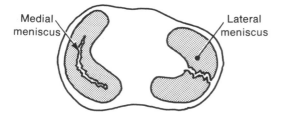

Figure 7.28.   Characteristic orientation of meniscal tears.

pain and swelling inhibit the quadriceps muscle.

Treatment

The knee should be immobilized if there is pain with motion. Painless knee motion does not require immobilization. Crutches should be used if there is swelling and weight bearing is painful. Quadriceps exercises may be initiated, and anti-inflammatory medication and/or analgesics should be provided. A tense effusion should be aspirated. If the knee is locked, manipulation may be attempted with adequate analgesia; rotation in flexion with a valgus stress may unlock the knee. However, it is not always necessary to attempt a manipulation. Spontaneous "unlocking" often occurs with immobilization and the use of analgesics.

While most meniscal tears do not heal, a peripheral tear often does. The knee with a peripheral tear may be immobilized for 4 weeks by medial and lateral splints with the knee flexed at 15° to 20°, or a limited motion brace set to allow motion between 20° and 60°. If the knee remains locked or symptoms of pain, giving way, and swelling persist, orthopaedic referral should be made to consider surgical removal or repair. This can be accomplished arthroscopically. Meniscal injuries with symptoms that can be successfully eliminated by modifying activity and avoiding activities that produce effusion, catching, or giving way do not require surgery. Patients must accept limited activity as return to full activity may reactivate symptoms. If return to activity after symptoms have abated does not cause recurrence of symptoms, then patients may proceed with the activity.

LIGAMENT INJURY

The ligaments are subject to external forces as well as those generated by muscular force. Contact forces occur in sporting events, in motor vehicle accidents, and at work. The history of the injury and the exact mechanism involved are helpful in the evaluation.

Clinical Characteristics

The degree of injury depends on the amount of force and the circumstances of support by muscles. First-degree sprain is a tear of the fibers of the ligament with no demonstrable instability or laxity. Second-degree sprain is a tear of ligamentous fibers with some loss of function but still no noticeable laxity. Third-degree sprain is a gross disruption of the fibers with demonstrable laxity. Within this third-degree injury, there are grades I, II, and III laxity. In grade I third-degree sprain, there is less than 5 mm opening of the joint surface with applied stress. In grade II there is less than 10 mm opening and grade III has greater than 10 mm opening.

All patients complain of pain at the time of injury. With first-degree, second-degree, and grade I third-degree injuries, they are able to walk or even to resume activities. The morning after injury there is moderate stiffness. The physical examination will detect tenderness in the area of the ligament. Either the attachment site or the area along the line of the ligament is tender. Stressing the ligament will cause pain in all and slight laxity in the grade I third-degree injuries.

Patients with grade II third-degree injuries manifest more difficulties and are not likely to continue with their activities. They may have an effusion, which suggests that some of the capsule as well as some of the ligament has been stretched. They will have more laxity on ligament testing.

Grade III third-degree injuries have gross and easily detectable laxity, and there is usually accompanying effusion. The development of ecchymosis in the area of the ligaments suggests a moderate tear with gross laxity. In this case, one should suspect that more than one ligament is involved. Patients may have a knee dislocation if they have grossly unstable ligaments with multidirectional laxity and a history of violent injury. A large percentage of knee dislocations are accompanied by popliteal artery injuries; therefore, vascular consultation and angiography are recommended. X-rays will show no evidence of injury or occasionally a small avulsion fragment from the site of ligament attachment.

Medial Collateral Ligament Injury

The medial collateral ligament is usually injured by a valgus force applied to the lateral aspect of the knee with the foot fixed. It may also be injured by a twisting mechanism. There is tenderness along the line of the ligament or at points of attachment, and grade I, II, or III laxity in the third-degree injuries. In the evaluation of a patient with medial or lateral collateral ligament injury, it is important to assess the presence of injury of the anterior or posterior cruciate ligaments. If cruciate ligament injury is suspected, orthopaedic referral should be obtained. It is also important to recognize that patients with medial (or lateral) instability in extension probably do not have an isolated ligament injury and these patients should also be referred for further evaluation and treatment.

Treatment. Isolated grade I and II injuries, without instability in extension, and without cruciate ligament injury, can be treated nonoperatively. The injured knee should be immobilized with commercially available immobilizers or medial-lateral plaster splints. This lessens pain and reduces strain on the ligament. Immobilization may continue for a period of 7 to 14 days, depending on the degree of injury and pain. As pain subsides, the knee should be mobilized because mobilized ligaments heal with greater strength than continuously immobilized ligaments.

The patient should be placed on crutches with weight bearing as tolerated. Crutches are discontinued when there is no limp with ambulation. Aspiration may be required if there is a tense effusion. Ice should be used to reduce swelling, and analgesics prescribed as necessary. When pain subsides and motion is full, whirlpool and bicycling are encouraged. Straight leg raising in the immobilizer is encouraged, followed by the use of weights when motion returns. The symptoms of a grade I injury may decrease rapidly and be at a point of strengthening in 2 weeks. A more severe injury will take at least 6 weeks before strength returns and the knee gains functional stability.

Grade III injuries can be treated nonoperatively, but because it is often difficult to detect associated injury, an orthopaedic consultation is recommended to assess the need for surgical intervention for these injuries.

Lateral Collateral Ligament Injury

The lateral collateral ligament is injured by a varus force from the medial side of the knee. Because the peroneal nerve travels around the fibular head, any force applied to the inner aspect of the knee may cause stretch of the peroneal nerve. Therefore, with suspected lateral collateral ligament injuries, the function of the peroneal nerve should be assessed at the time of initial examination.

Treatment. Isolated grade I and II third-degree injuries can be treated nonoperatively. As in the case of the medial collateral ligament, however, a grade III injury is best handled by the orthopaedic surgeon. Treatment of grade I and II injuries is the same as for medial collateral ligament injury, with initial immobilization, crutches, and analgesics followed by motion and weight bearing to a point of strengthening.

Anterior Cruciate Ligament Injury

The anterior cruciate ligament may be injured by either varus or valgus force that stretches the medial or lateral ligaments. An anterior cruciate ligament tear can result from a noncontact injury. There is a history of a twisting injury accompanied by a pop or a tearing feeling and a subsequent effusion. With this history and the finding of a hemarthrosis, there is approximately a 70% chance of injury to the anterior cruciate ligament.

The anterior cruciate ligament is the major restraint to anterior translation of the tibia on the femur. The quadriceps muscle antagonizes this restraint as the leg goes into extension. There is strain in the ligament in the last 20° of extension. A violent pull of the quadriceps, as in turning quickly or jumping, may rupture the anterior cruciate ligament. The ligament tightens in internal rotation; therefore, when the leg is forced into internal rotation there is strain on the anterior cruciate. There is also strain in extreme valgus and external rotation, as occurs in skiing, and the anterior cruciate may be injured along with the medial collateral ligament. Hyperextension, as might occur when stepping in a hole, forces the anterior cruciate against the intercondylar notch and may result in a tear.

Clinical Characteristics. The patient with a deficient anterior cruciate ligament falls into one of three categories. The first group is made up of individuals who function satisfactorily without the ligament. This includes some competitive athletes. This group is small, however, comprising less than 20% of the individuals.

Most individuals fall into a second category that requires modification of activities. High-risk activities that involve jumping are not usually possible. Volleyball and basketball are given up, but racquetball and tennis may be played. If the activities of tennis are difficult, the person may further limit activity to a level of bicycling, swimming, and jogging. The routine activities of daily living are done with little difficulty. The patient may have a giving way episode once or twice a year. With increased activity there is a high likelihood of injuring a meniscus, and at some point a giving way episode may be followed by meniscal symptoms that require

meniscal surgery. Some patients will be able to move up in the activity category by use of a stabilizing brace.

In the last category are those individuals who cannot function well without the ligament. These patients are bothered by multiple giving way episodes in the course of daily activities and are significantly limited in sports. A brace may be tried, but does not provide adequate stability and is difficult to use for daily living activity.

After the initial injury, most people fall into one of these categories within a period of 1 to 2 years.

Anterior Cruciate Ligament Examination

With a moderate degree of spasm and effusion the detection of anterior cruciate ligament laxity can be difficult (see also the section "Evaluation of the Patient with Knee Symptoms.") The Lachman test is more sensitive than the anterior drawer test because the anterior drawer may be negated by the pull of the hamstrings or spasm about the knee. The pivot shift test is difficult to elicit in the acutely injured, and even in follow-up examination if the patient learns to protect the knee and use the muscles to prevent subluxation of the tibia. X-rays usually do not provide evidence of injury; however, the finding of avulsion from the lateral tibial plateau (Segond fracture) is pathognomonic of an anterior cruciate ligament tear.

Treatment. Because of the difficulty in detecting anterior cruciate ligament injuries, in separating symptoms of instability from meniscal symptoms, and in determining need for reconstruction, the treatment of these injuries should be supervised by an orthopaedist. The treatment of acute anterior cruciate injury depends on the severity of injury. Patients with suspected injury or partial tear, i.e., hemarthrosis and consistent history but without significant demonstrable instability, may have a tense hemarthrosis requiring aspiration. The knee may be immobilized for comfort. Crutches should be used for non-weight bearing, or partial weight bearing if tolerated without pain. Follow-up examination should be at 5 to 7 days, and if laxity secondary to anterior cruciate ligament injury is not detected, quadriceps exercises may be initiated and the knee and leg rehabilitated. For patients with demonstrable instability but without associated meniscal, collateral ligament, or posterior cruciate ligament injury, the knee should be immobilized for comfort and crutches provided for the patient. Since the torn anterior cruciate ligament is not likely to heal, quadriceps setting may be initiated. Patients with associated ligament injury and/or meniscal injury should be referred immediately to an orthopaedist as surgical intervention may be necessary.

To rehabilitate the leg with anterior cruciate injury, quadriceps exercises are initiated first. More vigorous exercises, with progressive strengthening of the quadriceps and hamstring muscles, are initiated when swelling subsides and range of motion returns. Recovery from an initial episode may take 6 to 8 weeks. If there is not sufficient recovery in this time to allow the patient to ambulate or if swelling is not reduced, the patient should be examined for meniscal injury. Meniscal symptoms may develop in the first 6 months after injury; meniscal injury will require treatment.

If a patient successfully rehabilitates with strength equal to or better than the uninjured leg, a brace may be applied. The patient is allowed to return to sports, and will then find the appropriate level of activity and make necessary modifications according to life-style.

The patient who continues to have difficulties in the activities of daily living and is not engaged in any sporting activity, and the patient who has difficulties in the brace with absence of any meniscal injury, become candidates for reconstruction of the ligament. Those persons who are professional or competitive athletes may not want to wait for 1 year to find the category into which they will fall, and should be considered for immediate reconstruction.

Posterior Cruciate Ligament Injury

The posterior cruciate ligament is often injured by a force that is applied to the anterior portion of the tibia, as in a dashboard injury. The ligament may also be injured from medial or lateral forces that injure other ligaments.

Treatment. The posterior cruciate is considered a prime stabilizer of the knee; early operation on gross instability of the posterior cruciate ligament, particularly if accompanied by medial or lateral collateral ligament injuries, yields better results than nonoperative management. Avulsion of the ligament with a bony fragment is best treated by open reduction and fixation. Isolated grade I and II third-degree injury is compatible with normal life activities and can usually be treated nonoperatively. Because of the significant instability, the knee should be evaluated by an orthopaedic surgeon.

FRACTURES
Fractures of the Shaft of the Femur

Fractures of the shaft of the femur are life-threatening injuries. They are typically accompanied by considerable bleeding into the thigh and hypovolemia. The violent forces required to produce them may impact directly on the surface of the thigh, or may apply torque or angulation to the thigh. Like hip dislocations, femur fractures occur most commonly in motor vehicle accidents. These fractures are nearly always complete and markedly displaced, with overriding, angulation, and rotation of the distal segment on the proximal. Fractures may be transverse, oblique, spiral, or comminuted, and may be simple or compound.

Clinical Characteristics. Patients with fractures of the shaft of the femur often have other injuries. They may develop evidence of circulatory insufficiency shortly after injury. These patients do not move the extremity and, if conscious, complain of intense thigh pain that usually refers throughout the extremity. The thigh is swollen, and the portion of the extremity below the fracture site may be rotated and angulated. Tenderness, false motion, and crepitation are evident at the fracture site. Anteroposterior and lateral x-rays of the thigh will identify the fracture.

Treatment.   The patient must be quickly assessed for other injuries. Hypovolemic circulatory failure must be treated (see Chapter 1). The fracture must be splinted, preferably with a Thomas-type splint (see Chapter 10). Traction improves alignment and stability.

An orthopaedist should be responsible for definitive treatment of the fracture.

Fractures of the Tibial Condyles

The same forces that tear the collateral ligaments can fracture the contralateral tibial plateau, as well as tear the ipsilateral meniscus (Fig. 7.29). The lateral tibial plateau is fractured more commonly than the medial. Until they tear, the stressed ligaments act as a tension band directing compressive forces onto the opposite tibial plateau. If the bone is less resilient than the ligaments, it will fracture before the ligaments tear. Osteoporotic individuals are more likely to suffer plateau fractures than torn ligaments. Com-

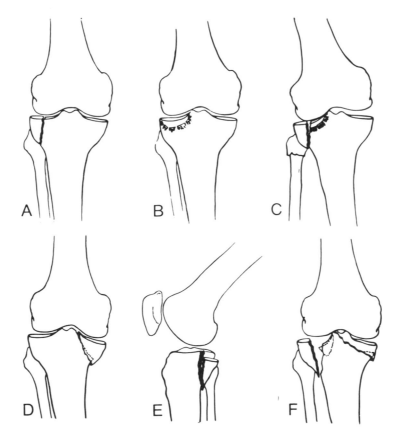

Figure 7.29.   Hohl classification of fractures of the condylar end of the tibia. *A*, undisplaced. *B*, local compression. *C*, split compression. *D*, total condylar compression. *E*, split. *F*, comminuted. (From Sisk TD. Fractures of the lower extremity. In: Crenshaw AH, ed. Campbell's operative orthopaedics, vol 3. 7th ed. St. Louis: CV Mosby Co, 1987:1654; and Hohl, M. Tibial condylar fractures. J Bone Joint Surg 1967;49A:1456.)

monly, they are women who fall from steps or ladders.

Clinical Characteristics. All patients with fractures of the tibial condyle complain of pain immediately at the time of injury. Pain persists and prevents weight bearing. Within the first few hours after injury, the joint capsule becomes tense with a hemarthrosis. The fractured condyle is tender and any manipulation that compresses that side of the joint causes an increase in pain. Ligaments on the opposite side of the joint may or may not be tender. X-ray will reveal the plateau fracture. A neurovascular examination should be performed as fractures of the tibial plateau may be associated with neurovascular injury. The peroneal nerve is particularly vulnerable. This injury is often associated with a fracture of the proximal fibula accompanying a tibial plateau fracture.

Treatment. Initial treatment should include arthrocentesis if there is a tense hemarthrosis. Fractures should be splinted in full extension. If the patient is not comfortable in full extension, however, this position should not be forced. Orthopaedic referral is recommended for definitive evaluation and treatment of these intraarticular fractures. If this is unavailable, minimally displaced fractures can be managed by the experienced primary care practitioner. Nonoperative treatment can be considered if there is no significant depression of the joint surface, less than 3 mm of separation or depression at the fracture line, and no associated collateral or cruciate ligament rupture.

A variety of treatment methods are appropriate for these minimally displaced fractures. In very reliable patients, a long-leg splint can be applied in full extension. The patient is placed on crutches and continues nonweight bearing until healing is evident. Isometric exercise can be carried out in the splint, then at 10 to 14 days the splint can be discontinued for active range of motion exercise. For less reliable patients, a long-leg or

cylinder cast is applied for 3 weeks, then range of motion is begun. Another method is to apply a cast brace primarily. This protects the fracture from compressive force but allows range of motion to the knee. (See Chapter 10 for details of cast technique.) In these injuries, healing usually occurs in 8 to 12 weeks. Weight bearing should be delayed until that time.

If the fracture line is displaced or depressed more than 3 mm, orthopaedic referral should be obtained for definitive evaluation and treatment. These fractures often require open reduction. The goal of treatment is to restore an anatomic joint surface, repair ligament injuries, and progress with early range of motion. Successful accomplishment of these goals reduces the risk of posttraumatic arthritis.

The intimate anatomic relationship between the condylar ends of the femur and tibia, and the sciatic nerve and popliteal vessels exposes these neurovascular structures to injury when there is juxtaarticular fracture of the knee. In addition, these fractures superficially resemble any of the other causes of a hemarthrosis. Thus, the primary care practitioner must consider this injury when evaluating a traumatic hemarthrosis because an unwary manipulation could result in displacement of an undisplaced fracture or neurovascular injury.

Fractures of the Condylar End of the Femur

These fractures usually result from an axial compression force with or without an angulatory force. The fractures in adults are of four kinds. Figure 7.30, *A* and *B*, shows fractures of the medial or lateral femoral condyle. The axial compression force, when accompanied by an angulatory force, usually fractures the condyle on the side of the angulation. Figure 7.30, *C* and *D*, shows T- or Y-shaped intracondylar fractures of the femur. Straight axial compression forces may fracture both condyles at once, driving

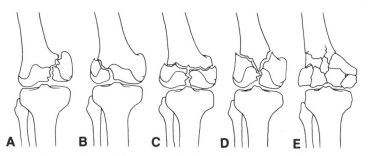

Figure 7.30. Fractures of the condylar end of the femur. *A*, fracture of the medial condyle. *B*, fracture of the lateral condyle. *C*, T-shaped intracondylar fracture. *D*, Y-shaped intracondylar fracture. *E*, comminuted fracture.

them proximally to each side of the femur. Figure 7.30*E* shows a comminuted fracture.

Clinical Characteristics. Except in the severely osteoporotic patient, the injuring forces are violent. Patients with these fractures complain of pain immediately at the moment of injury and are unable to bear weight. All patients with these injuries present with a tense hemarthrosis; some present with shortening or an angular deformity. The condylar end of the femur is severely tender. Firm palpation will often elicit bony crepitation. Evidence of neurovascular injury may be present. Anteroposterior and lateral x-rays of the knee will identify the fracture.

Treatment. The reduction must be precise. Any disturbance of the normal orientation of the condyles to one another will disrupt the joint mechanism, thus decreasing range of motion and increasing wear on the articular surfaces. Vascular injury requires immediate repair to avoid ischemic necrosis below the knee. An orthopaedist and perhaps a vascular surgeon must assume responsibility for treatment. The primary care practitioner should facilitate the treatment goals as follows. Assume every hemarthrosis is a fracture of the condylar end of the femur (or tibia) until proven otherwise. Examine sciatic nerve and vascular function whenever the distal end of the femur is tender or crepitant. If a neurovascular injury is evident, notify a vascular surgeon and/or an orthopaedist at once, and begin preparations for surgery. When neu-

rovascular function is intact, refer the patient to an orthopaedist and apply a long-leg splint (see Chapter 10). Ensure that neurovascular function is monitored until arrival of the orthopaedist.

Epiphyseal Fractures

Children and adolescents may sustain fractures of the distal femoral or proximal tibial epiphyses. Patients with these fractures may present with stable or unstable injuries. Injuries that produce ligament damage in the mature person may produce epiphyseal injury in the immature person. Fractures occur because the epiphysis is weaker than the ligament. Therefore, when stressing ligaments during an examination, be aware that opening may take place at the epiphyseal line and not as the result of ligament laxity. Stress x-ray will determine whether this is a ligamentous injury or a displacement through the epiphysis. Displaced fractures at either epiphysis may have accompanied popliteal artery injury. These injuries should be referred to an orthopaedist.

INJURY OF THE PATELLOFEMORAL ARTICULATION

To support body weight in the many activities of bipedal locomotion, tremendous force is exerted through the extensor mechanism of the knee. The patella is a sesamoid bone embedded in the quadriceps tendon. It enlarges the surface area of the tendon and increases its efficiency by shifting the line of pull of the muscle anteriorly. This improves leverage of the quadriceps in extending the knee. The patella also provides a cartilage-on-cartilage low coefficient of friction for a smooth glide of the quadriceps and maintains the tendon in a centralized track.

The large force needed to attain upright stance produces a large reaction force between the patella and its femoral articulation (Fig. 7.31). The patellofemoral joint reaction force increases as the knee is flexed and is least at full extension. The force across the patellofemoral articulation in stair climbing may be three to five times body weight, and a tremendous force is generated in squat exercises with heavy weights on the shoulder. To meet these demands, the articular cartilage on the undersurface of the patella is the thickest in the body.

The patella does not track in a straight line or have contact on the same surfaces throughout the range of motion. At full extension, the patella lies above the trochlea. Within 10° to 30° of flexion, the normal tibial internal rotation pulls the patella into the trochlea. By 60°, the midportion of the patella and midportion of the trochlea are in contact, and at 90°, the proximal portion of

the patella and the distal portion of the trochlea are in contact (Fig. 7.32).

These dynamic relationships also accommodate the normal valgus vector of the extensor mechanism. Because of the position of the hips, upright stance requires a valgus position of the knee joint. As a result of this angulation, there is a valgus vector to the muscles. The force of the body tends to bow the knee outward and this is resisted by the lateral musculature and the architecture of the trochlea and patella: the vastus lateralis muscle is stronger than the medialis, and the

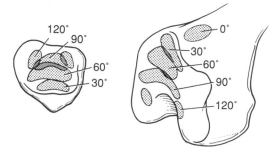

Figure 7.32. Contact areas from extension to flexion. (Adapted from Aglietti P, Insall JN, Walker PS, Trent P. A new patella prosthesis: design and application. Clin Orthop 1975;107:179.)

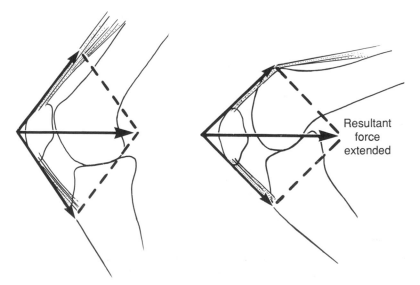

Figure 7.31. Reaction force across the patellofemoral joint increases with knee flexion. (Adapted from Ficat RP, Hungerford DS. Disorders of the patellofemoral joint. Baltimore: Williams & Wilkins, 1977:24.)

lateral portion of the trochlea and the lateral segment of the patella are larger than the medial.

The common problems with the patellofemoral mechanism result when these normal relationships and biomechanics are disturbed (Fig. 7.33). They can be subdivided into problems of stability, in which there is muscle insufficiency or exaggeration of the normal valgus alignment with excessive lateral pull; problems in which there is excessive force across the patellofemoral joint; or a combination of the above.

Examination of the Patellofemoral Articulation

When examining a patient with an injured patellofemoral articulation, it is important to differentiate the areas of pain. The pain associated with patellar problems is usually caused by peripatellar synovitis or synovial plica, which must be differentiated from medial joint line pain. Often, anterior swelling and inflammation extends to the anterior portion of the meniscus and may create symptoms mimicking meniscal derangement. This occurs when the swelling

impinges on the anterior meniscus as the knee is extended. Lateral knee pain may also be present. This is due to lateral synovitis, extension of the anterior swelling laterally, or hypertrophy of the lateral patellofemoral ligament. There is often palpable hypertrophy at the lateral patellotibial ligament. This may be tender or there may be tenderness at the insertion of the vastus lateralis at the superior patella. Some patients will have atrophy or actual dysplasia of the vastus medialis.

As noted above, the alignment of the femur and the arrangement of the muscle attaching to the tibia through the patella have a valgus angle. This is the quadriceps angle (Q angle). The Q angle is determined by measuring the angle formed by a line through the center of the patella and femur, and a line from the center of the patella through the tibial tubercle (Fig. 7.33). This does not exceed 15° in the normal individual.

Tightness in the lateral retinaculum can be demonstrated by attempting to lift the patella by the lateral edge. Inability to level the patella suggests tightness (Fig. 7.34). With the lateral structure held taut, palpate the lateral patellotibial and lateral patellofemoral ligaments (Fig. 7.35).

Observe the tracking of the patella from extension to flexion with the patient sitting. Normally the patella is positioned laterally in extension and at 10° of flexion, and by 30° of flexion should have moved medially into the trochlear groove. A patella that stays lateral through flexion is abnormal. A patella that starts laterally, becomes medial, then goes back to lateral (a C-shaped route) also is abnormal. When the patella goes from flexion to extension, there is a gentle lateral excursion at the end; an abrupt lateral excursion suggests abnormality. Swelling may be evident in the peripatellar soft tissue, but effusion is rare except in dislocation. In patients with recurrent subluxation or dislocation, there is apprehension with patellar

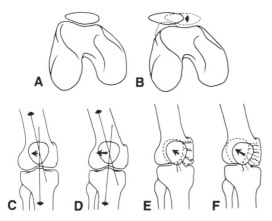

Figure 7.33. Anatomic peculiarities predisposing to recurrent patellar dislocation. *A*, normal, distal end of femur. *B*, flat anterior eminence of the lateral condyle. *C*, normal lateral vector during active extension. *D*, excessive lateral vector. *E*, normal medial retinaculum. *F*, lax medial retinaculum.

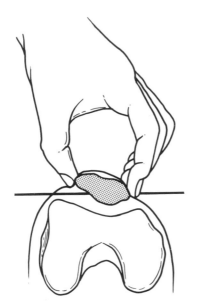

Figure 7.34. Testing for lateral tightness. (Adapted from Rosenberg TD, Kolowich PA. Complications of lateral retinacular release. In: Sprague III NF, ed. Complications in arthroscopy. New York: Raven Press, Ltd, 1989:146.)

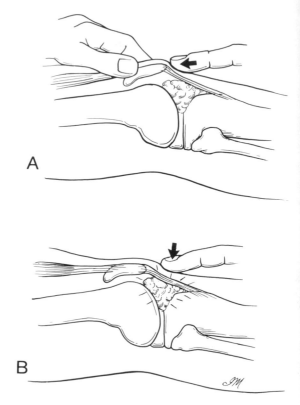

A

B

Figure 7.36. A, holding the patella and tilting it up isolates the patellar ligament and inferior pole of the patella from fat pad and synovium that may be tender. B, direct pressure over the ligament may elicit pain that is from the synovium and not the ligament.

motion, especially if a lateral push is applied to the knee cap.

Confusion can result when differentiating patellar tendinitis and fat pad synovitis. Direct pressure over the tendon will also contact the fat pad. It is helpful to isolate the tip of the patella by pressing on the superior patella and quadriceps tendon (Fig. 7.36), thereby lifting the inferior pole of the patella and palpating the patella at adjacent ten-

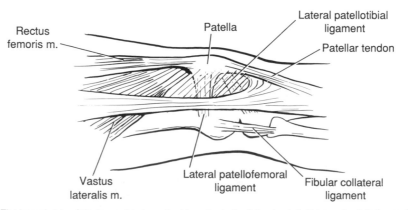

Figure 7.35. The lateral side of the knee. It is important to palpate the lateral patellotibial and patellofemoral ligament and the insertion of the vastus lateralis for their presence, tightness, and possible source of pain.

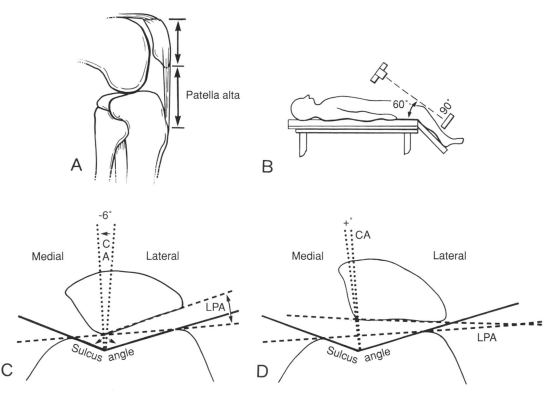

Figure 7.37. *A*, patella alta. *B*, X-ray beam directed across the top of the patella with varied angles to view the patella and trochlea. (Adapted from Carson WG Jr, James SL, Larson RL, Singer KM, Winternitz WW. Patellofemoral disorders: physical and radiographic evaluation. Part II. Radiographic examination. Clin Orthop 1984;185:182.) *C* and *D*, the lateral patellofemoral angle (LPA) is formed by a line on the femoral sulcus and a line on the lateral facet. An angle open laterally is normal (*C*) and a parallel or angle open medially suggests subluxation (*D*). The congruence angle (CA) is determined by a line bisecting the sulcus and a line drawn from the lowest point on the patella. The normal CA is $-6° \pm 11°$ (*C*). The sulcus angle is the angle of the trochlear surface measured from the highest point on the medial and lateral trochlea to the lowest midtrochlear point. The normal sulcus angle is 137° (*C*). (Adapted from Ficat RP, Hungerford DS. Disorders of the patellofemoral joint. Baltimore: Williams & Wilkins, 1977:46; Merchant AC, Mercer RL, Jacobsen RH, Cool CR. Roentgenographic analysis of patellofemoral congruence. J Bone Joint Surg 1974;56A:1395; and Laurin CA, Levesque HP, Dussault R, Labelle H, Peides JP. The abnormal lateral patellofemoral angle: A diagnostic roentgenographic sign of recurrent patellar subluxation. J Bone Joint Surg 1978;60A:58.)

dons rather than exerting pressure down on the fat pad.

X-rays in the lateral and skyline (tangential) projection are helpful in evaluating patellofemoral problems. On the lateral view, patella alta, a patellar tendon that is longer than the patella, can be determined by measuring the length of the patellar tendon and comparing this to the length of the patella. Any value over a 1.2:1 ratio may be considered patella alta (Fig. 7.37*A*). Skyline x-rays should be taken at 15°, 30°, 45°, and 60° to see the relationship between the patella and femur in varying degrees of flexion because abnormal tracking may be missed on a single view (Fig. 7.37*B*). These views will demonstrate lateral subluxation or abnormal tilt of the patella, and also dysplasia of the patella or trochlear groove. Various measurements are determined to demonstrate abnormal patella tilt or an incongruent articulation (Fig. 7.37*C,D*).

Instability of the Patella

Instability of the patellofemoral mechanism is usually associated with excessive lateral pull. In the mildest forms this may produce occasional momentary subluxation of the patella. In its most severe form, chronic recurrent or persistent dislocation of the patella may be seen. There is another group of patients in whom it is not possible to diagnose clear subluxation or malalignment, although many of these patients have other characteristic clinical signs that indicate their anterior knee pain is in fact secondary to functional instability of the patella.

Dislocation of the Patella

Some patients who suffer a dislocation of the patella do so as a result of a major acute injury, such as a direct impact on the patella driving it laterally. These patients may have no underlying anatomic abnormalities. Many patients, however, have one or more anatomic abnormalities that predispose to patella dislocation.

Certain patients with patellar dislocation have Q angles in excess of 20°. Some individuals, however, have Q angles greater than 20° and an otherwise normal mechanism and alignment, and may function well. The presence of a Q angle greater than 20° accompanied by excessive external rotation at the tibia and increased internal rotation at the hip is generally referred to as malicious malalignment, and patients with this condition more commonly have patellar dislocation. In patella alta, the increased length of the patellar tendon is inherently unstable as it allows the patella greater medial-lateral translation. It also allows the patella to ride high in the trochlea, where it is somewhat flatter, or even above the trochlea of the femur. Patients with a shallow trochlear groove or small, flat patella have substantially increased chance of dislocation. Finally, atrophy or dysplasia of the vastus medialis muscle also increases the relative strength of the lateral musculature and this can predispose to lateral subluxation.

Clinical Characteristics. Dislocation is manifested during a sudden motion, usually creating a valgus external rotation force. The patella slides over the lateral femoral condyle. The patella may spontaneously reduce or may be reduced by gradual extension of the leg. There is an accompanying moderate hemarthrosis. If the patient presents with a relocated patella and a moderate hemarthrosis, the history and appearance may suggest an anterior cruciate ligament injury, and medial tenderness may suggest medial collateral ligament injury. Tenderness that is localized to the medial or lateral patella and apprehension with lateral patella push should suggest patella dislocation. Anteroposterior and varus/valgus instability is absent. X-rays may show avulsion fractures from the medial patella, which usually do not require surgery. There may also be lateral femoral condylar fractures, and patients with these fractures should be referred to an orthopaedic surgeon.

Treatment. A tense hemarthrosis should be aspirated and the leg immobilized. With dislocation, quadriceps atony is common and it is difficult to begin quadriceps setting and isometric exercise until 1 to 2 weeks after injury. Immobilization for 2 weeks allows for some early healing of the medial retinaculum. After 2 weeks, quadriceps setting exercises can be initiated, and motion out of the immobilizer can be started if there is no pain with motion. Patients will continue to need the immobilizer for support because the quadriceps usually will not gain sufficient strength for independent activity until 6 weeks. Thereafter, quadriceps development is important. An acute dislocation does not require surgery unless the patella cannot be maintained in an anatomic position or loose bodies are present that could cause derangement of the joint.

Subluxation of the Patella

Subluxations occur with the same mechanism as dislocations. They are accompanied by a pop and some swelling, but not as severe as with a dislocation. Symptoms are compatible with continued activities or at least with walking. Treatment is the same; however, rehabilitation is shorter, swelling subsides after 1 week, and quadriceps strength returns by 4 to 6 weeks.

Some patients with a history of subluxation or dislocation and x-ray findings of patella dislocation may develop degeneration. This is called permanent subluxation. The patient experiences lateral knee pain when sitting and climbing stairs. Examination shows lateral patellar tenderness and tightness, and may show evidence of malalignment. X-ray will show degenerative changes in addition to changes of subluxation. Definitive treatment requires surgical intervention. In some patients adequate symptomatic relief can be achieved with relief of aggravating activity and the use of anti-inflammatory medication.

Anterior Knee Pain without Subluxation

The same valgus forces that produce subluxation may in some patients simply produce peripatellar knee pain. This has a more insidious onset and is usually related to athletic activities that involve turning, twisting, or running.

Clinical Characteristics. Pain usually occurs after the event or during the event, but allows the athlete to continue playing. The history may be that of the athlete having difficulties for long periods of time, but not severe enough to stop participation. There may be an acute episode in a quick turn. Often the symptoms are intermittent or only related to a certain sport. Effusion is uncommon, but there may be a feeling of swelling medially in the patella and fat pad area.

Pain with these episodes is related to the pull on the medial soft tissues by the lateral force, resulting in inflammation. In many instances, there is an associated synovial plica that is trapped between the patella and femur or against the medial femoral condyle. In other instances, the fat pad attached to the plica is pinched in the same area. The episode may not require medical treatment, but the condition may progress. The patient can continue to participate in sports after a brief period of rest.

Occasionally, symptoms are present with activities of daily living. Patients manifest difficulties in going up and down stairs, kneeling or squatting, and occasionally turning and twisting. They have crepitus in the knee and giving way. Crepitus in these instances usually comes from the swollen soft tissue. These patients may have some of the characteristics of dislocation. They may have hypermobility, some degree of vastus medialis dysplasia or underdevelopment compared with the lateralis, or tightness in the lateral retinaculum.

In those patients whose anterior knee pain and soft tissue swelling are caused by a direct blow, as in a fall or dashboard injury, there may be no manifestation of malalignment or dysplasia.

Treatment. Ice should be used after athletic events, and anti-inflammatory medications may be used for moderate symptoms. A period of rest is advisable if there is difficulty participating in sports. Patients should avoid activities that cause irritation, such as bending, squatting, and stair climbing. They should initiate a period of stretching the hamstrings and quadriceps muscles, especially when the symptoms occur at the time of the adolescent growth spurt. Quadriceps muscle strengthening exercises are important for developing the medialis muscle and maintaining a better muscular balance for the patella. This program is usually successful. Patellar bracing providing pressure to resist lateral subluxation may also be helpful. If after 6 months of nonoperative treatment or a long period of intermittent problems the patient still has pain with daily activity and is not able to participate in sports or exercise, evaluation by arthroscopy is indicated. Orthopaedic referral should be made.

Chondromalacia

As noted previously, there can be a large force across the patella in activities such as running or stair climbing. Cartilage that is subject to too much or too little force is likely to soften, producing the lesion known as chondromalacia. Chondromalacia can occur as the result of a direct blow, when a plica rubs against the medial inferior patella, or when high pressure is generated by doing squats with heavy weights. Chondromalacia can also occur in association with recurrent subluxation or dislocation or as a result of an isolated dislocation with damage to the cartilage surface. The softening may produce crepitus. The pain of chondromalacia is related to soft tissue inflammation and is usually peripatellar. Pain involving the patella itself does not become manifest until the cartilage is completely worn and there is bone-to-bone apposition between the patella and trochlea.

Excessive Lateral Pressure Syndrome

People who do not have full excursion of the patella can develop a lateral tightness that holds the patella tightly in the trochlea. Degeneration develops laterally on the patella and trochlea. There is no evidence of subluxation. This syndrome is called excessive lateral pressure syndrome.

This condition is characterized by lateral knee pain when sitting and climbing stairs.

Female patients are more commonly affected. Examination shows lateral patellar tenderness and tightness. X-ray changes will show lateral sclerosis and narrowing. As pain increases, the quadriceps weaken and degeneration extends into the medial and lateral compartments, resulting in complete degeneration.

Treatment of Chondromalacia and Excessive Lateral Pressure Syndrome

The problems occurring from chondromalacia or excessive lateral pressure syndrome may be alleviated by removing the source of pressure. This may be accomplished by discontinuing heavy weight lifting, or modifying the work environment to avoid climbing stairs and squatting. If symptoms persist despite force modification and use of anti-inflammatory medication, the patient should be referred to an orthopaedist.

SUGGESTED READINGS

Ewing JW, ed. Articular cartilage and knee joint function: Basic science and arthroscopy. New York: Raven Press, 1988.

Fulkerson JP, Hungerford DS. Disorders of the patellofemoral joint. Baltimore: Williams & Wilkins, 1990.

Insall JN. Surgery of the knee. New York: Churchill Livingstone, 1984.

Muller W. The knee—form, function, and ligament reconstruction. Berlin: Springer-Verlag, 1982.

CHAPTER 8

Leg and Ankle

Anthony K. Teebagy, M.D.

Essential Anatomy
BONES, JOINTS, AND LIGAMENTS
Tibia and Fibula and Their Articulations

The tibia and fibula are bound together proximally through a synovial joint called the tibiofibular articulation. This joint is located approximately 1 cm distal to the posterolateral joint line of the knee. The joint is reinforced by strong anterior and posterior ligaments.

Distally the tibia and fibula are joined through the tibiofibular syndesmosis. This is a ligamentous complex made up of the anterior inferior tibiofibular ligament and the posterior inferior tibiofibular ligament with the interosseous membrane (Fig. 8.1). These ligaments allow slight motion at both joints. The interosseus membrane joins the tibia to the fibula throughout the entire length of the fibula. The two bones, along with the interosseus membrane, form the anatomic barrier that separates the posterior compartments of the leg from the anterior and lateral compartments.

Ankle Joint

The distal tibia and fibula form a box-like frame that is commonly termed the "mortise." Following this carpentry terminology, the anatomic tenon is the dome of the talus, which fits into the mortise made up of the fibula and tibia (Fig. 8.2). Unlike a normal mortise and tenon joint, the ankle is not rigidly stable throughout its range of motion. Because the talus is wider anteriorly than posteriorly, the ankle is more stable in dor-

siflexion than in a plantar flexion. One of the best x-ray views of the ankle joint is the so-called "mortise view." This is done with the ankle in slight internal rotation and most clearly demonstrates the box-like configuration of the ankle joint (Fig. 8.3). The ankle joint is surrounded by a fibrous and synovial capsule.

There are several important stabilizing ligaments of the ankle. The syndesmotic lig-

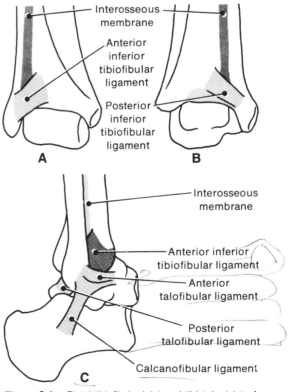

Figure 8.1. Distal tibiofibular joint and tibiotalar joint. *A,* anterior view. *B,* posterior view. *C,* lateral view.

231

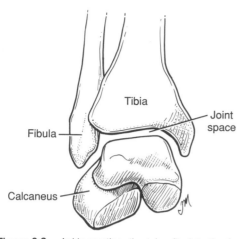

Figure 8.2. Ankle mortise; the talus fits into the frame comprised of the tibia and fibula.

amentous complex has been described above. It is responsible for maintaining the width of the mortise. When these ligaments are torn, the mortise widens and the talus becomes unstable. The deltoid ligament is a strong fan-shaped ligament medially. There are three lateral ligaments: the anterior and posterior talofibular ligaments and the calcaneofibular ligament (Fig. 8.1). The degree to which these ligaments are torn determines the degree of talar instability. Motion within the ankle joint is largely in the dorsiflexion, plantar flexion range. With disruption of specific ligaments, the ankle becomes unstable. This can be demonstrated by abnormally increased motion to abduction (eversion), adduction (inversion), or anterior stress.

Growth of the leg occurs at both ends of the tibia and fibula. Approximately 55% of the growth of the lower leg occurs at the proximal end of the bone and the remaining 45% at the distal end (Fig. 8.4). Any abnormality or injury that involves the growth plates should be referred to an orthopaedic surgeon as angular or length deformities may result.

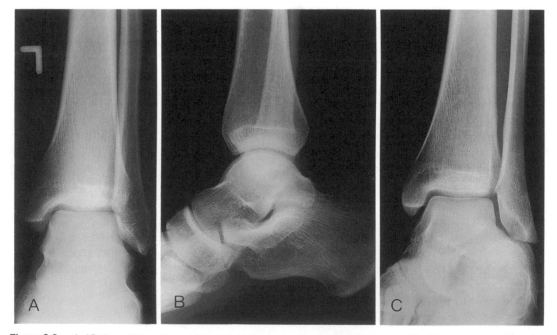

Figure 8.3. *A,* AP view of the ankle; overlap on the lateral aspect is a normal appearance. The lateral process of the talus is well seen. *B,* lateral view of the ankle; note the congruency of the distal tibia and the talar dome. *C,* mortise view of the ankle; note the symmetry of the joint space and the frame formed around the talus by the tibia and fibula. This film is taken with the ankle internally rotated 15°. An asymmetric joint space is abnormal and represents injury to the ankle ligaments.

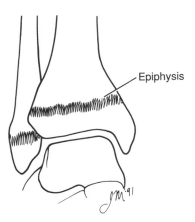

Figure 8.4. Location of growth plate at the distal tibia and fibula. Any suspected injury to the growth plate should be referred to an orthopaedic surgeon.

NEUROMUSCULAR ORGANIZATION
Muscle Compartments of the Leg

The bones and muscles of the leg are surrounded by a strong fascial sheath called the crural fascia. This fascial sheath is densely adherent to the tibia anteromedially and loosely adherent to muscles posteriorly. Fibrous septi that extend inward from the crural fascia and the interosseus membrane divide the leg into four compartments. These are the anterior compartment, the lateral compartment, the deep posterior compartment, and the superficial posterior compartment (Fig. 8.5). Contained within these compartments are various muscles, nerves, and blood vessels (Fig. 8.6). These compartments are relatively closed and because of the stout fascial envelope, increased pressure within these compartments caused by bleeding or posttraumatic edema can lead to necrosis of the structures within the compartment.

Nerves of the Leg

The sciatic nerve divides into two major nerve trunks above the popliteal fossa: the common peroneal nerve and the tibial nerve. The common peroneal nerve travels across the lateral head of the gastrocnemius and along the medial border of the biceps tendon, then curves laterally below the head of the fibula across the fibular neck. At about that point the common peroneal nerves divide into the superficial and deep peroneal nerves. The common peroneal nerve is securely fixed as it comes around the neck of the fibula. This fact, combined with its superficial location, render it prone to injury by a variety of mechanisms, including trauma

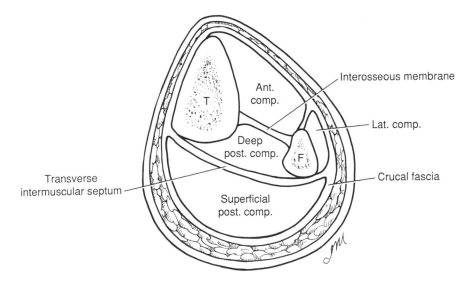

Figure 8.5. Cross-section of the leg: crural fascia and septa which divide the leg into four compartments.

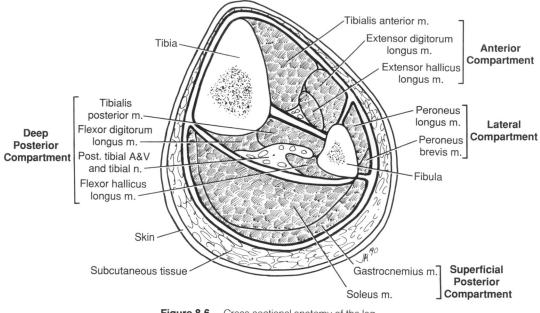

Figure 8.6. Cross-sectional anatomy of the leg.

to the proximal leg, especially on the lateral side, and pressure from tight casts or bandages about the knee. After branching, the superficial peroneal nerve travels to the lateral compartment, and the deep peroneal nerve to the anterior compartment. The tibial nerve passes medially between the two femoral attachments of the gastrocnemius muscle and continues distally into the deep posterior compartment. After branching, these nerves share the cutaneous innervation of the leg and foot (Figs. 8.7 and 8.8).

Muscles of the Leg and Their Innervations

The muscles of the anterior compartment are the dorsiflexors of the ankle and toes (Fig. 8.9A). They are all innervated by the deep peroneal nerve. These muscles include the tibialis anterior, the extensor hallucis longus, the extensor digitorum longus, and the peroneus tertius. The tendon of the tibialis anterior crosses the anteromedial aspect of the ankle to insert on the plantar surface of the medial cuneiform and base of the first

metatarsal. It functions as a powerful dorsiflexor of the ankle. The tendon of the extensor hallucis longus crosses the ankle just lateral to the tendon of the anterior tibialis and passes distally to insert on the dorsum of the base of the distal phalanx of the great toe. As its name implies, it extends the distal phalanx of the great toe. The extensor digitorum longus and the peroneus tertius share a common origin and separate as they become tendinous. They cross the anterolateral aspect of the ankle together. The peroneus tertius inserts on the dorsum of the base of the fourth and fifth metatarsals, and it acts as a weak ankle extensor. The extensor digitorum longus divides into four tendons, one to each of the lesser four toes, and functions to extend the distal phalanx of the lesser toes.

The muscles of the lateral compartment are the peroneus longus and peroneus brevis (Fig. 8.9B). They are pronators of the foot and evertors of the hindfoot. Both are innervated by the superficial peroneal nerve. They originate from the lateral surface of the fibula and pass as separate tendons around

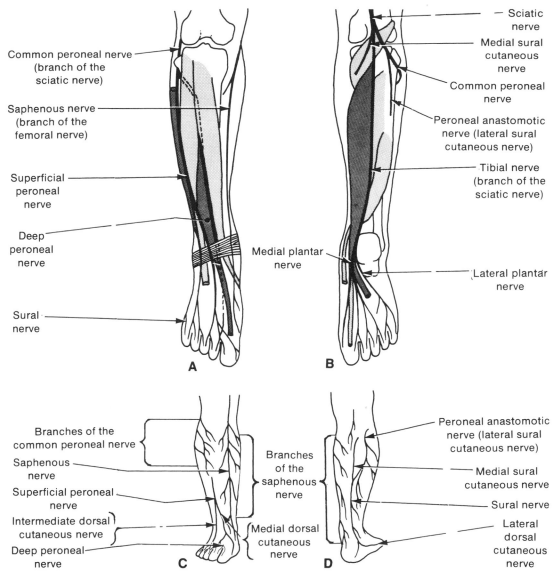

Figure 8.7. Nerves of the leg. *A* and *B*, major divisions. *A*, anterior view. *B*, posterior view. *C* and *D*, cutaneous nerves of the leg. *C*, anterior view. *D*, posterior view.

the lateral malleolus. The peroneus brevis inserts on the base of the fifth metatarsal. The peroneus longus rounds the cuboid and crosses the plantar aspect of the foot to insert on the medial cuneiform and base of the first metatarsal.

The three long muscles of the deep posterior compartment are all innervated by the tibial nerve (Fig. 8.10*A*). The flexor hallucis longus originates from the posterior surface of the fibula, passes around the medial malleolus and through the plantar aspect of the foot to insert on the base of the distal phalanx of the great toe. It flexes the distal phalanx of the great toe. The flexor digitorum longus originates from the posterior aspect

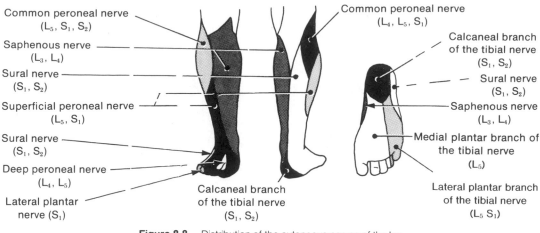

Figure 8.8. Distribution of the cutaneous nerves of the leg.

of the tibia and passes around the medial malleolus just posterior to the posterior tibialis tendon. It then divides into four tendons that pass through the plantar aspect of the foot to insert in the bases of the distal phalanges of the four lateral toes. These act to flex the distal phalanx of the lesser toes. The

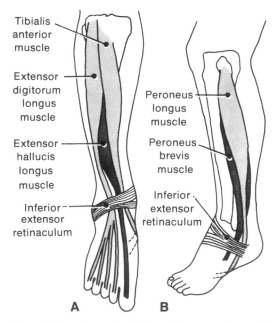

Figure 8.9. *A*, muscles of the anterior compartment. *B*, muscles of the lateral compartment.

tibialis posterior originates between the two flexor muscles from the tibia, fibula, and interosseus membrane, rounds the medial malleolus, and inserts on the plantar medial surface of the navicula, the plantar surfaces of the cuneiform bones, and bases of the second, third, and fourth metatarsals. This muscle is a powerful invertor and supinator of the foot.

The large muscles of the superficial posterior compartment are the strong plantar flexors of the ankle, the gastrocnemius, and soleus (Fig. 8.10*B*). The more superficial of the two, the gastrocnemius, originates from two attachments (one from each femoral condyle) and the deeper soleus originates from its broad attachment to the upper third of the tibia and fibula. Both merge to form the Achilles tendon, which inserts on the calcaneus. It should be recognized that the gastrocnemius originates above the knee joint, and therefore crosses the knee and the ankle as well as the subtalar joints. The plantaris muscle and its long narrow tendon cross the soleus and gastrocnemius from its origin on the femoral condyle to its insertion with the fibers of the Achilles tendon. The muscles of the deep and superficial posterior compartments are all innervated by branches of the tibial nerve.

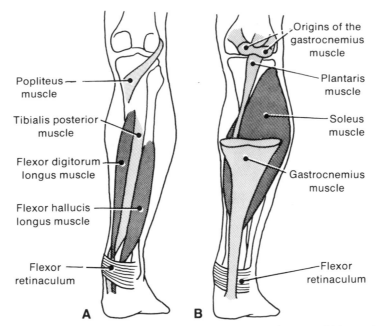

Popliteus — muscle

Tibialis posterior muscle

Flexor digitorum longus muscle

Flexor hallucis longus muscle

Flexor — retinaculum

A

Origins of the gastrocnemius muscle

Plantaris muscle

Soleus muscle

Gastrocnemius muscle

Flexor retinaculum

B

Figure 8.10.   *A*, muscles of the deep posterior compartment. *B*, muscles of the superficial posterior compartment.

Retinaculum of the Ankle.   Across the ankle joint, there are thickenings of the crural fascia called retinacula. These structures hold the long tendons to the ankle and foot in positions of mechanical advantage as they cross the ankle joint, preventing bowstringing as the muscles contract (Fig. 8.11).

Radiographic Evaluation of the Patient with Leg or Ankle Symptoms

When patients complain of difficulties in the leg or ankle, it is standard practice to include a radiographic examination in the patient's overall evaluation. The standard radiographs for the leg are the anteroposterior (AP) and lateral views, with the knee and ankle included on the same film. Abnormalities of the bone structure and alignment can be evaluated with these x-rays, and the angular relationship between the knee and ankle can also be visualized. Soft tissue abnormalities can often be noted and can be represented by soft tissue swelling or defects or both.

Standard ankle radiographs include the AP, lateral, and mortise views. The importance of the mortise view was discussed in the section on "Bone, Joints, and Ligaments."

Nontraumatic Conditions of the Leg and Ankle

There are a variety of torsional and angular deformities of the leg, ankle, and foot. There are also a variety of congenital aplasias in which complete bones or sections of bones are absent or hypoplastic; these have associated soft tissue deformities. The latter group of conditions are relatively uncommon and will not be discussed.

In the adult, the normal lower extremity is aligned so that a straight line can be drawn from the center of the femoral head, through the midportion of the knee, to the center of the talus, and into the second ray of the foot. The knee normally has 5° to 8° of valgus and the tibia is relatively straight, although there may be a few degrees of varus contour or, less often, valgus contour (Fig. 8.12). The

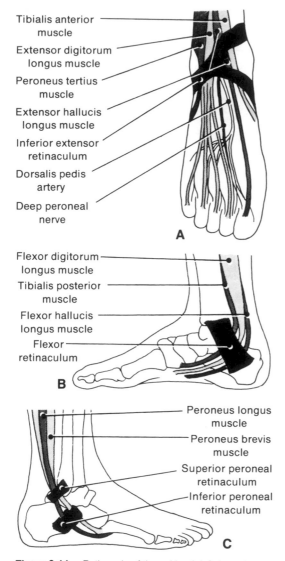

Tibialis anterior muscle
Extensor digitorum longus muscle
Peroneus tertius muscle
Extensor hallucis longus muscle
Inferior extensor retinaculum
Dorsalis pedis artery
Deep peroneal nerve

A

Flexor digitorum longus muscle
Tibialis posterior muscle
Flexor hallucis longus muscle
Flexor retinaculum

B

Peroneus longus muscle
Peroneus brevis muscle
Superior peroneal retinaculum
Inferior peroneal retinaculum

C

Figure 8.11. Retinacula of the ankle. *A*, inferior extensor retinaculum. *B*, flexor retinaculum. *C*, superior and inferior peroneal retinacula.

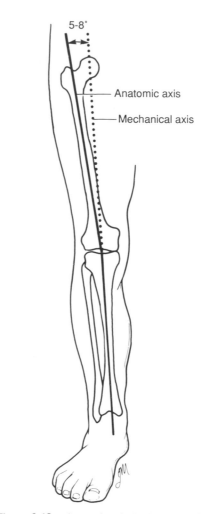

5-8°
Anatomic axis
Mechanical axis

Figure 8.12. Anatomic axis depicts an angle of 5° to 8° between the shaft of the femur and the shaft of the tibia. The mechanical axis is usally a straight line from the femoral head, through the center of the knee joint, to the middle of the ankle. Weight bearing is along the mechanical axis. Reconstructive surgery utilizes the anatomic axis.

alignment of the foot relative to the leg, or the foot progression angle, has a wide range of normal values from approximately 5° of internal rotation to 15° to 20° of external rotation. Postures that significantly exceed these "normal limits" are considered deformities.

In the infant, it is common to have more varus through the knee and tibia. The alignment of the foot to the leg may also have a relatively greater amount of internal rotation compared with the adult.

TORSIONAL DEFORMITIES

Patients with torsional deformities of the tibia usually present with intoeing or outtoeing deformities of gait, and this will be described in Chapter 9.

ANGULAR DEFORMITIES

Angular deformities may occur in the sagittal plane as well as the coronal plane. Tibia vara gives the appearance of bowlegs. This may be physiologic or pathologic. Physiologic tibia vara is usually noted from infancy to approximately 18 months of age. This is replaced by a variable amount of valgus from 18 months through the age of 5 to 6 years. At this point the knee will usually have assumed the normal adult value of 5° to 8° of knee valgus.

Pathologic tibia vara does not usually follow the above guidelines and frequently becomes progressively worse. This varus deformity may represent Blount's disease, in which there is an abnormality of the tibial growth plate, or it may be a manifestation of a vitamin D deficiency state, such as rickets. Radiographs of the knee in Blount's disease show a normal width of the growth plate, but there is an abnormality at the medial side. In vitamin D deficiency states, the growth plate will be abnormally wide. In pathologic tibia vara, referral to an orthopaedist is recommended.

Angular deformities in the sagittal plane include anterior and posterior angulation, and are usually noted at birth. These deformities often require specialized treatment and should be referred to the orthopaedist.

Posterior Angulation

The angle of the bow is directed posteriorly, but may be posteromedial, i.e., the apex of the angle is posterior or posteromedial. This may be due to the intrauterine position of the infant, resulting in tight anterior compartment musculature and limited plantar flexion of the ankle.

Treatment. Treatment is largely non-operative. Passive stretching of the tight musculature is required and occasionally a total contact orthosis is used. The deformity usually corrects by about age 4. A residual limb length discrepancy often results and, if necessary, an equalization procedure can be performed at the appropriate time. Osteotomy of the tibia and fibula is not indicated in this deformity.

Anterior Angulation

This direction of angulation is more serious, and referral to an orthopaedist is recommended. This angulation may be associated with congenital absence of the fibula, congenital pseudarthrosis of the tibia and fibula, or fibrous dysplasia.

In congenital absence of the fibula, treatment may range from limb length equalization procedures to an amputation of the foot. Congenital pseudarthrosis is believed to be associated with neurofibromatosis and requires specialized surgical procedures in an attempt to achieve lasting union.

Treatment of fibrous dysplasia is directed toward establishing pathologic diagnosis, then achieving union and protecting the limb from subsequent fracture.

CONGENITAL DEFORMITIES OF THE ANKLE

Congenital deformities of the ankle are complex and are intimately related to deformities of the foot. A definition and description of the direction of deformity will be described; however, a detailed discussion will be undertaken in Chapter 9. The four directions of deformity that can affect the ankle are the equinus, calcaneus, varus, and valgus. Equinus refers to the plantar flexed position of the ankle. This deformity can result from excessively tight gastrocsoleus muscle complex. Calcaneus is the dorsiflexed position of the ankle and can result from laxity of the gastrocsoleus muscles, tight anterior musculature, or a combination of both. Varus refers to a position in which the heel is pointing toward the midline of the body, and valgus to a position in which the heel is pointing away from the midline of the body. Combinations of deformity can occur, such as the equinovarus deformity of the clubfoot. These deformities can occur because of muscle imbalance, abnormal intrauterine position, or true bone or soft tissue dysplasia.

Traumatic Disorders of the Leg and Ankle

Traumatic disorders may be the result of repetitive minor trauma, often designated as overuse syndromes, or a single major traumatic event. Some conditions, such as compartment syndrome, may be associated with either category of trauma.

OVERUSE SYNDROMES
Shin Splints

Shin splints is a term that many people use, perhaps inappropriately, to refer to any pain in the leg occurring during or soon after exercise. In fact, like the term internal derangement of the knee, the term shin splints can refer to a number of different anatomic problems in the leg. In many cases specific diagnosis is difficult. Certain muscular activity or stretching is associated with muscle pain of varying severity and persistence. The term shin splints can be applied to this type of pain and is usually described as pain along the tibia with a varying location when the muscles of the anterior or deep posterior compartments are overstressed. Visible evidence of inflammation suggests that the pain syndrome represents myositis, periostitis, or musculotendinous strains or tears. Included in the differential diagnosis of shin splints are stress fractures, exertional compartment syndrome, and tenosynovitis.

Clinical Characteristics. The patient complains of pain over a muscle compartment near the tibia. Pain may be referred to the foot or into the knee. Movements that stretch or work the affected muscle increases the pain. Palpation over the affected muscle group and the adjacent tibia will elicit tenderness. Slight swelling and redness may be visible over the affected muscle and its tibial origin.

These symptoms often occur in athletes who change their running surfaces and/or types of shoes, alter their techniques, or participate in intensive hard training. They may also be noted in nonathletes performing activities to which they are unaccustomed, such as walking up a large hill or numerous stairs. If a technetium bone scan is performed to rule out stress fractures, it may show diffuse increased uptake along the tibia (in cases of periostitis), but not the intense local uptake of a stress fracture. Sometimes the differentiation is not very clear. In soft tissue cases, the bone scan will be normal.

Treatment. Minimal pain and tenderness need not require a restriction of activity, if symptoms abate readily or do not progress.

When pain is quite intense and/or inflammation visibly evident, the provoking activity should be avoided until recovery is well advanced. Ice is the safest applied analgesic during the first 2 or 3 days. Thereafter, heat or ice may be used, whichever is more comforting. Stretching and mild exercise may begin as soon as visible evidence of inflammation has subsided. The provoking activity should be resumed gradually.

In some cases foot abnormalities, such as excessive pronation, can be the cause of shin splints, and orthotic devices can be beneficial in these patients.

Stress Fractures

Stress fractures may occur in either the tibia or the fibula. They usually will occur after prolonged and repeated loading, as in long distance or cross-country running or repeated jumping. Many times the individual is not properly conditioned prior to participating in the inciting activity. Tibial stress fractures typically occur in the upper two-thirds of the bone, although they may occur at the junction of the middle and distal third as well. Fibula stress fractures usually occur 5 to 7 cm above the tip of the lateral malleolus.

Clinical Characteristics. The patient typically complains of pain in the affected leg during or soon after the repeated load which subsides with rest after a variable length of time. When feeling well again, the patient (often an athlete) will resume the activity, and symptoms will recur. Local tenderness and some swelling are noted over the fracture site.

Differential diagnosis includes shin splints, exertional compartment syndrome, and tenosynovitis. Radiographs will often be negative when initially performed. Technetium bone scanning can confirm the diagnosis before radiographs become positive.

Treatment. Treatment of tibial stress fractures consists of cessation of the inciting activity for approximately 6 to 8 weeks, and then gradual return at a pace that is below the level which causes pain. Patients who have pain even with walking, or those who will not comply with the required decreased level of activity, should be casted with a short-leg walking cast for 4 to 6 weeks, allowing healing to progress. After that time, a progressive return is allowed, as described above.

Bone scanning can be utilized in those patients who require a expeditious diagnosis or who do not seem to be progressing as expected. Follow-up radiographs should be obtained. Nonunion of the fracture is a possibility in those patients who persist in running "through the pain," and this may present treatment problems that require consultation with an orthopaedic surgeon.

Stress fractures of the fibula can be effectively treated in the same fashion.

Compartment Syndrome

Compartment syndrome is the result of increased volume within one or more compartments of an extremity because of increased blood flow or swelling. The anatomic compartments are surrounded by dense fascial layers that have little capacity for stretch. Consequently, bleeding or edema that would increase the potential volume of the tissue within the compartment will lead to increased pressure rather than actual distention of the compartment, which rapidly reaches its limit due to the inelasticity of the fascial envelope. Compartment syndromes of the lower extremity may be acute or chronic and related to exertion.

Acute Compartment Syndrome. Acute compartment syndromes may result from a single traumatic event to the lower leg, including fractures and crush injuries. They may also result from disruption of arterial blood flow, as in vascular injuries. These are surgical emergencies and the diagnosis must be sought in any extremity that is subjected to trauma. Evaluation for compartment syndrome involves a motor, sensory, and circulatory examination of the extremity.

Clinical Characteristics. The early and most dramatic characteristics of acute compartment syndrome are severe pain in the leg, tense swelling of one of more compartments with associated tenderness, extreme pain with passive motion, and with stretching of the musculotendinous units in the involved compartment. Paralysis of active motion of toes or ankle, paresthesia or anesthesia of the dorsum of the foot where there is peroneal nerve involvement, or sole of the foot, if there is tibial nerve involvement, usually present much later in the course of compartment syndrome. The arterial pulse is usually present until very advanced stages of the syndrome and should not be included as a criteria for diagnosis. Of course, a pulseless extremity does indicate an interruption of blood flow and requires immediate surgical consultation. The diagnosis of compartment syndrome is not always clear in the injured extremity. Often it is difficult to distinguish the pain from the underlying injury, i.e., a fracture versus the development of pain from a compartment syndrome. Consequently, once the question of compartment syndrome is raised, immediate referral to an orthopaedist is required so that the patient can be rapidly evaluated. The decompression of involved compartment is accomplished by fasciotomy. This treatment is successful if performed early.

Chronic Exertional Compartment Syndrome. Chronic exertional compartment syndromes are often more difficult to diagnose than the acute syndrome and usually do not present as surgical emergencies.

Clinical Characteristics. Symptoms of exertional compartment syndrome are not unlike the symptoms of other stress-induced problems in the lower leg. These include pain in the lower leg when running or during repeated jumping. Some patients may even have pain with fast walking. As muscles are exercised, they increase their volume and blood flow. This results in increased pressure, which may actually decrease blood flow, leading to a relative lack of oxygenation, increased lactic acid production, and further swelling. Subsequently, pain of a dull quality develops and will usually resolve with a few minutes of rest; other symptoms include a feeling of weakness and paresthesia. The location of symptoms will help define which compartment is affected, with the anterior compartment being the most common. Often the patient will have a history of blunt trauma to the soft tissues or a previous fracture of the affected extremity.

Treatment. The diagnosis and treatment of true exertional compartment syndrome are invasive and therefore it is worthwhile to initially treat the patient with conservative measures. This first consists of conditioning the muscles to the increased demand with stretching and strengthening of the extremity, and a slow progression to the desired activity. If these prove ineffective, a bone scan to rule out stress fracture and periostitis is performed and will be normal in the case of exertional compartment syndromes. The diagnosis is confirmed with pressure measurements of the compartments during exercise and the "cool-down" period. Specific criteria have been elaborated for the diagnosis. If these criteria are met, surgical release is in-

dicated. Since the measurements and treatment are invasive, referral to an orthopaedist is recommended when conservative measures fail to relieve symptoms. Rarely, a patient with exertional compartment syndrome will unwittingly attempt to run through the pain. This can result in an acute compartment syndrome, in which the symptoms do not resolve with rest, and immediate referral is required as emergency decompression may be necessary.

Tenosynovitis

The long tendons to the foot and their synovial sheaths are vulnerable to irritation where they pass under the retinacula at the ankle. Activity that requires prolonged repetitive movement of a tendon is most likely to provoke its inflammation. The tibialis anterior and posterior, and the peronei longus and brevis are most commonly involved.

It is important to note that occasionally patients with systemic disease, such as rheumatoid arthritis or a collagen vascular disease, will present with a localized tendosynovitis as a manifestation of their generalized illness. When evaluating a patient, this fact must be considered in a differential diagnosis.

Clinical Characteristics. Pain is felt over the affected tendon and may refer into that portion of the foot distal to it: tibialis anterior to the anteromedial aspect of the ankle and dorsum of the foot; tibialis posterior to the posteromedial aspect of the ankle and medial plantar aspect of the foot; peronei to the posterolateral aspect of the ankle and lateral aspect of the foot. Tenderness to palpation, visible fullness, and often a creaky crepitation are evident over the tendon where it passes beneath the retinaculum. Movement or action of the tendon usually causes pain. This includes passive stretching of the tendons as well as active function of the inflamed tendons.

Treatment. Specific treatment depends on the severity of the symptoms. In general, rest, ice, and anti-inflammatory agents are used. While mild ambulation may continue, activities requiring prolonged repetitive motions should be avoided. Any activity that causes the symptoms should be avoided. When symptoms are so severe that even level walking produces symptoms, or if mild symptoms continue beyond 2 to 3 weeks, a 4- to 6-week period with a short-leg walking cast should then be used to provide complete rest of the tendon. Ice should be used until the visible signs of inflammation have disappeared, and oral anti-inflammatory agents can be helpful until the tenderness has resolved.

As symptoms are resolving, a physical therapy program consisting of stretching and strengthening the involved tendons should be employed to avoid recurrence.

POSTERIOR HEEL AND ANKLE PAIN

The primary care practitioner will usually encounter one of four common causes of posterior heel and posterior ankle pain. These include Achilles tendinitis, posterior calcaneal bursitis, retrocalcaneal bursitis, and calcaneal apophysitis (Sever's disease).

Achilles Tendinitis

The retinacular fascia surrounding the Achilles tendon can become irritated whenever the Achilles tendon is subjected to uncustomary repetitive stress, such as hiking or jogging. Although commonly known as Achilles tendinitis, the inflammation more frequently involves the paratenon surrounding the Achilles tendon. In severe or chronic cases, the tendon itself can become inflamed. The physical findings and treatment of tendinitis and paratendinitis are identical. The inflammation can occur from running or competing in shoes with heels lower than street shoes or training shoes. In addition, people with hyperpronating feet are at increased risk for developing Achilles tendinitis or paratendinitis.

Clinical Characteristics. The patient complains of pain in the back of the heel and leg which worsens when the Achilles tendon is stretched or worked. Tenderness and swelling will be noted approximately 3 to 4 cm above the tendon's insertion on the calcaneus.

Treatment. Treatment is directed toward reducing the inflammation, reducing the stress on the Achilles tendon, and increasing the flexibility of the gastrocsoleus complex. Specifically, oral anti-inflammatory medications, a heel lift of ½ inch, and a stretching and strengthening physical therapy program are prescribed. Often, complete rest by way of a short-leg walking cast for 4 to 6 weeks is initially necessary to reduce the inflammation. A soft orthotic device with a navicular pad and a ⅛-inch medial wedge can be of benefit in those patients whose feet tend to hyperpronate and who have recurrent symptoms.

Retrocalcaneal Bursitis

Retrocalcaneal bursitis is an inflammation of the retrocalcaneal bursa located between the posterior superior border of the calcaneus and the Achilles tendon. This may develop following activity requiring repetitive dorsiflexion/plantar flexion of the ankle.

Clinical Characteristics. The patient complains of heel pain worsened by dorsiflexion of the ankle. There is tenderness just anterior and superior to the insertion of the Achilles tendon on the calcaneus. Swelling and redness may be evident in this location or at the Achilles tendon insertion itself. X-rays may show a protuberance on the superior posterior aspect of the calcaneus; this is known as Haglund's disease.

Treatment. Weight bearing is minimized and, when necessary, a ½-inch elevation of the heel is utilized. Hot or cold compresses may afford some relief. Oral anti-inflammatory medication and occasionally steroid injection may speed the remission. In chronic or recurrent cases, orthopaedic referral should be considered for surgical treatment, which may include excision of the prominent tubercle and removal of the retrocalcaneal bursa.

Posterior Calcaneal Bursitis

Posterior calcaneal bursitis is inflammation of a subcutaneous bursa superficial to the insertion of the Achilles tendon. It is irritated by friction of the upper border of the heel counter of the shoe. This can result from laceless shoes and loafers (which must fit closely to the heel), or high-heeled shoes.

Clinical Characteristics. The patient complains of posterior heel pain and a tender bump on the back of the heel. This bump is an inflamed and swollen bursa. As in retrocalcaneal bursitis, radiographs may show a protuberance on the superior posterior aspect of the calcaneus.

Treatment. Ideally, open-heeled shoes or sandals should be used until the inflammation subsides. Local injection of the bursa with corticosteroid may speed remission, but should be used with caution as it may weaken the tendon. Oral anti-inflammatory medications can also decrease the inflammation. When shoes with heel counters are again worn, the counter should be less convex and its upper border should be soft. A posterior wedge can be cut away from the posterior counters of the shoe and soft leather sewn across the defect (Fig. 8.13). Alternatively, a U-shaped pad can be placed between the heel and the counter to relieve the irritated prominent area. In chronic or recurrent cases, orthopaedic referral is indicated for possible surgical treatment, which might include ostectomy of the prominent tubercle or calcaneal osteotomy.

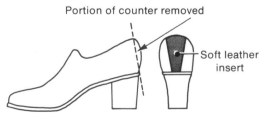

Portion of counter removed

Soft leather insert

Figure 8.13. Insertion of soft leather into the back of the heel counter.

Calcaneal Apophysitis (Sever's Disease)

This overuse syndrome occurs in active prepubertal children. The calcaneal apophysis is longitudinally aligned with the fibers of the gastrocsoleus complex and therefore subject to shearing stresses by the forceful repetitive action of these muscles.

Clinical Characteristics. The child will limp and complain of heel pain, worsened by heel strike on hard surfaces and by running. The tenderness will be localized over the insertion of the Achilles tendon. Radiographs will often show partial fragmentation and sclerosis of the calcaneal apophysis, but this can also be seen in many asymptomatic patients. The radiographs will help rule out other causes of the pain.

Treatment. Mild symptoms, present only during increased activity, should be treated by restriction of the activity until the tenderness resolves. Children with symptoms severe enough to be present when walking, or those children who will not alter their activity should be treated with a 2- to 4-week period in a short-leg walking cast. During and following resolution of the acute symptoms, a ¼-inch heel lift for 3 to 4 months and physical therapy aimed at stretching and strengthening the Achilles complex can help prevent recurrence.

TENDON DISRUPTIONS

In general, tendon disruptions about the foot and ankle are relatively uncommon events. The disruption may be caused by a direct laceration, a sudden force applied to the tendon, or a gradual intrinsic degeneration of the tendon. In the first instance, the diagnosis should be made at the time of evaluation of the laceration. The patient will demonstrate weak and usually painful motion when testing the action of the specific tendon involved. Following a sudden force, the patient will again demonstrate painful and weak action of the specific tendon, and a palpable gap may be noted along the course of the tendon if examined before significant swelling occurs. Gradual disruption may be more difficult to diagnose. The patient will complain of ankle and foot fatigue, and a progressive foot or ankle deformity may be noted.

The posterior tibialis tendon disruption is most commonly the result of gradual deterioration. Disruption of the anterior tibialis tendon is usually the result of a laceration because of its anterior and relatively vulnerable position. Disruption of the peroneal tendons is rarely caused by either trauma or deterioration. The etiology of Achilles tendon ruptures is most commonly the result of a sudden force applied to the plantar flexed ankle.

Disruption of the Achilles tendon will be discussed in this chapter; the other tendon disruptions will be discussed in Chapter 9.

Achilles Tendon Rupture

Rupture of the Achilles tendon is usually the result of forced dorsiflexion against a plantar flexed foot.

Clinical Characteristics. The typical patient is over 25 years old and sustains the injury during an athletic event. The athlete notices a snap in the back of the heel, often stating that it felt as if a stick may have struck the back of the ankle or lower leg. Activities in which this most often occurs are diving, tennis, and basketball. Any activity in which the patient may suddenly "toe off" or land on his toes after a jump can cause the excessive load.

In addition to the typical history, the diagnosis is made on the basis of three diagnostic signs on physical examination. The first is a palpable defect noted between 2 to 6 cm above the Achilles insertion on the calcaneus. The second is weak active plantar flexion against resistance. The third and pathognomonic finding is a positive Thompson squeeze test. This test is performed with the patient prone and the knees bent at 90°. Squeezing the calf will produce a definite plantar flexion of the ankle in the normal ex-

tremity; however, in the extremity with the ruptured Achilles tendon, plantar flexion will be absent. Comparison with the normal side is important to convince the examiner of the difference. Occasionally, radiographs can delineate the tendon rupture or may demonstrate a bony avulsion from the calcaneus. The diagnosis, however, can be made clinically by history and physical examination (Fig. 8.14).

Treatment. Treatment of Achilles tendon rupture is controversial. There are many advocates for operative treatment and many advocates for nonoperative treatment. Nonoperative treatment consists of the application of a long-leg cast with the knee in 45° of flexion and the ankle in gravity equinus. Gravity equinus is the amount that the ankle will naturally assume when the knee is bent over the edge of a table. This is continued for 4 weeks, followed by a short-leg cast with the ankle in gravity equinus for another 4 weeks. Following this, the patient obtains a 1-inch heel lift, which is gradually decreased by ¼ inch per week for the next 4 weeks. During the period in a heel lift, a physical therapy program, including active dorsiflexion and gentle resistive plantar flexion, is begun and continued until the ankle regains normal strength.

Operative treatment consists of surgical approximation of the disrupted tendon. The postoperative treatment is identical to the nonoperative treatment.

It has been shown that surgical treatment has the benefit of slightly increased resistance to fatigue and decreased rate of rerupture. The risks of surgery include anesthesia, infection, and wound problems. It is probably appropriate to recommend surgery in very active individuals who wish to remain very active.

Rupture of the Gastrocnemius Muscle or the Plantaris Tendon

Included in the differential diagnosis of Achilles tendon rupture is a partial tear of

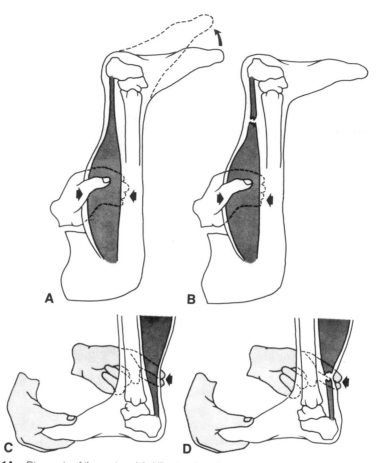

Figure 8.14.   Diagnosis of the ruptured Achilles tendon. *A*, normal. *B*, ruptured. *C*, normal. *D*, ruptured.

the gastrocnemius muscle, usually at the medial muscle aponeurotic junction. The patient may have the same history as the patient with Achilles tendon rupture, but the classic physical findings will be absent and the tenderness will be noted medially approximately midway between the knee and ankle. This can be treated with an elevated heel after the tenderness has resolved. Care should be taken to assure that no compartment syndrome develops.

Rupture of the plantaris has a very similar history and physical examination as the partial tear of the gastrocnemius, and it is treated in a similar manner.

Major Traumatic Injuries to the Leg and Ankle

The prognosis of lower extremity injuries depends heavily on the integrity of the circulation. Patients with preexisting arterial and/or venous insufficiency are at much higher risk for infection as well as poor soft tissue and bone healing. This increased risk is also seen in patients with diabetes. This contingency bears emphasis because inexperienced clinicians may have a tendency to overlook these facts in their preoccupation with the details of the injury. It is also important to note that the presence of an acute vascular injury or compartment syndrome significantly impairs the patient's prognosis. The neurologic and circulatory status of any injured extremity must be evaluated, and patients with compromised vascular or neurologic function should be referred immediately.

In addition, the following injuries should be referred whether or not obvious arterial, venous, or neurologic injury has occurred: (*a*) extensive muscle contusion, (*b*) unstable sprains and dislocations, and (*c*) compound (open) fractures and avulsions of the integument.

Evaluation and treatment of specific injuries will be described.

CONTUSIONS OF THE LEG
Anterior Compartment

Because the crural fascia is tough and tense over the anterior compartment, severe contusion and crush injuries such as a lower extremity caught between the bumpers of two cars, can result in a compartment syndrome. Bleeding and edema into the confined anterior compartment can increase the tissue pressure to such an extent that ischemic necrosis of the muscle occurs. Because the skin over the anterior aspect of the leg is tightly bound to the crural fascia, it also tolerates swelling poorly, and contusions of the anterior skin commonly lead to necrosis of the central zone of the contused skin. The clinician must minimize swelling and closely watch for signs of anterior compartment muscle ischemia.

Treatment. Any associated abrasions must be scrubbed as free of ground dirt as possible, using a surgical scrub brush, under local anesthesia. The extremity must be elevated moderately above heart level. Too little elevation will allow the swelling to continue; too much elevation will decrease the hydrostatic pressure of the arteriovenous gradient. Toe-gripping exercises should be repeated every few minutes to encourage ve-

nous and lymphatic return. Ice packs should be applied over the injury for the first 24 to 48 hours. The leg should not be bound, as this will increase compartment pressure externally. Dorsiflexion of the ankle and extension of the toes should be attempted every 30 minutes for the first 12 hours, and several times daily thereafter. Any decline in apparent strength or significant increase in pain with the effort suggests muscle ischemia. Pain alone can inhibit extensor tone, but many patients who are made aware of the importance of the test will generate a stronger movement with a well-perfused muscle than with an ischemic muscle. The inability to discriminate a sharp point from a dull touch over the dorsum of the foot can also suggest increased compartment pressure because of the pressure on the nerves. If at any point muscle ischemia or nerve compression is suspected, an orthopaedist must be consulted to evaluate the patient for compartment measurements or to consider fasciotomy. As swelling and pain subside, active stretching and working exercises of the anterior compartment are begun. The patient should avoid ambulation during the first 48 hours, except for bathroom needs, and then ambulation should be non-weight-bearing with crutches. Partial weight bearing may begin when non-weight-bearing ambulation and active exercises have been performed for 24 hours without increase in pain or swelling.

Posterior Compartment

Contusions to the posterior compartment are less subject to the danger of muscle ischemia, and restorative treatment can proceed more rapidly; however, the principles above must be kept in mind. In the posterior compartment, the muscles to observe closely are those that plantar flex the ankles and toes. Active working and stretching exercises and weight bearing as tolerated can usually begin after 24 to 48 hours of ice and elevation. Vigorous running and exposure to further contusion should be avoided until healing is complete, as repeated intramuscular bleeding can lead to myositis ossificans.

FRACTURES OF THE SHAFTS OF THE TIBIA AND FIBULA

The tibia is fractured more frequently than any other long bone. Fractures of the tibia and fibula can occur anywhere along the length of the bones. Fractures may be open (compound) or closed (simple), displaced or undisplaced, angulated or not angulated, stable or unstable. Fractures of the tibia and fibula can be associated with acute compartment syndromes, and diligent following of the neurovascular condition, as noted above, is mandatory. It is important to categorize tibia and fibula shaft fractures with each of the above descriptions to help with treatment decisions, and to communicate information to a consulting orthopaedist.

A closed fracture is a fracture in which the skin of the lower leg is not broken. An open fracture is classified according to the degree of skin disruption, and whether or not there is significant soft tissue loss, blood vessel disruption, or gross contamination (Table 8.1). Open fractures should be covered with antiseptic solution and a bulky sterile dressing, splinted, and transferred to the care of an orthopaedic surgeon. The wound and fracture ends will then be thoroughly irrigated and debrided, and the fracture will be treated with casting, external fixation, or open reduction and internal fixation. A vascular surgeon will be consulted if vascular injury is present. Displacement of less than 50% in either anteroposterior or lateral planes is adequate reduction, and angulation of less than 10° in the anteroposterior plane or less than 5° in the lateral plane is usually acceptable.

Stability of the reduction is a function of the configuration of the fracture, the degree of comminution, and extent of periosteal

Table 8.1.
Open Fracture Classifications[a]

Grade	Wound	Comment
I	<1 cm	This is usually a low-energy injury in which the skin defect is frequently caused by the bone piercing the skin from inside to outside, rather than from penetrating trauma
II	>1 cm but <10 cm	Moderate-energy trauma, without gross contamination
III	>10 cm	High-energy trauma; this grade is also attributed to injuries with any size wound where there is marked skin loss, periosteal stripping, gross contamination (as in farm injuries), vascular compromise, or segmental bone injury

[a] Adapted from Chapman MW. The role of intramedullary fixation in open fractures. Clin Orthop 1986; 212–27, 1986 and from Gustilo RB, Anderson JT. Prevention of infection in the treatment of one thousand and twenty-five open fractures of long bones: retrospective and prospective analyses. J Bone Joint Surg 1976; 58A:453–458, with permission.

disruption. A useful definition of an unstable fracture is one in which acceptable position and length cannot be easily maintained with a well-applied cast immobilizing the joint above and below the fracture. Usually short oblique fractures are less stable than transverse fractures. Comminuted fractures are often unstable. Unstable fractures should be referred to an orthopaedic surgeon.

Careful neurovascular evaluation must be performed and repeated at frequent intervals on all extremities that have sustained a tibial and/or fibular fracture. An acute compartment syndrome can result in loss of function of the extremity. Compartment syndromes can occur in any or all of the four compartments of the lower leg, and evaluation as previously described in the section on "Contusions of the Leg" is mandatory. If any question of compartment syndrome exists, immediate referral to an orthopaedist is required, and fasciotomy may be indicated.

Role of the Primary Care Practitioner

The primary care practitioner should evaluate and describe the injury. A neurovascular examination should be performed initially and repeated frequently. Open wounds should be dressed and the limb placed in a splint, without tight circular bandages, and ice applied to the injured extremity. Prompt consultation with an orthopaedic surgeon should be the routine.

In some cases, it is appropriate for an experienced practitioner to definitively treat tibial shaft fractures. These would include noncomminuted, closed fractures in which a satisfactory position is present initially, or in which a stable acceptable position can be obtained with closed manipulation and cast application. The extremity must have a normal neurovascular examination. Acceptable position and angulation are noted above.

A long-leg cast is applied with the knee in 30° to 45° of flexion. Radiographs taken after reduction must confirm acceptable position. The patient is admitted to the hospital, and the limb is elevated with ice packs over the fracture site. Frequent neurovascular examinations are performed to ensure that no compartment syndrome is developing. After 48 hours, the patient may begin non-weight-bearing ambulation. The long-leg cast is kept on for 4 to 6 weeks and is followed by a patellar tendon-bearing cast for the next 4 to 6 weeks. The patient can often be at a partial weight-bearing status at this point. A short-leg cast is then applied for an additional 4 to 6 weeks, with weight bearing as tolerated. If healing has not occurred by this time, referral to an orthopaedist is recommended. Should a compartment syndrome start to develop after the cast is applied, the cast is split along the medial and lateral sides, and the top half is discarded, effectively leaving a posterior splint. If the examination does not improve rapidly, prompt referral is mandatory.

Fibular shaft fractures in the proximal two-thirds of the bone are most commonly the result of a direct blow. Uneventful healing is the usual case. The ankle should be included in the radiographs and clinical examination to ensure that there is no injury. Also, careful examination for a compartment syndrome is performed. If there is no ankle injury by examination and by x-ray, and the neurovascular examination is normal, a short-leg walking cast is applied largely for comfort. The fracture will usually heal even without the cast. The patient should be instructed to keep the extremity elevated for at least 48 hours with ice packs, frequently move the toes and check them for color and sensation, and return if any problems develop. The cast is kept on for a 4- to 6-week period.

ANKLE INJURIES
Ankle Sprains

Ankle sprains are common injuries seen in every emergency department. They occur in athletes and nonathletes. Ankle sprains are commonly misunderstood and underestimated by both primary care physicians and the patients who sustain them.

The most common mechanism of injury that produces ankle sprains is a supination or inversion force. This occurs when the foot turns under the ankle after walking or running on uneven surfaces, or during an athletic event when the upper body is twisted over the planted foot, or when landing on the inverted foot after a jump. This results in stretching or tearing of the ligaments of the lateral side of the ankle. The most common ligament injured is the anterior talofibular ligament, with more prolonged or severe stress, the calcaneofibular ligament, and rarely, the posterior talofibular ligament can be torn. The fibulocalcaneal ligament is also more commonly injured if the ankle is in the

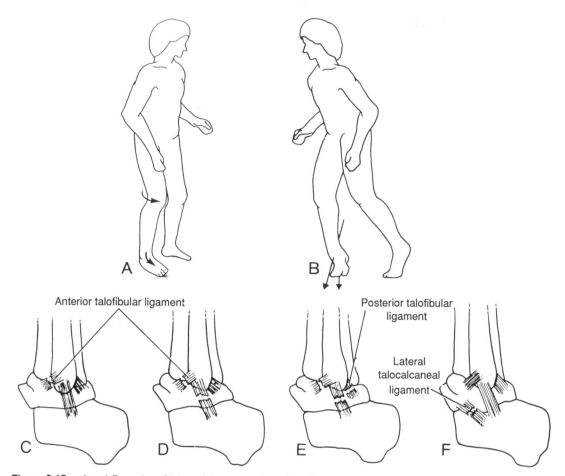

Figure 8.15. *A* and *B*, modes of injury. *A*, by convention, deformities are measured from distal as related to proximal. Therefore, in this supinated foot, as the leg internally rotates on the planted foot, the foot is relatively externally rotated. Thus, this is a supination external rotation injury. *B*, plantar flexed foot is forced into supination. *C–E*, sequence of injury to the ligaments based on severing of the force producing the injury. *F*, the lateral talocalcaneal ligament may also be injured and can contribute to subtalar instability, which may follow ankle sprains.

dorsiflexed position at the time of injury (Fig. 8.15).

Clinical Characteristics. Examination of a patient with an ankle sprain reveals a variable amount of swelling and tenderness over and about the lateral malleolus. The severity of the injury can often be estimated by the history. Mild sprains will allow the patient to walk soon after the injury, whereas severe injuries will be such that the patient cannot immediately walk. The amount of swelling is often an indication of the severity

of the injury as well. If a person is examined within a few minutes of the injury, location of the tenderness over the specific anatomic region of the various ligaments can help the examiner determine which ligaments have been injured (Fig. 8.16). However, in most instances, by the time the patient is examined the swelling and tenderness is diffuse, and determination of the specific ligaments injured is more difficult.

Tests for ankle instability, such as the anterior drawer and varus stress tests, can as-

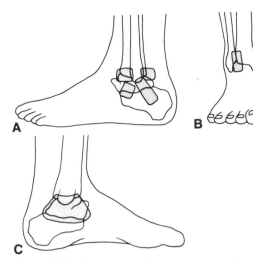

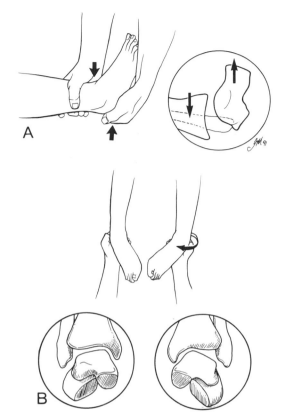

Figure 8.16. Examination of the ankle: zones of tenderness of the individual ligaments. *A*, the lateral ligaments. *B*, the anterior-inferior tibiofibular ligament. *C*, the deltoid ligament.

sist in determining the severity of ligamentous disruption if performed prior to the onset of severe swelling, or soon after the swelling has diminished (Fig. 8.17).

Radiographic studies are necessary to rule out fractures of the malleoli, talus, and foot. In reviewing the ankle radiographs, it is important to specifically look for certain bony injuries that can occur following the inversion stress. These include osteochondral fracture of the talus, fractures of the lateral process of the talus, fractures of the posterior tubercle of the talus, fractures of the anterior process of the calcaneus, and fractures of the base of the fifth metatarsal (Fig. 8.18). Treatment of these injuries will be discussed in Chapter 9.

Treatment. If radiographs are negative, initial treatment is aimed at controlling the swelling and pain about the ankle. This is accomplished by splinting the foot and ankle in a neutral position. A simple posterior plaster splint often breaks down within a day or two and is not recommended. A U-shaped short-leg stirrup splint extending around the ankle, heel and midfoot, over a bulky compressive dressing, provides comfortable,

Figure 8.17. *A*, anterior drawer test: while holding the tibia steady, the heel is grasped and directed forward. A lateral radiograph is taken and will show 3 mm or greater anterior displacement if positive. *B*, varus (inversion) stress test: both heels are grasped and a supination force is applied. Mortise radiographs are taken of both ankles. A difference in the talar of 10° or greater is an indication of significant lateral ligament injury.

sturdy immobilization (Fig. 8.19). This is applied with the ankle in neutral position, often with the patient prone and the knee flexed. The foot is wrapped with a cotton roll, if available, and cotton padding, as if a cast were to be applied. A splint is then made of 4- or 5-inch plaster, depending on the patient's size, and applied in a stirrup fashion using 10 to 12 thicknesses of plaster. This is held in place by an elastic bandage applied without excessive tension around the entire dressing.

Ice is then applied for 20 minutes every 4 hours, and strict elevation above the heart is

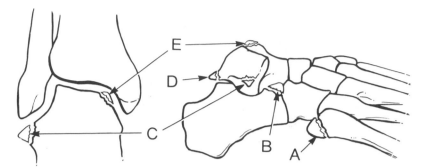

Figure 8.18. Schematic of fractures occasionally missed during a twisting injury to the ankle. *A*, base of the fifth metarsal. *B*, anterior process of the calcaneus. *C*, lateral process of the talus. *D*, posterior tubercle of the talus. *E*, osteochondral fracture of the talus.

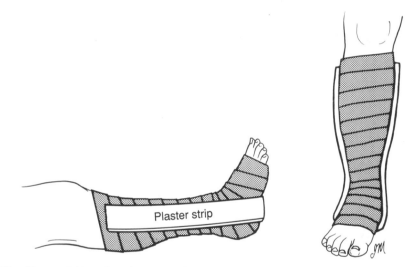

Plaster strip

Figure 8.19. Stirrup splint is preferred over posterior splint by the author. Details for application are noted in the text.

observed. The patient is encouraged to move the toes in the dressing. Three to 5 days following the injury, the patient returns and the dressing is removed. Usually the swelling has resolved substantially, and a reexamination is performed in an attempt to localize the ligaments injured and to reassess the stability of the ankle.

The treatment of ligamentous disruptions is controversial. Many authors recommend minimal treatment and suggest range of motion exercises and ambulation "as tolerated." The other extreme is routine operative repair of injuries involving several ligaments. Most ankle sprains can be treated successfully with nonoperative measures. The exception would be the grossly unstable ankle, either at the time of injury or on subsequent follow-up. Obvious instability of the ankle would be noted on inversion and/or anterior stress. Operative repair is especially considered in the competitive or serious recreational athlete.

After removal of the initial dressing, if the ankle is still markedly tender and range of motion is very painful, the patient is placed is a short-leg walking cast for 4 weeks. Physical therapy follows with range of motion exercises, peroneal strengthening, and proprioceptive training. Once range of motion is normal and ankle strength returns, the patient may return to normal activities.

For many patients, return to activity can be hastened by physical therapy after the initial dressing is removed. The competitive or serious recreational athlete is usually willing to devote the time and effort to such therapy. This consists of early range of motion exercises, the use of electrical stimulation to decrease swelling, and sequential compressive dressings. Once the swelling is under control and range of motion approaches normal, peroneal strengthening is begun. This is followed by proprioceptive training, and the use of an Aircast or similar brace is begun to start the return to athletics. The athlete can progress with rehabilitation as comfort allows. A return to athletic activity is allowed when the patient feels the ankle is at least 90% recovered and is able to perform the usual demands of the activity.

In milder ankle sprains in which the patient can walk painlessly soon after the sprain, a more progressive return is indicated. Patients who have sustained ankle sprains should be advised that residual tenderness, propensity to swell after activity, and pain on inversion of the injured ankle commonly persists for 6 weeks and may be present for 6 or more months following the injury.

Patients who have chronic problems with ankle instability should be referred to an orthopaedist for evaluation, and the possibility of reconstructive surgery.

Eversion ankle sprains are much less common than inversion injuries. Patients with these will present with medial tenderness; these sprains involve injury to the deltoid ligament. Eversion injuries are frequently accompanied by injuries to the syndesmotic ligament or fractures of the fibula, and these must be carefully evaluated. The treatment philosophy is similar to inversion injuries, in which control of swelling is followed by immobilization and physical therapy.

Fractures of the Ankle

Fractures of the ankle are common injuries. The fracture pattern is the result of the forces applied to the ankle at the time of injury. Fractures may involve the distal fibula alone, or occur in combination with a fracture or ligamentous injury of the medial ankle. Fractures that involve the medial malleolus alone are uncommon, and a careful search for additional injury on the lateral side of the ankle must be performed. This should include radiographs of the entire leg, as a fibula fracture may occur anywhere along the length of the bone. Also a tear of the interosseous ligament will often occur in certain fracture patterns, especially those with a more proximal fibula fracture and a medial malleolar fracture.

Clinical Characteristics. The examination of a patient who has sustained an ankle fracture includes a thorough examination of the skin and the neurovascular status of the injured extremity. The location of the tenderness and the areas of swelling will give clues to which portions of the ankle have sustained either bony or ligamentous injury. Any gross deformity in the alignment of the ankle can be a sign of a fracture or dislocation, and severe displacement should be reduced immediately if the skin or neurovascular structures are at risk.

Radiographs are necessary and should include AP, lateral, and internal oblique views to visualize the ankle mortise. In cases where there is a medial fracture but no obvious lateral fracture, or in cases where there is lateral tenderness but not lateral fracture, radiographs of the entire leg should be performed to check for a more proximal fibula fracture.

The specific pattern of injury at the ankle is largely a function of the direction of forces applied to the ankle and foot at the time of injury. Pronation injuries may be associated with an abduction force or an external rotational force. Those associated with an abduction force produce either a ligamentous tear of the deltoid ligament or an avulsion fracture of the medial malleolus. The fibula fracture is often comminuted and appears as a crush-type injury. Those associated with an external rotational force produce a similar medial lesion, but the interosseous ligament is often torn and the fibula fracture is often spiral, with the spike of the distal fragment noted anteriorly (Fig. 8.20).

Supination injuries may be associated

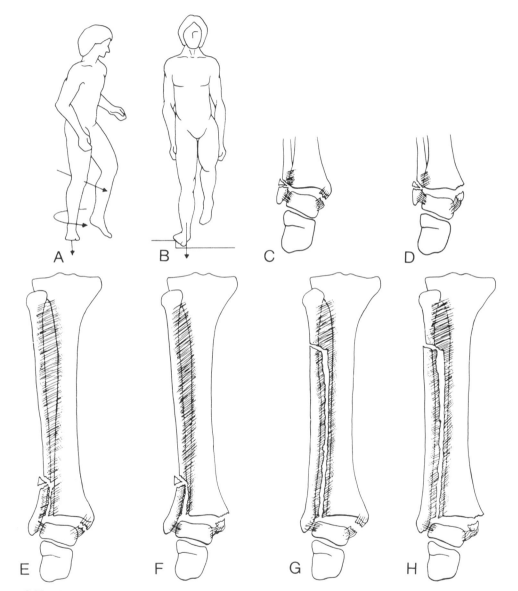

Figure 8.20.   Pronation injuries of the ankle. *A* and *B*, modes of injury. *A*, extremity rotates internally on the fixed foot. Since the foot is distal to the leg, by convention, the foot is considered externally rotated in relation to the leg. *B*, the foot is forced into pronation by weight taken on the lateral aspect of the forefoot. *C* and *D*, the medial injury may be ligamentous or involve a fracture of the medial malleous. The fibula fracture is frequently comminuted. *E–H*, the fibula fracture can occur at any level, with an accompanying tear of the interosseous membrane up to the level of the fracture. Note that the medial injury can be either ligamentous or bony.

with an adduction or an external rotational force. In adduction injuries, the medial fracture is often vertical and the fibula fracture is an avulsion type. In external rotational injuries, the medial malleolus is often avulsed and the fibula sustains a spiral fracture, usually at the joint line and with the spike of the distal fragment noted posteriorly (Fig. 8.21).

Axial compression forces can produce dramatically comminuted fractures of the tibial plafond (Fig. 8.22).

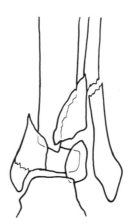

Figure 8.22. Axial compression injury produces severe disruption and fragmentation of the distal tibia. These injuries are very difficult to treat. (From Mast J. Reduction techniques in fractures of the distal tibial articular surface. Techniques in Orthopaedics, vol 2. Frederick, MD: Aspen Publishers, Inc, 1987:30, with permission.)

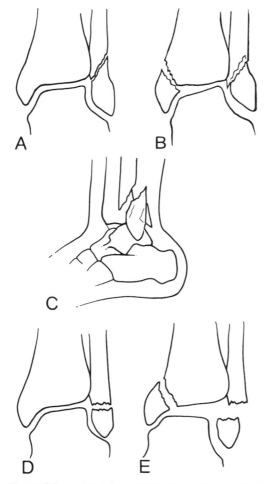

Figure 8.21. *A* and *B*, supination injury with external rotation produces a spiral fibula fracture with or without an accompanying fracture of the medial malleolus. *C*, lateral view of supination, external rotation injury. *D* and *E*, supination injury with the foot in adduction results in an avulsion fracture of the fibula with or without a fracture of the medial malleous.

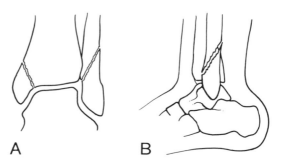

Figure 8.23. Acceptable reduction of an ankle fracture results in virtually an anatomic position on the mortise radiograph, and less than 3 mm displacement of the nonarticular portion of the fibula; fracture on the lateral view.

Treatment. It has been shown that displacement of the talus within the mortise of 1 to 2 mm reduces the area of contact force between the tibia and talus by 42%.[a] Consequently, this dramatically increases the degree of force on the remaining articular joint. These abnormal stresses can predispose to traumatic arthritis over time. Because of this predisposition, anatomic restoration of displaced fractures and/or dislocations of the ankle is a routine goal of treatment. Fortu-

[a]Ramsey PL, Hamilton W. Changes in tibio-talar area of contrast caused by talar shift. J Bone Joint Surg 1976;58A:356–357.

nately, the techniques of open reduction and internal fixation have improved substantially and if closed treatment cannot provide anatomic reduction, it can now be safely and almost routinely achieved by surgical means.

An anatomic result is one in which the subchondral plate of the tibia is continuous and does not show more than 1 mm of step-off or displacement on any radiographic view of the ankle. The subchondral margin of the fibula likewise should show less than

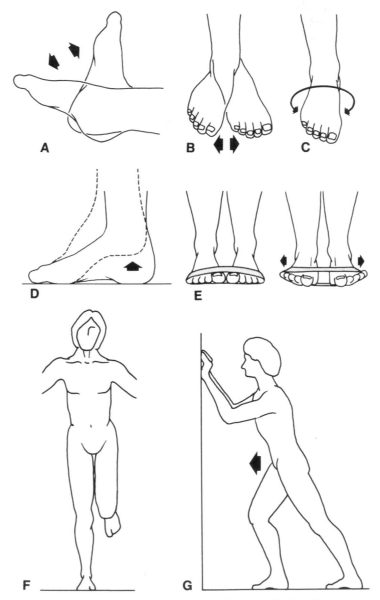

Figure 8.24. Range of motion and strengthening exercises of the foot and ankle. *A*, active movement of the tibiotalar joint by alternate dorsiflexion and plantar flexion. *B*, active movement of the subtalar, intertarsal, and tarsometatarsal joints by alternate supination and pronation. *C*, active movement of the tibiotalar, subtalar, intertarsal, and tarsometatarsal joints by circling the foot. *D*, repeated elevation onto the toes, standing. *E*, pronation against elastic resistance. *F*, balancing on one foot. *G*, heel cord stretching.

1 mm of step-off or displacement. The joint space between the talus and the tibia and fibula should be symmetrical on the mortise view, and the displacement of the nonarticular portion of the fibula less than 3 mm on the lateral radiograph (Fig. 8.23). Any result of a closed reduction that does not meet these criteria should be referred to an orthopaedist for possible internal fixation.

From a practical standpoint, this means that all fractures or fractures with ligamentous injury that occur on both sides of the ankle joint are best managed by consultation with an orthopaedist. Closed treatment of bimalleolar injuries require a specific reduction and casting technique, and subsequent displacement often occurs.

When a fracture apparently involves the fibula alone, it is important to be sure that there is no medial tenderness or widening of the medial joint space, which indicates a deltoid ligament injury. When there is no medial injury and the displacement of the non-articular portion of the fibula is less than 3 mm on the lateral view, the fracture can be treated with a short-leg walking cast for 6 weeks. A follow-up radiograph should be obtained at 2 weeks to ensure that no displacement occurs. To achieve range of motion and strengthening, physical therapy should follow the removal of the cast (Fig. 8.24).

SUGGESTED READINGS

D'Ambrosia R, Drez D Jr. Prevention and treatment of running injuries. Thorofare, NJ: Charles Slack, Inc, 1982.

Lovell WW, Winter RB, eds. Pediatric orthopedics, vol 2. 2nd ed. Philadelphia: JB Lippincott Co, 1986.

Mann RA: Surgery of the foot. 5th ed. St. Louis: The CV Mosby Co, 1985.

Rockwood AR Jr, Williams KE, King RE. Fractures in Children, vol 3. Philadelphia: JB Lippincott Co, 1984.

Rockwood CA Jr, Green DR. Fractures in adults, vol 2. 2nd ed. Philadelphia: JB Lippincott Co, 1984.

Torg JS, Vegso JJ, Torg E.: Rehabilitation of athletic injuries. Chicago: Yearbook Medical Publishers, 1987.

CHAPTER 9

Foot

Thom A. Tarquinio, M.D.

Essential Anatomy
BONES, JOINTS, AND LIGAMENTS

In this discussion, the foot will be divided into the hindfoot, midfoot, and forefoot. The hindfoot consists of the talus, the calcaneus, and the articulation between them, called the subtalar joint. The midfoot includes the navicular, cuboid, and three cuneiforms. The forefoot is comprised of the metatarsals and phalanges of the toes. The seven bones of the hindfoot and midfoot are collectively referred to as the tarsal bones (Figs. 9.1 and 9.2).

Hindfoot

The talus is divided into the larger posterior portion called the body and the rounded anterior end called the head, joined by the neck of the talus (Fig. 9.2). Because the talus is largely covered with articular cartilage, there is limited access for vascular supply. The main blood supply to the body of the talus enters at the level of the neck. Therefore, a displaced fracture through the neck of the talus may lead to loss of blood supply to the body, resulting in avascular necrosis of the talus. The talus articulates superiorly, medially, and laterally with the distal tibia and fibula at the ankle joint, inferiorly with the calcaneus at the subtalar joint, and anteriorly with the navicular at the talonavicular joint.

The largest bone of the foot is the calcaneus (Fig. 9.2), which articulates with the talus above and the cuboid at its anterior end. The calcaneus has a large posterior por-

tion called the tuberosity, which serves as the site of insertion of the Achilles tendon. The superior surface of the calcaneus is covered by three areas of articular cartilage forming the posterior, middle, and anterior facets of the subtalar joint. The subtalar joint is a very stable articulation because of the corresponding irregular bony surfaces of the calcaneus and talus plus the strong talocalcaneal interosseous ligament. On the anterolateral aspect of the hindfoot, just in front of the lateral malleolus, is a sulcus between the calcaneus and talus called the tarsal sinus. The plantar, medial, and lateral surfaces of the calcaneus serve as the site of origin of several intrinsic muscles of the foot. The plantar aspect of the calcaneus also serves as the origin for the strong plantar ligaments of the foot, including the long plantar ligament, plantar calcaneocuboid ligament, and plantar calcaneonavicular ligament. Because of the longitudinal arch of the foot, these plantar ligaments are under tension during weight bearing and aid in maintaining the longitudinal arch. Although the calcaneus sits beneath the talus in the posterior aspect of the subtalar joint, the anterior ends of the talus and calcaneus diverge. Because of this divergence, the anterior end of the talus lies medial and slightly superior to the anterior end of the calcaneus.

Midfoot

The proximal surface of the navicular is cup-shaped to articulate with the head of the talus. Distally, the navicular articulates with

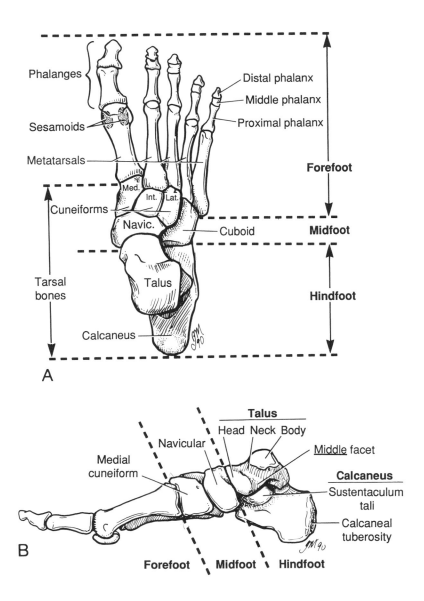

Figure 9.1. *A*, bones of the foot (superior view)—forefoot, midfoot, hindfoot. *B*, bones of the foot (medial view).

the three cuneiform bones. The navicular sits at the apex of the medial longitudinal arch and is supported in this position by the strong spring ligament (calcaneonavicular ligament) and the posterior tibial tendon. The importance of the posterior tibial tendon in supporting the midfoot medially is shown by the severe flatfoot deformity that devel-

ops after spontaneous rupture of this tendon. The cuboid articulates with the anterior end of the calcaneus on the lateral side of the midfoot and distally with the bases of the fourth and fifth metatarsals. The calcaneocuboid joint and the talonavicular joint together form the transverse tarsal joint. Because of the obliquity between the subtalar

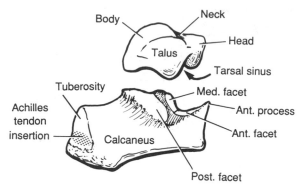

Figure 9.2. Lateral view of hindfoot.

joint and the transverse tarsal joint, the midfoot is flexible in pronation and becomes rigid (stable) in supination. The importance of this will be discussed under the section "Biomechanics of Gait."

The three cuneiform bones are called the medial, middle, and lateral cuneiforms or the first, second, and third cuneiforms, respectively. The cuneiforms provide the articulation for their correspondingly numbered metatarsal bases. The relatively transverse tarsometatarsal joints are collectively referred to as the Lisfranc joint. The second metatarsal base extends slightly more proximally than the remaining metatarsal bases and is the keystone of the Lisfranc joint, providing increased stability across the tarsometatarsal joint complex.

Forefoot

The five metatarsals are each composed of a base that articulates with a tarsal bone, a shaft, and an enlarged rounded distal end called the metatarsal head. The distal end of the metatarsal head provides the articular surface for the proximal phalanx of the toe, and the plantar surface of the metatarsal head is a major weight-bearing surface of the foot. Beneath the first metatarsal head are the medial (tibial) and lateral (fibular) sesamoid bones, which are incorporated into the flexor hallucis brevis tendon. The metatarsal heads are connected by the transverse metatarsal ligaments. The relative lengths of the individual metatarsals are variable. Because of the plantar inclination of the metatarsals as seen from the lateral view, a longer metatarsal will be directed further plantarward and therefore may be subjected to greater weight-bearing forces. Therefore, the anatomic variability in the length of the metatarsals may cause or contribute to metatarsalgia. The great toe has only two phalanges (proximal and distal), whereas the second, third, and fourth toes have three phalanges (proximal, middle, and distal). The fifth toe may have either two or three phalanges.

Accessory Ossicles of the Foot

There are several accessory ossicles or separate ossification centers of the foot which can be symptomatic or may be mistaken for a fracture (Fig. 9.3). The os trigonum and the os vesalianum are present in approximately 10% of adolescents and may be misdiagnosed as avulsion fractures. An accessory navicular bone on the medial side of the foot is a common cause of symptoms. These ossicles may fuse to their adjacent bone in adulthood.

MUSCLES OF THE FOOT

Active motion of the joints of the foot and active support of the foot during stance and gait are provided by the extrinsic and intrin-

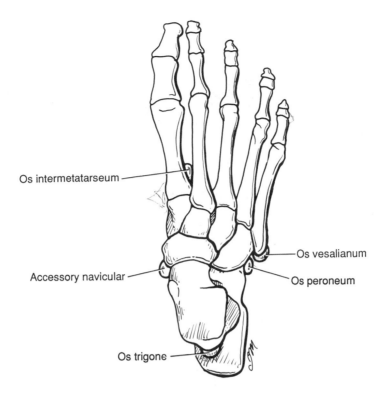

Os intermetatarseum

Os vesalianum

Accessory navicular

Os peroneum

Os trigone

Figure 9.3.   Accessory ossicles of foot.

sic muscles of the foot and leg. The extrinsic muscles (Fig. 9.4), described in the preceding chapter, arise in the leg and their tendons insert on the tarsals, metatarsals, and phalanges of the toes. The long extensor tendons (anterior tibial, extensor hallucis longus, extensor digitorum longus, and peroneus tertius) can be individually palpated on the dorsum of the foot and may be involved in pathologic conditions such as tendinitis, ganglion cysts, or tendon rupture. The posterior tibial, flexor digitorum longus, and flexor hallucis longus tendons coursing behind the medial malleolus, as well as the peroneal tendons laterally, may also be affected by tendinitis or tendon rupture. The posterior tibialis is the major supinator of the foot and is largely responsible for the dynamic support of the arch of the foot. This important tendon can be palpated just at the posterior edge of the medial malleolus and

then along the medial side of the hindfoot and midfoot.

The intrinsic extensor muscles of the foot include the extensor digitorum brevis (which dorsiflexes the proximal phalanges of the medial four toes and occasionally the small toe) and the four dorsal interossei. The plantar intrinsics of the foot function as a group to provide flexion of the metatarsophalangeal joints and extension of the interphalangeal joints of the toes. Therefore, if intrinsic function is lost, the metatarsophalangeal joints will extend and the interphalangeal joints will flex due to extrinsic tendon pull, and a hammertoe or claw toe will occur. The intrinsic muscles on the plantar aspect of the foot are arranged in layers along with the tendons of the long extrinsic flexors. These layers of the foot have significance for surgical procedures on the foot and are shown in Figure 9.5.

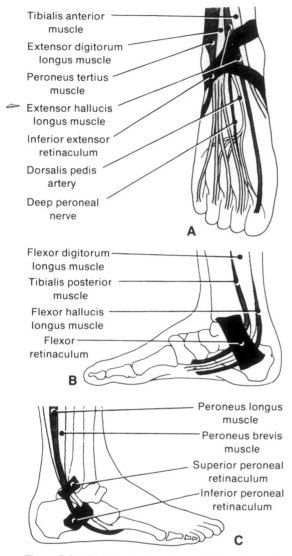

Tibialis anterior
muscle

Extensor digitorum
longus muscle

Peroneus tertius
muscle

Extensor hallucis
longus muscle

Inferior extensor
retinaculum

Dorsalis pedis
artery

Deep peroneal
nerve

A

Flexor digitorum
longus muscle

Tibialis posterior
muscle

Flexor hallucis
longus muscle

Flexor
retinaculum

B

Peroneus longus
muscle

Peroneus brevis
muscle

Superior peroneal
retinaculum

Inferior peroneal
retinaculum

C

Figure 9.4. Extrinsic tendons of foot. *A*, dorsal view. *B*, medial view. *C*, lateral view.

INNERVATION AND BLOOD SUPPLY

The posterior tibial nerve courses behind the medial malleolus and then gives off medial calcaneal branches, which supply sensation to the heel and a branch to the abductor digiti minimi. The posterior tibial nerve then continues deep to the abductor hallucis muscle and divides into the medial and lateral plantar nerves (Fig. 9.6). These nerves then innervate the plantar intrinsic muscles and supply sensation to the remaining sole of the foot.

The medial plantar nerve supplies innervation to the medial half of the sole of the foot as well as the medial three and one-half toes, whereas the lateral plantar nerve supplies the lateral portion of the sole of the foot and the lateral one and one-half toes. The medial plantar nerve also supplies the innervation to the following intrinsic foot muscles: adductor hallucis, flexor hallucis brevis, flexor digitorum brevis, and the first lumbrical. The lateral plantar nerve innervates the following intrinsic foot muscles: quadratus plantae, abductor digiti minimi, adductor hallucis, all interossei, and the lateral three lumbricals. The sensation to the remainder of the foot is provided by the sural, saphenous, superficial peroneal, and deep peroneal nerves, as indicated in Figure 9.7.

Circulation to the foot is derived from the posterior tibial artery and anterior tibial artery. The posterior tibial artery (Fig. 9.8*A*) curves behind the medial malleolus and then courses deep to the abductor hallucis muscle, where it divides into the smaller medial and larger lateral plantar arteries. The lateral plantar artery yields the plantar metatarsal arteries, which terminate in the common and digital arteries to the toes. The anterior tibial artery (Fig. 9.8*B*) becomes the dorsalis pedis artery just distal to the ankle joint, at which level it lies just lateral to the extensor hallucis longus tendon. The dorsalis pedis artery gives rise to the deep plantar artery and the arcuate artery and then terminates as the first dorsal metatarsal artery.

Biomechanics of the Foot
DEFINITIONS OF FOOT POSTURE (FIG. 9.9)

The hindfoot is said to be in equinus when the talus and calcaneus are plantar flexed (for example, heel cord tightness). The hindfoot is said to be in a calcaneus position when the talus and the calcaneus (the bone) are dorsiflexed (for example, loss of gastroc-

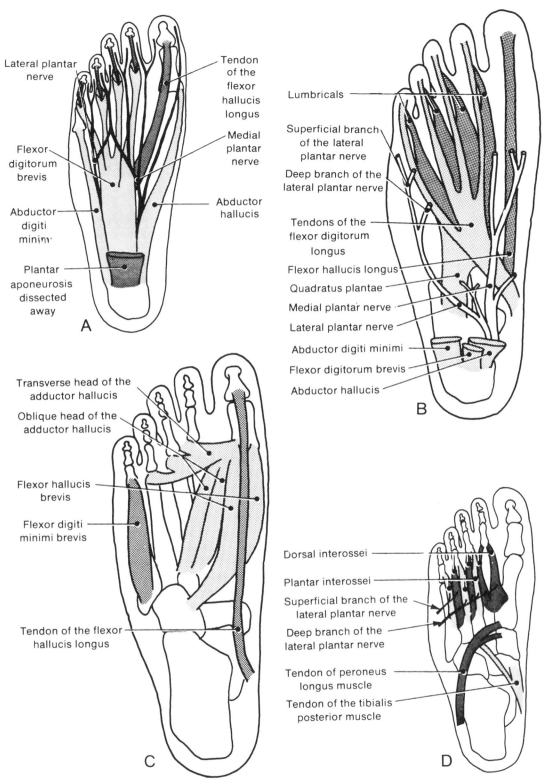

Figure 9.5. Intrinsic muscles of foot. *A*, first layer (most superficial). *B*, second layer. *C*, third layer. *D*, fourth layer (most deep).

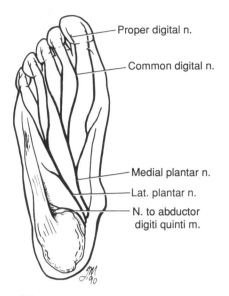

Figure 9.6. Branches of posterial tibial nerve on plantar aspect of foot. (Adapted from Baxter DE, Thigpen CM. Heel pain—operative results. Foot Ankle 1984;5(1):16–25.)

soleus function after polio). Viewing the heel from behind, the hindfoot is in varus or inversion if the heel is inclined so that the heel pad is medial to the ankle. The hindfoot is in valgus or eversion when the heel is inclined so that the heel pad is lateral to the ankle.

The terms used to describe the position of the forefoot and midfoot are used inconsistently in the literature. The following definitions of the position of the midfoot and forefoot are the most commonly used terms and will be used in the remainder of this chapter. When viewing the foot from the bottom, the metatarsals should approximately be in line with the hindfoot. Forefoot adduction means the metatarsals are angled medially toward the midline of the body when compared with the hindfoot. Metatarsus primus varus refers to adduction of the first metatarsal only, thereby increasing the angle between the first and second metatarsal shafts. Forefoot abduction means that the metatarsals are deviated laterally when compared with the hindfoot. If the forefoot is rotated around its long axis, so that the sole of the foot is turned toward the midline of the body, the forefoot is said to be in inversion, varus, or supination. If the sole of the foot is rotated around its long axis so that the sole of the foot is turned away from the midline of the body, the forefoot is said to be in eversion, valgus, or pronation.

Motion of the ankle, hindfoot, midfoot, and forefoot are all interconnected. As the normal foot goes into plantar flexion at the ankle, the hindfoot automatically goes into varus and the forefoot supinates (Fig. 9.9*G*). As the ankle dorsiflexes, the hindfoot goes into valgus and the forefoot everts (Fig. 9.9*H*). Metatarsus adductus may occur alone or in association with forefoot varus (supination). In the sagittal plane, the foot is in

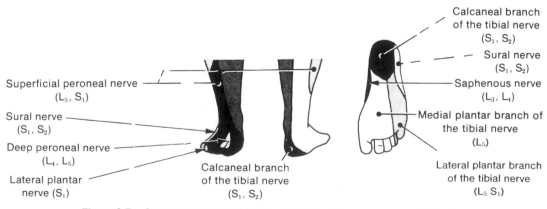

Figure 9.7. Sensory innervation of foot by peripheral nerve and nerve root distribution.

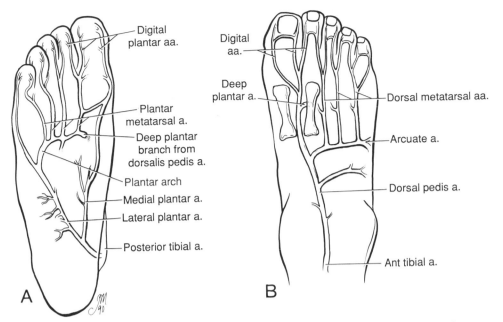

Figure 9.8. Circulation of foot. *A*, branches of posterior tibial artery. *B*, branches of anterior tibial artery.

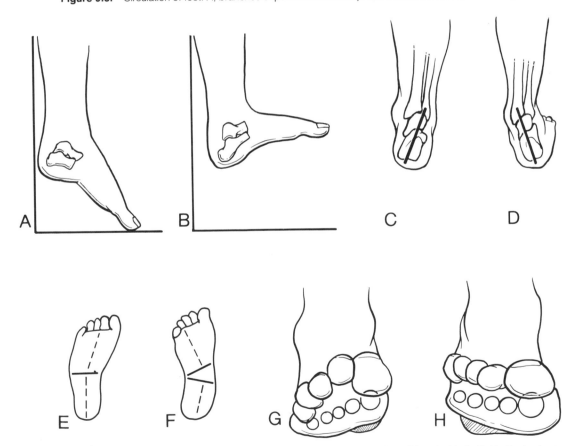

Figure 9.9. Postures of the foot. *A*, equinus. *B*, calcaneus. *C*, hindfoot varus (viewed from behind). *D*, hindfoot valgus (viewed from behind). *E*, metatarsus adductus (viewed from sole of foot). *F*, metatarsus abductus (viewed from sole of foot). *G*, forefoot suppination (varus). *H*, forefoot pronation.

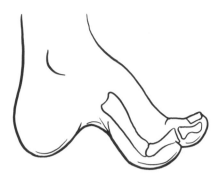

Figure 9.10. Cavus (high arch) foot. This deformity may be caused by calcaneus position of hindfoot (Fig. 9.9*B*) and/or equinus position of forefoot.

cavus if the forefoot is plantar flexed more than normal when compared with the calcaneus (Fig. 9.10).

BIOMECHANICS OF GAIT

The gait cycle during normal walking is divided into the stance phase and swing phase for each foot. Each foot is in stance phase for about 65% of the cycle and swing phase for 35% of the cycle. Both feet are on the ground for 30% of the gait cycle (double-limb support) during normal walking, but during running there is no period of double-limb support. Stance phase is further subdivided into three phases: (*a*) heel strike to foot flat, (*b*) period of foot flat, (*c*) heel raise to toe-off.

First Phase

As the heel strikes the ground, the anterior tibial and long toe extensors are active, allowing controlled plantar flexion and preventing foot slap. As the body weight progresses over the foot, the foot is loaded and passively goes into pronation. The posterior tibial and the foot intrinsics are silent during this phase and provide no support for the foot. As previously mentioned, the transverse tarsal joints are flexible in the pronated position, allowing the foot to adapt to the ground during the first phase of stance.

Second Phase

During the second phase of gait, the foot is flat on the ground and the ankle passively dorsiflexes as the tibia passes forward over the fixed foot. The gastrocsoleus complex fires at this point to limit the forward motion of the tibia, which allows the knee to passively extend. At this time, the posterior tibialis and the foot intrinsics begin to function actively, causing the foot to supinate and the heel to invert. This supinated position of the foot provides stability to the foot in preparation for push-off. In a patient with an equinus contracture, the ankle cannot dorsiflex so there is increased pressure beneath the forefoot during this phase of gait. This may result in metatarsalgia or forefoot plantar callosity. If the posterior tibial tendon is not functioning (due to paralysis or tendon rupture), the foot cannot actively be converted to the stable supinated position. Push-off then occurs with the foot in the flexible pronated position, resulting in foot strain and pain.

Third Phase

During the third phase of gait, the heel raises off the ground as body weight is progressively increased on the forefoot. The posterior tibialis and the foot intrinsics progressively supinate the foot to provide a more rigid structure for push-off. The windlass effect of the plantar fascia also assists in supination of the foot and elevation of the plantar arch during push-off, as the metatarsophalangeal joints passively extend when the patient "walks over" the metatarsophalangeal joints (Fig. 9.11). The triceps surae, peroneals, and long toe flexors all actively fire at this point to assist in push-off. During this phase of gait, the vertical load on the forefoot is greater than body weight.

BIOMECHANICS OF RUNNING

With the recent popularity of running for exercise, the primary care physician will be

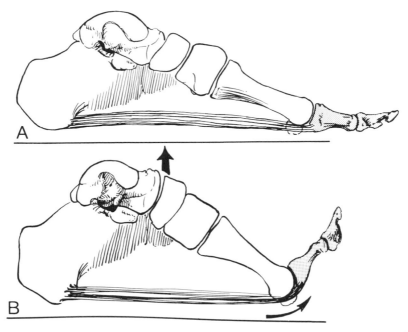

Figure 9.11. Windlass mechanism—when toes are dorsiflexed, the plantar aponeurosis becomes tight. This raises the longitudinal arch and assists in creating a stable supinated foot for push-off. (From Mann R, ed. Surgery of the foot. 5th ed. St. Louis: The CV Mosby Co, 1986:11, with permission.)

seeing more injuries or symptoms related to running. The gait cycle as just described for walking is altered when running. There is no longer a period when both feet are on the ground, and instead there is a period of time when both feet are off the ground. The pronation to supination seen during walking still occurs, but this change in position occurs much more rapidly when running. Also, the peak vertical loads when running can reach many times body weight. Because of the rapid change of position of the foot and the increased vertical loads, the patient may develop symptoms in the foot not seen during normal walking.

Evaluation of the Patient with Foot Symptoms
PHYSICAL EXAMINATION

The examination of the foot will be somewhat different when evaluating a toddler for in-toeing, a young adult following specific trauma, and a geriatric patient with chronic foot pain. However, there are basic principles that are important and should be understood for any foot examination. The foot must always be examined in non-weight-bearing (sitting), standing, and walking positions.

For most clinical problems, the examination begins by observing the feet with the patient sitting and the feet hanging over the side of the examination table. Observation will reveal any obvious swelling, color change, fixed deformity such as a rigid flat-foot, or evidence of superficial infection. The skin is examined for changes such as corns and calluses, plantar warts, or areas of ulceration. Temperature and pedal pulses are evaluated by palpation, or Doppler studies if clinically indicated. Next, the range of motion of the ankle, subtalar joint, midtarsal joints, and metatarsophalangeal joints and toes is evaluated. Motor, sensory, and deep tendon reflex examination is performed while the patient is sitting. Careful palpation will reveal areas of tenderness, and accurate location of tenderness based on a knowledge of anatomy is extremely important.

The patient is asked to stand and the overall alignment of the legs evaluated. Leg length is evaluated by checking for a level pelvis during stance. Thigh and calf atrophy may be observed during stance. As the patient stands, the amount of heel inversion or eversion and the height of the plantar arch are observed.

Next, the patient is asked to perform toe raises and the foot is observed to make sure that normal inversion of the heel and supination of the foot occur. The patient is then asked to ambulate and any limp is evaluated. The examiner also checks for in-toeing or out-toeing. The examiner should try to determine whether the foot normally pronates during initial stance phase and then supinates at push-off.

Last, because many foot deformities may result in unusual patterns of shoe wear, the patient's shoes should be evaluated.

RADIOGRAPHIC EVALUATION

Some foot complaints may be adequately evaluated without x-rays, but the primary care physician should be aware of certain radiographic studies that often are helpful in evaluating foot symptoms. Routine radiographs are satisfactory in the evaluation of most foot disorders (Fig. 9.12). Anteroposterior (AP), lateral, and oblique views are necessary for the evaluation of trauma, suspected osteomyelitis, or tumors. Standing AP and lateral radiographs provide valuable information in disorders such as flatfeet, hallux valgus, and some congenital abnormalities. The Harris axial view is useful in the evaluation of the calcaneus and talocalcaneal coalition. Technetium bone scans are useful in suspected cases of osteomyelitis or

stress fractures when plane radiographs are normal or equivocal. Computed tomography (CT) scan of the hindfoot often provides more information about the os calcis, talus, ankle joint, and subtalar joint than can be obtained with plane radiographs or conventional tomography. The indications for magnetic resonance imaging (MRI) of the foot are still being developed, but MRI is useful in evaluating soft tissue disorders such as tendinitis or tendon rupture and soft tissue tumors.

Nontraumatic Conditions of Childhood

Flatfeet and in-toeing are the two most common pediatric foot disorders. Most cases can be evaluated and definitively treated by the primary care physician. There are also a few less common pediatric foot deformities that should be recognized by the primary care physician, although they will require referral to the orthopaedic surgeon.

IN-TOEING

Although in-toeing frequently needs no specific treatment, the physician must understand the causes and explain the natural history of the deformity to the patient's parents. The foot progression angle is used to document the presence and magnitude of in-toeing (Fig. 9.13). The foot progression angle has a wide range of normal, from 5° of turning in to 20° of turning out. Although the patient will present with a chief complaint of turning in of the feet, it is important to remember that the etiology may be abnormal rotation of the femur or the tibia. In-toeing may be caused by one or more of the following: (*a*) increased femoral anteversion, (*b*) increased internal tibial torsion, and (*c*) metatarsus adductus. Each of these entities has specific physical findings, natural history, and treatment options, and each will be discussed separately.

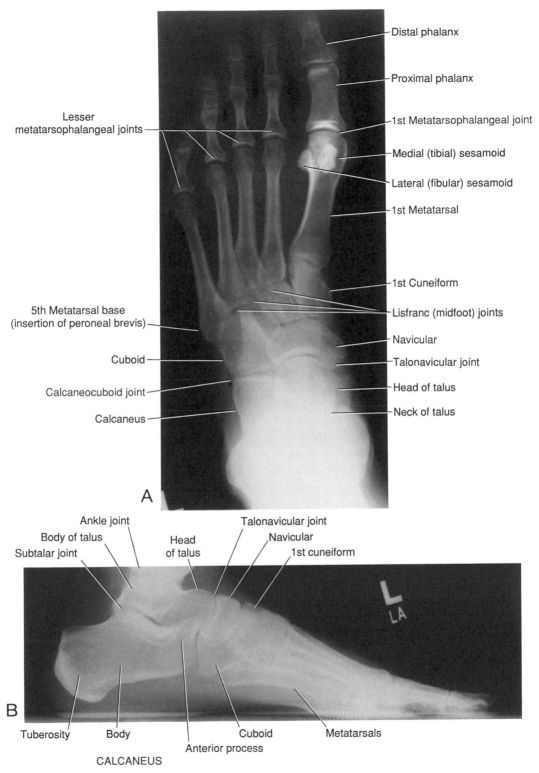

Distal phalanx

Proximal phalanx

1st Metatarsophalangeal joint

Medial (tibial) sesamoid

Lateral (fibular) sesamoid

1st Metatarsal

Lesser metatarsophalangeal joints

1st Cuneiform

Lisfranc (midfoot) joints

5th Metatarsal base (insertion of peroneal brevis)

Navicular

Talonavicular joint

Cuboid

Calcaneocuboid joint

Head of talus

Calcaneus

Neck of talus

A

Ankle joint

Body of talus

Subtalar joint

Head of talus

Talonavicular joint

Navicular

1st cuneiform

Tuberosity

Body

Anterior process

Cuboid

Metatarsals

B

CALCANEUS

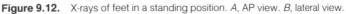

Figure 9.12. X-rays of feet in a standing position. *A,* AP view. *B,* lateral view.

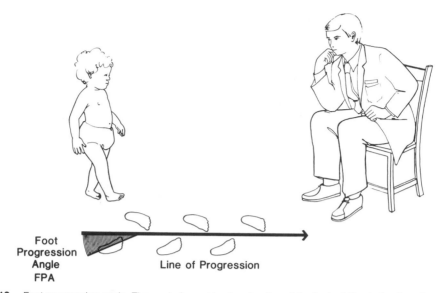

Figure 9.13. Foot progression angle. The angle formed by the direction of the foot relative to the line of progression of gait. (From Staheli LT. Torsional deformity. Pediatr Clin North Am 1986;33:1373–1383, with permission.)

Femoral Anteversion

Femoral anteversion is the angle of the femoral neck relative to the femoral condyles in the sagittal plane (Fig. 9.14). In the average adult standing with the femoral condyles directed straight ahead, the femoral necks angle forward about 15° to enter the acetabula. Normal infants may have up

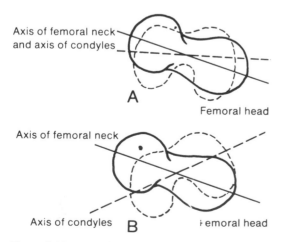

Figure 9.14. Anteversion of the femur. *A*, normal axis. *B*, the axial twist of anteversion.

to 45° of anteversion, which gradually decreases to an average of 15° during adolescence. If the amount of anteversion is increased, the hip will have more internal rotation and less external rotation. This will allow increased internal rotation of the entire leg during gait, thus causing in-toeing. Due to soft tissue contracture, normal infants may have much more external rotation of the hips than internal rotation. Normally, an older child will have slightly more external rotation than internal rotation of the hips, measured with the child in the prone position and the knees flexed (Fig. 9.15). If a patient is found to have more than 70° of internal rotation of the hips and less than 30° of external rotation of the hips, then femoral anteversion is causing or contributing to the in-toeing.

Treatment. Various devices such as twister cables, external rotation (Denis-Browne) splints, and shoe wedges have been used in the past to treat femoral anteversion. However, these are either ineffective or may cause secondary deformities, such as excessive external tibial torsion or foot deformi-

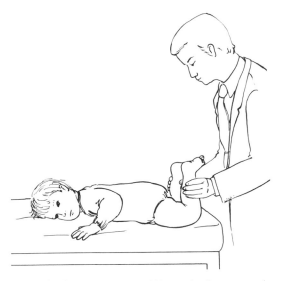

Figure 9.15. Measurement of hip rotation in prone position. (From Straheli LT. Torsional deformity. Pediatr Clin North Am 1986;33:1373–1383, with permission.)

ties, and are rarely indicated. The parents can be reassured that most femoral anteversion resolves by adolescence and that there is no effective nonoperative treatment. It should be explained to the parents that femoral anteversion has not been shown to cause back pain, hip pain or hip arthritis, flatfeet, or any problems with sports participation. Femoral anteversion plus abnormal external tibial torsion, however, may cause patella malalignment and subsequent knee symptoms. In the rare case of severe femoral anteversion persisting in late childhood, only derotational osteotomies of the femurs

will change the anteversion and correct the in-toeing, and orthopaedic referral will be necessary.

Internal Tibial Torsion

Tibial torsion is the angular relationship of the medial and lateral malleoli to the coronal plane of the knee. This is best measured as the thigh-foot angle with the child prone (Fig. 9.16). If the transmalleolar axis and therefore the foot are internally rotated compared with the thigh, then internal tibial torsion is present. If the foot and ankle are externally rotated to the thigh, then external tibial torsion is present. The range of normal tibial torsion is quite variable and up to 20° of internal tibial torsion is normal in infants. The transmalleolar axis normally becomes more externally rotated during childhood, resulting in 15° to 20° of external tibial torsion by adolescence. If internal tibial torsion persists, the ankle joint will be internally rotated compared with the knee and in-toeing will result. During gait, the child with in-toeing secondary to femoral anteversion will be noted to have both patellae turned inward toward each other (because the inward rotation occurs at the level of the hips), whereas in a child with internal tibial torsion, the feet will turn in but the patellae will not (because the inward rotation occurs below the knees).

Treatment. Internal tibial torsion, like femoral anteversion, improves spontane-

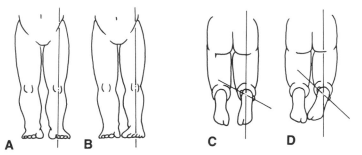

Figure 9.16. Tibial Torsion. *A*, normal axis *B*, the axial twist of internal tibial torsion. *C*, normal thigh-foot angle. *D*, thigh-foot angle in internal tibial torsion.

ously with growth and usually only reassurance is needed rather than active treatment. Special shoes, shoe wedges, and casts are ineffective in treating internal tibial torsion, but in severe cases an external rotation splint may be indicated. If internal tibial torsion remains significant (thigh-foot angle greater than 20°) by 6 to 8 months of age, orthopaedic referral is then indicated for possible treatment with an external rotation splint. If severe internal tibial torsion persists, orthopaedic referral is indicated for possible tibial osteotomies.

Metatarsus Adductus

The final cause of in-toeing is metatarsus adductus, a deformity of the foot itself. In patients with metatarsus adductus, the alignment of the legs will be normal from the hips down to and including the hindfoot. However, the forefoot will be adducted or turned inward referable to the hindfoot (Fig. 9.9E). This is best seen when the foot is examined from the bottom. Normally, the lateral border of the foot will form a straight line from the heel to the fifth toe. In metatarsus adductus there will be a break or curve at the midfoot such that, even with the entire leg and hindfoot directed straight ahead, the forefoot will turn in toward the midline of the body.

Treatment. Metatarsus adductus is a very common positional deformity of the newborn and, unless associated with a deformity of the hindfoot (such as a true clubfoot), it usually corrects with growth and stretching. Parents should be instructed to perform passive stretching exercises with each diaper change. When the infant is 1 to 3 months old, the metatarsus adductus is again evaluated as to severity and also to flexibility, which is measured by how easily the foot can be passively overcorrected by the examiner. If significant metatarsus adductus persists to the age of 4 to 6 months, it can usually be corrected by manipulation and serial corrective casts. The proper molding of these corrective casts is difficult to per-

form, and because of potential skin problems, the author feels that these children should be referred to the orthopaedic surgeon for cast treatment of persistent metatarsus adductus.

FLATFEET

Flatfeet or pes planus is generally divided into the very common and rarely symptomatic flexible flatfoot and the uncommon but symptomatic rigid flatfoot. The differentiation between a flexible and rigid flatfoot is made by physical examination. In both types of pes planus there is loss of the normal plantar arch when the child stands. However, in a flexible flatfoot there will be a normal arch when the patient is sitting with the feet hanging over the side of the examination table and when the patient stands on tiptoes. Also, a flexible flatfoot will have normal motion of the subtalar joint. The patient with flexible flatfeet will often have other findings of increased ligamentous laxity (e.g., hyperextension of the knee or elbow) or a history of being double-jointed. In children up to the age of 2, the fat pad on the medial side of the foot may give a false appearance of a flatfoot when the toddler is standing. Flexible pes planus is usually bilateral, often hereditary, and as mentioned above, usually asymptomatic.

Longitudinal studies of large groups of children have shown that some flexible flatfeet will gradually develop a plantar arch without treatment. The author is not aware of any study that has shown significant statistical difference in arch development in children with flexible flatfeet treated with orthoses versus simple observation. Therefore, orthotic treatment of asymptomatic flexible flatfeet is not usually recommended. However, orthotic devices may decrease symptoms in a child with flexible flatfeet who has discomfort in the legs or feet.

In contrast to flexible pes planus, the rigid flatfoot is usually symptomatic. The rigid flatfoot will be flat with loss of the arch even when the child is non-weight bearing or standing on tiptoes. The rigid flatfoot has limited or absent motion of the subtalar joint. Peroneal muscle spasm is also frequently noted on physical examination, and hence the term "peroneal spastic flatfoot" is used interchangeably with rigid flatfoot. The most common cause of a rigid flatfoot is a tarsal coalition or fusion between the calcaneus and either the talus or navicular. The radiographic diagnosis of tarsal coalition is sometimes difficult and may require conventional tomography, CT scanning, or MRI evaluation, in addition to routine x-rays.

Treatment

Any pathology involving the subtalar joint, such as arthritis, infection, or trauma, may result in a rigid flatfoot and must be considered in the differential diagnosis. If symptoms of a tarsal coalition persist after conservative treatment with immobilization, orthoses, and anti-inflammatory medication, surgery is often indicated. Therefore, patients with rigid flatfeet should be referred to the orthopaedist for evaluation.

NEWBORN FOOT DEFORMITIES

Significant foot deformities in the newborn will usually be referred to the orthopaedic surgeon, but these congenital deformities must first be recognized by the primary care physician. These include talipes equinovarus (clubfoot), calcaneovalgus foot deformity, and congenital vertical talus.

Talipes Equinovarus

Talipes equinovarus is a congenital foot deformity in which the heel is in equinus (plantar flexed) and varus, and the forefoot is adducted (Fig. 9.17). The initial treatment is stretching combined with either corrective taping or corrective casting. This manipulative treatment of clubfoot is much more effective when started immediately. Therefore, the orthopaedic surgeon should be consulted promptly so that treatment can begin in the newborn nursery. The foot is then treated by serial manipulation and cast-

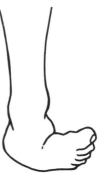

Figure 9.17.   Talipes equinovarus (clubfoot).

ing, often for several months. If manipulation and casting is not successful in completely correcting the foot, surgery may be necessary. Surgery may be performed as early as 3 or 4 months of age, but at other times will be delayed until the child is 1 to 2 years old.

Calcaneovalgus Foot

The calcaneovalgus foot presents with dorsiflexion of the ankle and eversion and abduction of the forefoot (Fig. 9.9, *B* and *F*). In severe cases, the dorsal surface of the foot will be resting on the anterolateral aspect of the lower leg. Although this deformity may initially look as severe as a clubfoot, its prognosis is much better. A calcaneovalgus foot will usually respond within 1 to 3 months with simple passive stretching exercises. The parents are taught to stretch the foot down out of the dorsiflexed position and inward toward the midline of the body with each diaper change. In a severe case that does not correct well by the age of 2 to 3 months with passive stretching exercises, manipulation by the orthopaedic surgeon and corrective cast may be necessary. Surgery is almost never required for a calcaneovalgus deformity of the foot.

Vertical Talus

A rare but severe congenital foot deformity is a congenital vertical talus. In this deformity, the navicular is dislocated onto the dorsal surface of the talus, forcing the talar head down into a plantar flexed position. The Achilles tendon is tight, pulling the calcaneus into a plantar flexed position also. This results in a rigid flatfoot with a rounded appearance on the sole of the foot caused by the displaced head of the talus. This uncommon deformity should be referred to the orthopaedic surgeon immediately. Manipulation may partially correct the deformity, but surgery is usually necessary to gain a satisfactory correction of this foot deformity.

CAVUS FOOT

The foot with a high arch and a plantar flexed forefoot is called a cavus foot (Fig. 9.10). This foot deformity is frequently associated with hammertoes or claw toes and may or may not be symptomatic. A cavus foot should alert the physician to the possibility of an underlying neurologic disorder. Neurologic causes of a cavus foot include Charcot-Marie-Tooth disease, diastematomyelia, myelomeningocele, and polio. Therefore, examination of the spine and a careful neurologic examination, as well as a family history, are necessary in the evaluation of a patient with a cavus foot. Because of the plantar flexed forefoot and the claw toes, there is frequently pain in the plantar aspect of the metatarsal heads. This pain may be relieved with orthoses and metatarsal pads or shoe modifications. Severe cases should be referred to the orthopaedist for consideration of surgical correction of the foot deformity.

Nontraumatic Conditions in Adulthood

Pain and deformity are the most common complaints in adults presenting with a nontraumatic foot problem. The patient will usually relate symptoms to the hindfoot, midfoot, or forefoot and toes, and this section of the chapter will be subdivided on this basis. After the history is obtained, examination of the foot is performed following the principles previously described. At this point, a differential diagnosis is established and further evaluation and treatment planned. Radiographic evaluation, e.g., routine x-rays, bone scan, CT scan, or MRI, may then be appropriately ordered. For some foot disorders, blood tests may be helpful. Certain systemic diseases, such as diabetes or inflammatory disorders, may affect the foot and will be discussed separately.

HINDFOOT PAIN

One of the most common foot complaints is heel pain. The pain will usually be localized to the posterior aspect or the plantar surface of the heel. Less frequently, the medial or lateral side of the heel may be symptomatic. Common causes of posterior heel pain, such as Achilles tendinitis and calcaneal bursitis, were discussed in the previous chapter. Pain on the plantar aspect of the heel is usually due to plantar fasciitis. Pain on the medial side of the heel may arise from the subtalar joint or the posterior tibial tendon. Lateral-sided heel pain may arise from subtalar joint pathology or a disorder of the peroneal tendons. A differential diagnosis of heel pain may therefore be developed by history alone, based on the location of the pain. Several common causes of heel pain are discussed below.

Plantar Fasciitis

An extremely common complaint is plantar heel pain secondary to plantar fasciitis. The patient will typically localize the pain to the distal medial aspect of the plantar surface of the heel pad at the site of origin of the plantar fascia. The pain is most severe when the patient first stands up in the morning or stands after prolonged sitting during the day. The pain may gradually worsen toward the end of the day and is usually relieved when the patient lies down at night.

The most dramatic physical finding is tenderness to palpation on the plantar aspect of the heel in the anteromedial aspect of the

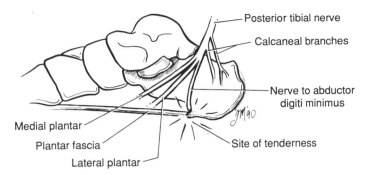

Figure 9.18.   Plantar fasciitis. Note site of tenderness on plantar aspect of heel at origin of plantar fascia off calcaneus. Also note course of nerve to abductor digiti minimi. (Adapted from Baxter DE, Thigpen CM. Heel pain—operative results. Foot Ankle 1984;5(1):16–25.)

heel pad, at the site of origin of the plantar fascia (Fig. 9.18). An x-ray may be normal or may show a plantar calcaneal spur. In addition to plantar fasciitis, other terms used to describe this syndrome include heel spur syndrome or plantar heel pain syndrome. The pain may result from inflammation or microtearing of the origin of the plantar fascia from the os calcis. Some orthopaedists believe this syndrome is caused by entrapment of the nerve to the abductor digiti minimi on the plantar surface of the os calcis. The plantar calcaneal spur is more likely to be a radiographic result of the trauma and inflammation than the cause of the pain. This distinction is important because some patients falsely believe their pain is caused by the spur and therefore can only be relieved by surgical excision of the spur. In truth, the pain of plantar fasciitis will often be improved with oral anti-inflammatory medications, passive stretching exercises, rest, heel pads or heel cups, or physical therapy. Resistant cases may require steroid injection into the area of maximum tenderness and the use of orthoses which should be prescribed by a consulting orthopaedic surgeon.

With the above conservative treatment measures, at least 90% of patients will have satisfactory pain relief. The small remaining group of patients require orthopaedic referral for consideration of surgery. Several different operative approaches have been used in the treatment of this disorder. These include simple plantar fascial release, excision of the heel spur, neurolysis of the nerve to the abductor digiti minimi, or a combination of these procedures.

Subtalar Joint Pathology

Hindfoot pain should alert the physician to carefully evaluate the subtalar joint on physical examination and radiographic studies. By allowing inversion and eversion of the heel, subtalar joint motion allows the foot to accommodate to uneven ground. Therefore, a patient being evaluated for hindfoot pain should be specifically questioned about pain or difficulty walking on uneven ground. If such history is present, subtalar joint pathology should be suspected. When asked to localize the pain, the patient with subtalar joint pathology will often grasp the heel from behind with the thumb and index finger below both malleoli. The pain may be felt medially or laterally or on both sides of the hindfoot. On physical examination, the range of motion of the subtalar joint will be decreased or painful. Subtalar joint motion is examined with the ankle in dorsiflexion to lock the talus into the ankle mortise. The heel is grasped by the examiner's hand and rocked into inversion and eversion. The symptoms and signs of pathology involving the subtalar joint are nonspecific and may be seen with inflammatory arthritis, posttraumatic arthritis, loose bodies, tumors, or tarsal coalitions. In addition to routine radiographs, the Harris axial view and CT scanning are helpful in evaluating the subtalar joint.

Posterior Tibial Tendon Dysfunction

Dysfunction of the posterior tibialis may occur with tenosynovitis, partial tendon rupture, complete tendon rupture, or avulsion of the insertion of the tendon into the navicular. Disorders of the posterior tibial tendon may result in pain anywhere along the course of the tendon, from above the medial malleolus, to the posteromedial side of the ankle, to the medial side of the midfoot. Recently, it has been recognized that the posterior tibial tendon can degenerate and spontaneously rupture. The diagnosis of a ruptured posterior tibial tendon is rarely made at the time of rupture, and the primary care physician should be aware of the existence of this entity and the typical physical findings (Fig. 9.19). In addition to pain, there may be soft tissue swelling along the course of the tendon. When the posterior tibialis does not function, the foot loses its active supination and a flatfoot deformity may develop. The patient is unable to stand on tiptoes on the affected side or can do so only with pain. Normally, the heel will actively invert when the patient stands on tiptoes,

but with posterior tibial tendon dysfunction, the heel will remain in valgus when the patient stands on tiptoes. Active inversion of the foot against resistance will be decreased in posterior tibial tendon dysfunction, although the anterior tibialis and the long toe flexors may combine to give the appearance of active function of the posterior tibial tendon. Routine x-rays are not helpful, although an MRI study may show the tendon abnormality.

Conservative treatment for this problem includes nonsteroidal anti-inflammatory medications, physical therapy, and the use of an ankle brace. An orthotic device may be prescribed by a consulting orthopaedic surgeon. If rupture of the posterior tibial tendon is suspected, referral should be made to an orthopaedic surgeon for further treatment.

MIDFOOT PAIN

Pain restricted to the area of the midfoot is relatively uncommon compared with pain in the hindfoot or forefoot. An accessory navicular (Fig. 9.3) may cause pain from shoe pressure or from stress to the posterior tibial tendon as it passes around the accessory navicular. In addition to local tenderness over the accessory navicular, the foot may be hyperpronated. An orthosis and nonsteroidal anti-inflammatory medications may relieve symptoms related to stress on the posterior

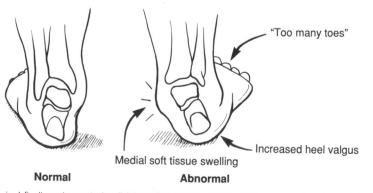

Normal   **Abnormal**

"Too many toes"

Medial soft tissue swelling

Increased heel valgus

Figure 9.19. Physical findings in posterior tibial tendon rupture. Note soft tissue swelling behind medial malleolus and increased heel valgus. Because of forefoot abduction, "too many toes" will be visible on affected side compared to normal side when both feet are viewed from behind.

tibial tendon. Steroid injections around the insertion of the posterior tibial tendon are generally contraindicated because of the increased risk of tendon rupture. A short-leg walking cast for 3 to 4 weeks may relieve the pain of a symptomatic accessory navicular. If conservative treatment does not relieve symptoms, excision of the accessory navicular may be indicated.

Another cause of pain in the midfoot is a tarsal boss, which is an osteophyte on the dorsum of the midfoot. This osteophyte is usually small but easily palpated on the dorsum of the foot and may be tender on palpation. The tarsal boss may be painful from direct shoe pressure or from tendinitis resulting from irritation of the extensor tendons by the osteophytes. Shoes with a softer, better-padded tongue may be successful in relieving the pain from the dorsal osteophytes. Surgical excision of a tarsal boss is occasionally necessary.

The dorsum of the midfoot is a common site for ganglion cysts, which are another cause of midfoot pain. The soft tissue mass can be aspirated, yielding the typical jelly-like material of a ganglion cyst, thereby confirming the diagnosis. After aspiration of the cyst, it can be injected with a small amount of steroid preparation. An asymptomatic ganglion cyst does not necessarily need to be surgically excised, but a symptomatic ganglion cyst can usually be excised under local anesthesia.

Plantar fibromatosis is a locally aggressive, frequently bilateral process that occurs as a painful mass involving the plantar fascia. Initially there may be tenderness along the entire course of the plantar fascia, and the patient may be seen before development of palpable nodules. As the process continues, however, one to several soft tissue masses develop along the course of the plantar fascia. Although not a malignant process, plantar fibromatosis may recur following surgical excision. The incidence of recurrence is decreased by surgically excising a large margin of normal plantar fascia rather than simply excising the individual fibrous nodules.

Aseptic Necrosis of the Navicular (Köhler's Disease)

This occurs for unknown reasons (perhaps akin to those of Legg-Perthes disease) in prepubertal schoolchildren. The child limps and complains of pain along the inner aspect of the foot. Physical examination will demonstrate tenderness over the medial aspect of the midfoot and pain during active or passive supination of the foot. X-ray may confirm the diagnosis eventually but may be normal if the child is first seen early in the course of the illness. Any child who complains of midfoot pain should be followed at biweekly intervals with this diagnosis in mind until pain remits or the x-ray confirms necrosis or is normal six weeks after the first consultation.

Treatment. Treatment with a cast is often necessary. It is recommended that an orthopaedic consultation be obtained at this point since healing is often difficult to judge.

FOREFOOT PAIN

Pain in the forefoot, with or without deformity, is probably the most common foot complaint for which patients will seek medical attention. Several common disorders involving the metatarsals, metatarsophalangeal joints, and toes will be seen by the primary care physician.

Hallux Valgus

The major cause of pain and deformity on the medial side of the forefoot is hallux valgus, which is a deviation of the great toe toward the lateral side of the foot (Fig. 9.20). This angular deformity occurs at the level of the metatarsophalangeal joint. This is associated with an exostosis or prominence of the medial aspect of the first metatarsal head. There also may be an overlying bursa, prone

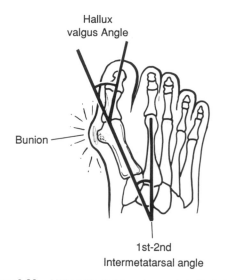

Hallux
valgus Angle

Bunion

1st-2nd
Intermetatarsal angle

Figure 9.20. Hallux valgus. Lines demonstrate the hallux valgus angle and the first-second intermetatarsal angle.

to inflammation. Hallux valgus is more common in female patients, and there is often a positive family history. Metatarsus primus varus refers to angulation of the first metatarsal shaft away from the second metatarsal shaft, and predisposes to the development of hallux valgus and a bunion. Hyperpronation of the foot may also predispose the patient to the development of hallux valgus.

Hallux valgus may be painful because of the development of bursitis or soft tissue inflammation over the bunion caused by shoe pressure. Conservative treatment for hallux valgus therefore begins with shoe modification. Many women prefer to wear "fashionable shoes," which often have high heels and a pointed toe. The pointed toe of the shoe forces the great toe into further valgus and the high heel causes the body weight to be borne more directly by the already symptomatic forefoot. In addition to pain over the bunion, hallux valgus may cause a secondary deformity of the second toe. The valgus position of the great toe may result in an overriding second toe. The second toe is therefore pushed up against the inside of the shoe and may become symptomatic.

Treatment. These patients should wear shoes with a wider toe box and flat heels. The shoe should be made of soft leather without seams over the bunion. If the patient has increased pronation, the shoe should have a good arch support or an orthosis should be added to the shoe to decrease pronation. Exercises and night splints are generally not helpful in the treatment of hallux valgus. Patients who have significant symptoms from hallux valgus in spite of shoe modifications should be referred to an orthopaedic surgeon for evaluation for surgical correction.

Hallux Rigidus

Hallux rigidus, an uncommon but often disabling disorder of the great toe, is an unusual type of degenerative joint disease involving the first metatarsophalangeal joint. Unlike degenerative joint disease of other joints, it is often seen in young adults and may even occur in teenagers. Hallux rigidus, more common in male than female patients, usually occurs spontaneously, although there may be a history of a specific injury. Examination reveals palpable, tender osteophytes dorsally on the first metatarsal head (Fig. 9.21), rather than medially as in a bunion. The range of motion of the first metatarsophalangeal joint is decreased, and dorsiflexion is especially limited and painful. X-rays show the osteophytes on the first metatarsal head as well as the base of the

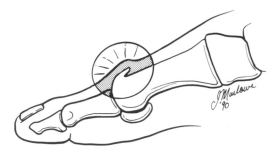

Figure 9.21. Hallux rigidus. Prominent dorsal osteophyte on first metatarsal head seen on lateral radiographic view.

proximal phalanx, and varying degrees of sclerosis and loss of the joint space of the first metatarsophalangeal joint. Rest, nonsteroidal anti-inflammatory medications, and a stiff-soled shoe may provide some relief, but often surgical treatment is required.

Lesser Metatarsal Pain

Pain in the area of the second through the fifth metatarsals (the so-called lesser metatarsals) may have many causes. The term metatarsalgia is sometimes used nonspecifically to denote any pain in the area of the lesser metatarsals. However, the author prefers to use the term metatarsalgia specifically to describe pain beneath the metatarsal heads that is caused by abnormal weight distribution among the metatarsal heads. Common causes of lesser metatarsal pain include stress fractures, metatarsalgia, Morton's neuroma, and synovitis of the metatarsophalangeal joints.

Stress Fracture. Stress fractures, also called fatigue fractures or march fractures, may occur when a bone is subjected to mechanical stresses of unusual severity. This might occur in an individual who starts a new exercise program or rapidly increases the exercise level. Stress fractures are common in the lesser metatarsals, although they also commonly occur in the calcaneus, tibia, fibula, and femur. Bone will remodel in response to the increased mechanical demands, but a stress fracture may occur before the bone can adequately reinforce itself. If a patient presents with pain, swelling, and tenderness over the shaft or neck of one of the lesser metatarsals, a history of increased activity should be sought by the physician. X-rays may show periosteal new bone formation, sclerosis across the metatarsal shaft, or a radiolucent fracture line, but may also be normal. If a stress fracture is suspected and x-rays are normal, repeat x-rays may show a stress fracture in 2 to 3 weeks. A technetium bone scan is the most sensitive technique for early diagnosis of a stress fracture, and a bone scan will often be "hot" before x-ray changes are seen. A stress fracture of a lesser metatarsal may be treated with crutches and decreased activities, but if very symptomatic, the patient should be placed in a short-leg walking cast for 3 to 6 weeks. Once the cast is removed, it is important that the patient be advised to return to the prior activity level on a very gradual basis.

Metatarsalgia. If one metatarsal head is subjected to increased weight-bearing stress, pain may occur beneath that metatarsal head. This may occur if one metatarsal is longer or more plantar flexed than adjacent metatarsals. A hammertoe may cause metatarsalgia because the top of the shoe will press the toe down, which will secondarily depress the metatarsal head (Fig. 9.22), and also because the involved toe will not share the weight-bearing function with the metatarsal head. Less common causes of metatarsalgia include a tight heel cord and the habitual use of high-heeled shoes. If one metatarsal head bears more than its fair share of weight over a long period of time, the skin beneath the metatarsal head may become thickened and hyperkeratotic, resulting in a corn or callus, also called a plantar keratosis (Fig. 9.23).

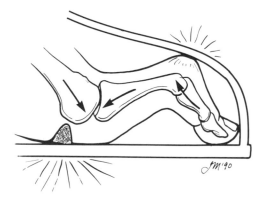

Figure 9.22. Hammertoe causing pain over top of proximal interphalangeal joint of toe and beneath the metatarsal head. Either area may also develop a hyperkerototic lesion (corn or callus). (Adapted from Mann R, ed. Surgery of the foot. 5th ed. St. Louis: The CV Mosby Co, 1986, with permission.)

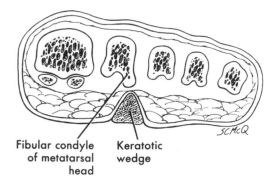

Figure 9.23. Plantar keratosis. Hyperkerototic lesion (corn) develops secondary to abnormally high weight bearing pressure by underlying metatarsal head. (From Crenshaw AH, ed. Campbell's orthopedics. 7th ed. St. Louis: The CV Mosby Co, 1987, with permission.)

It is important to understand that a corn or a callus beneath the metatarsal head is a response to increased pressure by the metatarsal head. It is therefore not possible to permanently cure a patient's pain by shaving or

removing the callus. Unless something is done to more equally distribute weight bearing, the callus will always recur. However, temporary relief of symptoms can be obtained by carefully debriding the plantar keratosis with a scalpel, stopping before bleeding occurs. Corn plasters with acid should be avoided as they can cause ulcerations. Modifications of the shoe with an orthosis, metatarsal pads, and lower heels may be the only treatment required for mild metatarsalgia. In severe cases, surgical realignment of the metatarsal may be required in order to balance the weight bearing among the metatarsal heads.

Morton's Neuroma. A common cause of forefoot pain is an interdigital neuroma, called a Morton's neuroma, which begins as an entrapment of the common digital nerve between the metatarsal heads (Fig. 9.24). The most common locations are between the third and fourth metatarsal heads or be-

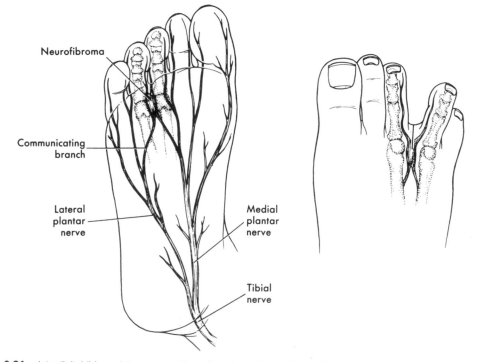

Figure 9.24. Interdigital (Morton's) neuroma. (From Crenshaw AH, ed. Campbell's orthopedics. 7th ed. St. Louis: The CV Mosby Co, 1987, and redrawn from McElvenny RY. J Bone Joint Surg 1943;25:675, with permission.)

tween the second and third metatarsal heads. This entrapment of the nerve will lead to an inflammatory process, and with time there will be edema, perineural fibrosis, and demyelination of the nerve. The patient commonly complains of pain on the plantar aspect of the forefoot, beneath the metarsal heads, or at the distal portion of the fat pad at the base of the toes. The pain is often poorly localized and may radiate to the toes or occasionally proximally up the foot. There may be a sensation of catching or clicking between the metatarsal heads, and the patient may also complain of tingling or paresthesias of the toes.

The symptoms of a Morton's neuroma are usually worse with shoe wear and relieved by shoe removal. The key to the diagnosis is tenderness between the metatarsal heads, rather than directly beneath the metatarsal head as seen in metatarsalgia. Routine x-rays are normal, although in rare cases an MRI study may be helpful in diagnosing a neuroma. Treatment includes shoes with a wider toe box and a soft sole, metatarsal pads or an orthosis, nonsteroidal anti-inflammatory medications, and steroid injections. The injection is given through a dorsal approach between the involved metatarsal heads. The needle is passed between the metatarsal heads and the steroid preparation is infiltrated in the plantar aspect of the foot. If severe symptoms persist, surgical excision of the neuroma may be performed, although reported rates of persistent pain following surgery have ranged as high as 30%.

Aseptic Necrosis of the Second Metatarsal Head (Freiberg's Disease). For unknown reasons (perhaps akin to Legg-Perthes and Köhler's diseases), the head of the second metatarsal may undergo aseptic necrosis in adolescence. The young person will complain of forefoot pain, worsened by weight bearing and extreme movements of the second metatarsophalangeal joint. Examination reveals tenderness of the second metatarsal head and often a visible and ten-

der swelling over the dorsum of the metatarsal head. X-ray confirms the necrotic process within 2 to 3 weeks of the onset of symptoms.

Treatment. If the pain is significant, then the foot may be immobilized in a short-leg walking cast, the plantar surface of which extends beyond the toes. When the cast is removed, the patient must be taught range of motion and strengthening exercises for the ankle and foot.

Synovitis of the Metatarsophalangeal Joint. The second metatarsophalangeal joint (and less frequently, the third metatarsophalangeal joint) may develop synovitis, which is present in patients as pain and swelling in the area of the involved metatarsophalangeal joint, sometimes with swelling of the involved toe. The patient may or may not have a history of a preexisting hammertoe of the involved toe. Physical examination will reveal tenderness directly over the metatarsophalangeal joint and pain with range of motion of the joint. X-rays may be normal, or may show joint space widening initially. Subsequent x-rays may show subluxation or complete dislocation of the metatarsophalangeal joint. Nonsteroidal anti-inflammatory medications and metatarsal pads may be helpful. If the joint progresses to subluxation or dislocation, surgical correction will usually be necessary.

Lesser Toe Pain

Other than pain radiating into the toes from a Morton's neuroma, pain in the lesser toes is usually due to shoe pressure on a deformed toe. Common deformities are hammertoes, claw toes, and mallet toes, which may be dynamic (occurring only during gait) or fixed deformities (Fig. 9.25). These toe deformities have a variety of etiologies, including muscle imbalances, cavus feet, excessively pronated feet, and improper shoe wear. Initially skin changes may be absent, but eventually the patient will develop corns over the dorsum of the proximal interpha-

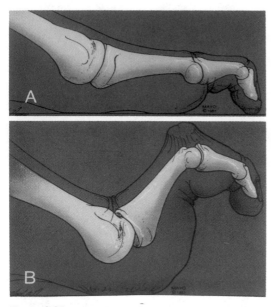

Figure 9.25.   *A*, mallet-toe. Flexion deformity of DIP joint. *B*, clawtoe. Accentuated hammertoe deformity with hyperextension at metatarsophalangeal joint and flexion at PIP and DIP joints. (From Johnson KA. Surgery of the foot and ankle. New York: Raven Press, 1988, with permission.)

langeal (PIP) or distal interphalangeal (DIP) joint, or at the tip of the toes. As mentioned in the section on "Metatarsalgia," hammertoes and claw toes may also result in calluses beneath the metatarsal heads.

The most effective form of conservative treatment of these toe deformities is a change in shoe wear. The toe box should be rounded rather than pointed and high heels avoided. Extradepth shoes provide increased height of the toe box so that the deformed toes do not strike the inside of the shoe. If the toe deformity is not rigid, metatarsal pads or an orthosis may provide relief of symptoms. The corns over the toes may be treated by the patient with a pumice stone after bathing or may be shaved with a scalpel by the physician. Donut pads with a hole in the center often aid in the relief of symptoms when applied over the corn on the toe. Foot pads with chemical agents to dissolve the corn are to be avoided because of the possibility of skin breakdown. Because these

corns develop in response to shoe pressure on the deformed toe, they cannot be surgically excised without a recurrence unless the toe deformity is corrected. Surgical treatment of these toe deformities, including resection of underlying bony prominences and surgical realignment of the toes, is indicated when conservative treatment fails.

Another cause of pain in the lesser toes is an interdigital corn or soft corn. As already mentioned, corns are caused by pressure on the skin from underlying bone. In soft corns, there is pressure between bony prominences of adjacent toes, usually the condyles of the PIP joints. The corn that subsequently develops becomes softened by moisture between the toes and may macerate or ulcerate. Once the soft corn macerates, it may also become secondarily infected. Soft corns are much more painful than the more common hard corns on the dorsum of the toes. Conservative treatment with lamb's wool or pads between the toes is usually not satisfactory. Surgical excision of the underlying bony prominence will result in spontaneous resolution of the soft corn and relief of pain.

Onychocryptosis (Ingrown Toenail)

Onychocryptosis, more commonly called ingrown toenails, refers to embedded nail margins usually involving the great toe that become infected and quite symptomatic. On rare occasions, this process can involve the lesser toes. Onychocryptosis is more common if the normal convexity of the nail is exaggerated. Toenails should be cut straight across and the corners allowed to extend beyond the nail groove. If the distal corner of a nail is trimmed back, the verge of the nail groove may swell over the nail in response to the dependent position of the feet and the stresses of weight bearing. With growth of the nail plate, the new distal angle will cut into the swollen verge of the nail groove. Infection may occur, resulting in a paronychia. Efforts to trim the corners of an embedded nail plate inevitably create a deep spicule, which then hooks into the verge of the nail groove and prevents the nail margin from being delivered except by surgery.

Treatment.   In a mild case, warm soaks, elevation, and antibiotics may be successful. The edge of the nail margin is gently elevated from the nail groove, and a small piece of cotton placed beneath the nail edge. It may then be possible for the distal end of the embedded nail margin to grow beyond the end of the nail groove.

In severe cases with advanced infection, surgical treatment is necessary. The basis of surgical treatment is to remove the embedded nail plate under block anesthesia at the base of the toe (Fig. 9.26, *A* and *B*). A short incision is made proximally at the base of the nail. A small straight hemostat is gently placed under the embedded edge of the nail. The nail edge is then grasped with the hemostat and twisted upward to allow removal of the involved nail edge. The exposed matrix is covered with bacitracin ointment so

that the dressing will not be adherent when it is changed. The patient is seen back again at 24 hours and the dressing is changed. The patient usually has much less swelling and tenderness, and is able to perform daily dressing changes and warm soaks at home.

If the nail has a deep convexity, or in recurrent cases, it is necessary to ablate the edge of the nail matrix in addition to removing the edge of the toenail (Fig. 9.26, *C* through *E*). This results in a narrower and less convex toenail which is less likely to become embedded. Ablation of the matrix can be performed either surgically or chemically. The surgical procedure consists of removal of a wedge-shaped segment of nail matrix and underlying soft tissue down to the periosteum of the distal phalanx. It is imperative that the germinal matrix at the proximal end of the nail is completely removed. The wound can then be dressed open with a nonadherent dressing, or the free skin edge may be loosely reapproximated toward the remaining edge of the toe nail. Some physicians remove only the nail plate itself and then ablate the nail matrix chemically.

Foot Manifestations of Systemic Diseases

Many systemic inflammatory processes, including rheumatoid arthritis, gout, psoriasis, and Reiter's syndrome, frequently affect the foot. Diabetes mellitus can result in severe limb-threatening and life-threatening complications in the foot. The diverse clinical manifestations of these disorders, as well as the diagnosis and medical treatment, are beyond the scope of this chapter. However, certain aspects are so important to the area of the foot that they will be discussed.

Rheumatoid Arthritis

The forefoot is frequently affected by rheumatoid arthritis, which often involves the metatarsophalangeal joints. Rheumatoid arthritis may cause severe hallux valgus, with a lateral deviation or valgus deformity of the lesser toes as well. The lesser toes

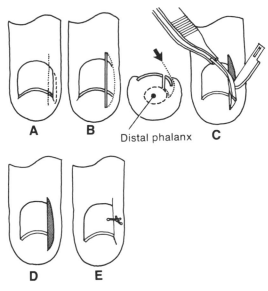

Figure 9.26.   Surgical treatment of onychocryptosis. *A* and *B*, partial excision of nail plate (nail matrix left intact). *C* through *E*, permanent ablation of nail edge by surgical excision of nail matrix. (From Johnson KA. Surgery of the foot and ankle. New York: Raven Press, 1988;121:128.)[1]

often dislocate at the metatarsophalangeal joints, causing prominence of the metatarsal heads on the plantar aspect of the foot. This may lead to disabling, intractable plantar keratoses that make ambulation very painful. Rheumatoid nodules may also develop on the plantar aspect of the forefoot, further adding to the difficulty in weight bearing. The midfoot joints are less commonly involved, but the subtalar joint is relatively frequently affected. Inflammation of the subtalar joint causes pain with inversion and eversion and may result in a progressive hindfoot valgus deformity and peroneal spastic flatfoot.

Local treatment of the foot in rheumatoid arthritis includes orthoses to control the hindfoot and to relieve weight bearing beneath the prominent metatarsal heads. Local steroid injections into the joints of the foot or into rheumatoid nodules are also helpful. If severe deformity of the foot is present, surgery may be necessary. Surgery of the hindfoot and midfoot usually involves fusion of the subtalar joint, triple arthrodeses, or localized fusion of involved midfoot joints. Surgery of the forefoot usually includes resections of the lesser metatarsal heads with resection, fusion, or implant arthroplasty of the first metatarsophalangeal joint and correction of the hallux valgus.

Gout

The diagnosis of gouty arthritis may be obvious when the patient presents with a sudden onset of severe pain and swelling of the first metatarsophalangeal joint, referred to as podagra. However, the presentation of gouty arthritis may be subacute and less severe, and may also involve other joints of the foot. In these cases, the diagnosis of gouty arthritis may not be entertained. Occasionally, patients with gout may also present as having inflammatory tenosynovitis of the foot. The definitive diagnostic test for gouty arthritis is evaluation of joint fluid under a polarizing microscope, where negatively bi-refringent crystals are seen. X-rays early in the course of gouty arthritis will be normal except for possible soft tissue swelling. With chronic gout, there may be joint destruction, juxtaarticular erosions, and tophaceous deposits in the soft tissue. In addition to medical treatment with anti-inflammatory medications and hyperuricemic agents, occasionally it may be necessary to surgically debride chronic tophaceous deposits, especially if they are spontaneously draining or secondarily infected.

Reiter's Syndrome

Involvement of the foot is common with Reiter's syndrome. The heel is the most commonly affected site in the foot, and patients with Reiter's syndrome may present with pain on the plantar aspect of the heel or posteriorly at the insertion of the Achilles tendon. X-rays may be normal or may show fluffy soft tissue calcifications on the plantar or posterior aspect of the calcaneus. Inflammation of the metatarsophalangeal joints may also occur in Reiter's syndrome. The clinical findings in the forefoot include the occurrence of sausage toes. Local treatment of foot symptoms include oral anti-inflammatory medications, local steroid injections, physical therapy, heel pads, and orthoses.

Psoriasis

Psoriatic involvement of the foot is generally limited to the toes. In addition to the typical psoriatic nail changes, the PIP and DIP joints of the toes are most frequently affected. The radiographs may show severe destruction of these joints, often with a great deal of bone resorption.

Diabetes Mellitus

Complications of diabetes mellitus in the foot can be quite disabling, very expensive in terms of medical care and lost wages, and sometimes limb-threatening. Neuropathic ulcers on the foot can occur with trivial trauma or without any history of trauma.

Foot ulcers in a diabetic patient may quickly progress to deep abscess formation, osteomyelitis, and gangrene, even with proper treatment. The best treatment with regard to neuropathic ulcers is prevention. The diabetic patient must be taught the importance of proper foot care and proper foot hygiene. The patient should visually inspect the feet on a regular basis. The patient must never walk barefoot or wear shoes without socks, even for short distances. New shoes must be broken in very gradually. Soaking the feet in hot water or exposure to heat from a radiator can cause devastating burns to a diabetic foot with a peripheral neuropathy. Corns or calluses should never be trimmed by the patient with a razor. The patient should notify the physician immediately if any skin breakdown or evidence of infection occurs.

If a diabetic foot ulcer occurs, a team approach, including the internist, orthopaedist, vascular surgeon, and orthotist, may be necessary for successful treatment. Systemic antibiotics based on deep cultures, surgical debridement when indicated, protection from weight bearing, vascular surgical evaluation, and local wound care may all be necessary to promote healing of diabetic ulcer. Superficial neuropathic ulcers that have not progressed to osteomyelitis or deep abscess will usually heal with this conservative approach. Custom-molded shoes with soft accommodative inserts may prevent recurrence of the ulcer. Surgical correction of a bony deformity may be necessary to prevent recurrence of the ulcer.

If deep abscess or osteomyelitis is present, aggressive surgical debridement and drainage is needed. This should be performed in the operating room with adequate anesthesia, as failure has often occurred with attempted drainage or local debridement at the bedside. If gangrene is present, at least partial amputation is necessary. If vascular evaluation reveals a treatable lesion, revascularization may be indicated. This may promote healing of an ulcer, and if amputation is necessary, it may allow a more distal amputation level.

In addition to neuropathic ulcers, diabetic patients may develop a Charcot arthropathy of the foot. This complication of diabetes is more difficult to diagnose than a diabetic ulcer, and early treatment is much more successful than late treatment. Because of the associated peripheral neuropathy, subluxation of joints with collapse and fragmentation of bone may occur. This process usually involves the midfoot, but the hindfoot and forefoot may be affected. The end result is a severely deformed, stiff foot with bony prominences. These bony prominences and the stiff foot make shoe fitting and ambulation very difficult. The deformity may often lead to skin ulceration and deep infection.

It is imperative for the primary care physician to be aware of this complication, as early treatment may prevent the progressive deformity. The early manifestations of a Charcot foot are swelling, erythema, and warmth of the foot; this presentation may be identical to cellulitis and the patient is often treated with antibiotics alone. The initial x-rays are normal, but when repeated several weeks later there is already severe bony destruction. Early protection from weight bearing with bed rest and cast may prevent the progressive deformity. Therefore, the author believes that the orthopaedic surgeon should be consulted early in the treatment of suspected cellulitis of the foot in a diabetic patient to rule out an early Charcot foot. Once the deformity has occurred, custom-molded shoes with soft inserts may prevent skin breakdown. However, surgery may be necessary to resect bony prominences or to fuse the affected joints.

Traumatic Disorders of the Foot

The foot is subject to a variety of injuries, including contusions, sprains, fractures, dislocations, and lacerations, many of which can be definitively treated by the primary care physician. In any case of trauma with neurovascular compromise, immediate referral to an orthopaedic surgeon or vascular surgeon is necessary. The discussion that follows is based on the assumption of an intact neurovascular status to the foot.

CONTUSIONS

Any type of blunt trauma can result in a contusion of the foot. If there is a history of significant trauma or severe swelling and pain, x-rays are indicated to rule out a fracture or dislocation. If the x-rays are normal, the initial treatment is elevation and a compression dressing. Within 2 to 3 days, at least partial weight bearing should be possible and activity level can be progressed as tolerated. Physical therapy is helpful if significant stiffness of the foot occurs following a contusion. After severe crushing injuries to the soft tissue, prolonged disability is possible and intensive physical therapy and anti-inflammatory medications may be necessary.

SPRAINS

The bony configuration and strong ligaments make sprains of the foot uncommon compared with sprains of the ligaments of the knee or ankle. When sprains of the foot do occur, they usually involve the tarsometatarsal joint. These patients present with a history of a weight-bearing, twisting injury to the foot, and pain across the midfoot. X-rays will be negative. Initial treatment is the same as for contusions, but if significant pain or inability to bear weight persists, casting should be considered. Often 2 to 3 weeks in a short-leg walking cast with weight bearing as tolerated will allow the ligament sprain to heal and lessen the long-term disability. After cast removal, physical therapy will usually be needed to regain range of motion and strength.

DISLOCATIONS

Dislocations of the foot are relatively uncommon. A subtalar dislocation occurs when the talus remains within the ankle joint, but the calcaneus and the rest of the foot are displaced either medially or laterally off the talus. The foot is markedly deformed clinically and the skin may be stretched tightly over the convex side of the deformed foot. Immediate reduction may be necessary to prevent skin necrosis and will decrease pain. If an orthopaedic surgeon is not readily available, the primary care physician may have to attempt the closed reduction under intravenous sedation and analgesia. The hip and knee are flexed and then longitudinal traction applied to the forefoot and heel. The physician then tries to reposition the foot out of its medially or laterally displaced position. If reduction of the subtalar joint can be obtained, it is usually stable due to the complex bony configuration of the subtalar joint. The ankle and foot are immobilized in well-padded splints. The patient should be referred to an orthopaedic surgeon for evaluation for associated fractures and for follow-up care.

Dislocations through the level of the tarsometatarsal joints generally do not occur without fractures. This so-called Lisfranc fracture-dislocation will be discussed in the section on "Fractures."

Dislocations of the metatarsophalangeal joints and interphalangeal joints of the toes are relatively uncommon. They are treated with closed reduction by longitudinal traction in the same fashion as when they occur in the corresponding joints in the hand.

FRACTURES
Fractures of the Talus

Twisting injuries to the foot may result in a variety of fractures of the talus. Talar dome fractures and lateral process fractures (Fig. 9.27) clinically appear similar to ankle sprains, but their treatment is significantly different from the treatment of an ankle

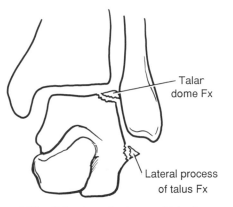

Figure 9.27. Talar dome fracture and lateral process fracture of talus can both clinically mimic an ankle sprain.

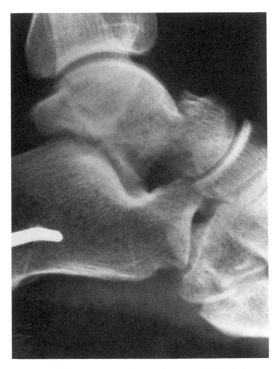

Figure 9.28. Fracture of neck of talus and circulation to talus. (From Rockwood CA, Green DP. Fractures of the talus in fractures in adults, vol 2. Philadelphia: JB Lippincott Co, 1984:1737, with permission.)

sprain. If these talar fractures are nondisplaced, they should be treated with nonweight bearing in a short-leg cast for 4 to 6 weeks, followed by a short-leg walking cast for an additional 4 weeks. Follow-up x-rays are necessary to ensure that the fracture heals. If these fractures are displaced, patients should be referred to an orthopaedic surgeon because immediate surgical fixation or removal of the fracture fragment may be indicated.

Fractures through the neck of the talus (Fig. 9.28) are serious injuries because they may interrupt the blood supply to the body of the talus, which enters at the level of the talar neck. This leads to avascular necrosis of the talus. Therefore, all fractures of the neck of the talus should be referred to an orthopaedic surgeon.

Fractures of the Calcaneus

The calcaneus is subject to avulsion fractures on the lateral side of the tuberosity and fractures of the anterior process, both of which clinically may appear identical to ankle sprains (Fig. 9.30). Nondisplaced avulsion fractures can be treated in a short-leg walking cast for 4 weeks, followed by a course of physical therapy. Nondisplaced anterior process fractures are treated in a

short-leg cast, non-weight bearing, for 4 weeks, followed by a short-leg walking cast for 4 weeks. Displaced fractures of the anterior process and displaced fractures of the tuberosity should be referred to an orthopaedic surgeon.

Much more serious than the small avulsion fractures are fractures of the calcaneus occurring through the tuberosity and the articular surface of the subtalar joint (Fig. 9.30). These fractures usually occur in a fall from a height, or occasionally in a motor vehicle accident. The fracture is often comminuted and is accompanied by severe pain and marked swelling. These fractures often yield a poor clinical result and historically have been treated by elevation and casting. However, in the past few years there has been an increased interest in open reduction

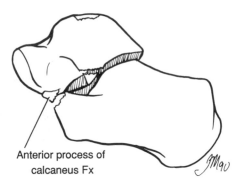

Figure 9.29. Fracture of the anterior process of the calcaneus can clinically appear identical to an ankle sprain.

and internal fixation of these serious fractures. Many authors report good results with this operative treatment. Therefore, patients with these severe fractures of the os calcis should be placed in a well-padded splint with the lower extremity elevated, and referred to an orthopaedic surgeon for initial treatment.

Fractures of the Midfoot

Acute fractures of the navicular, cuboid, and cuneiform bones are uncommon. They usually are small avulsion fractures from twisting injuries and can be treated in a short-leg walking cast for 3 to 6 weeks. Rarely, a crush-type injury or high-energy trauma may result in a complete fracture through the body of one of the midtarsal bones. These are more serious injuries that

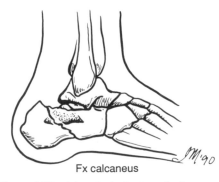

Fx calcaneus

Figure 9.30. Intraarticular fracture of calcaneus.

may be associated with subtle subluxations or dislocations of the tarsometatarsal joints; they should be splinted and referred to an orthopaedic surgeon.

Fractures of the Forefoot

Fractures of the metatarsals and toes are very frequent and many can be definitively treated by the primary care physician. An isolated fracture of the shaft of a single metatarsal is rarely displaced significantly and can be treated in a short-leg walking cast for 4 to 6 weeks. Fractures of the shafts of two or more metatarsals may be unstable and may require operative treatment. Therefore, orthopaedic consultation should be obtained when multiple metatarsal shafts are fractured. A common fracture is an avulsion fracture of the base of the fifth metatarsal caused by sudden pull of the peroneal brevis tendon. Some textbooks suggest that this fracture be treated in a comfortable shoe, but the author has found that these patients are more comfortable if they are placed in a short-leg walking cast. In rare cases, this fracture will result in a painful nonunion and referral to an orthopaedic surgeon may be necessary. If the fracture of the fifth metatarsal occurs through the proximal diaphysis rather than through the base, it is called a Jones' fracture and is much more likely to go on to delayed union or nonunion. Particular caution is indicated when treating fractures of the bases of the second, third, and fourth metatarsals. These fractures, especially when multiple, may be associated with dislocation of the tarsometatarsal joints, the so-called Lisfranc fracture-dislocation. This very serious injury may at times be difficult to diagnose and is usually difficult to treat. If a Lisfranc fracture-dislocation is present or suspected, referral to an orthopaedic surgeon is urgent.

Fractures of the phalanges of the toes are usually caused by a crush-type injury or kicking a hard object while barefoot. Fracture of the lesser toes are successfully treated by taping to adjacent toes. Reduction is indicated if there is marked angular or rotatory deformity. This reduction can be performed by traction under a Xylocaine block, and the toe is taped to an adjacent toe. Taping is usually continued for 2 to 3 weeks. Nondisplaced fractures of the great toe are best treated by a short-leg walking cast with a toe plate for 3 to 4 weeks. Displaced fractures of the great toe and fractures of the great toe that extend into the metatarsophalangeal joint or interphalangeal joint should be referred to an orthopaedic surgeon. In these fractures, open reduction and internal fixation is sometimes necessary to decrease the chance of posttraumatic degenerative arthritis.

SUGGESTED READINGS

Crenshaw AH, ed. Campbell's operative orthopedics. St. Louis: The CV Mosby Co, 1987.

Jahss M. Disorders of the foot and ankle. Philadelphia: WB Saunders Co, 1991.

Mann R, ed. Surgery of the foot. 5th ed. St. Louis: The CV Mosby Co, 1986.

Tachdjian MO. Pediatric orthopedics. 2nd ed. Philadelphia: WB Saunders Co, 1990.

Wu, KK. Foot orthoses. Baltimore: Williams & Wilkins, 1990.

CHAPTER 10

Mechanical Therapeutics (Casts, Splints, Traction)

John J. Monahan, M.D.

Orthopaedic treatments are essentially mechanical, whether done to a patient or by a patient. They apply forces to support, stabilize, or reconstruct disrupted structures, or to mobilize and strengthen stiffened, weakened structures. Details of manipulation and exercise for each area of the body are described in chapters related to those topics. This chapter presents general principles of treatment with specific attention to reduction of displaced injuries, application of casts and splints, traction, and rehabilitation.

Closed Treatment of Fractures and Dislocations

TIMING OF REDUCTION

All dislocations must be reduced as soon as possible, otherwise pain remains intense. Neurovascular injury is more likely the longer the joint is allowed to remain dislocated. Open fractures and dislocations always require immediate irrigation, debridement, reduction, and immobilization to minimize the risk of infection. Closed fractures do not constitute an emergency unless there is neurovascular injury or impending skin breakdown. Fractures should, however, be reduced as soon as possible since swelling of the extremity increases for hours following the fracture. This hemorrhage and transudate makes the muscle tissue indurated and inelastic. The longer reduction is delayed, the more difficult the reduction. If reduction cannot be accomplished relatively promptly, it is sometimes better to delay reduction for several days rather than to attempt manipulation of a severely swollen, edematous extremity that will be difficult to reduce and for which external immobilization will be difficult to maintain. During this waiting period, the extremity should be elevated and its neurovascular status carefully monitored.

STANDARDS OF REDUCTION

No reduction is required if there is no significant displacement or if the displacement is of little consequence. Avulsion fractures usually do not require reduction.

Any displacement is unacceptable when it threatens skin or neurovascular structures, disrupts the continuity of a joint surface, or delays healing. For example, displaced tibial fractures threaten the tight overlying skin. A significant number of all elbow and knee fractures and/or dislocations are associated with neurovascular complications. Displaced ankle fractures or dislocations can threaten adjacent neurovascular structures and skin integrity.

The degree of axial displacement that is acceptable varies with the nature of the injury, the age of the patient, and the bone involved. In an adult with a tibial and fibular fracture, an attempt should be made to correct more than 1 cm of shortening. In a child's fractured long bone, it is desirable to allow some axial shortening. This compensates for the usual accelerated growth of the fractured bone. Unless the long bone is shortened by axial displacement, the extremity will ultimately grow undesirably longer than the uninjured extremity. Therefore, for children it is reasonable to allow 1 cm of overriding for tibial or humeral fractures, and 1 to 1.5 cm for femoral fractures. In other instances, axial displacement should be corrected because it may delay healing or alter muscle balance and can create subluxation at joints between paired bones.

Angular deformity in mature bone has limited "remodeling" potential. Mild deformity, i.e., 5° to 10°, in a long bone is generally acceptable. Angular deformity near a joint in the plane of the major joint motion is more acceptable than a similar deformity at the midshaft of the bone. For example, in an elderly patient with a fractured neck of the humerus, 30° of varus deformity can be accepted. Thirty degrees of deformity in a fracture of both bones of the radius and ulna in the same patient would not be acceptable. Angulation of long bones changes the orientation of the articular surfaces of adjacent joints. In weight-bearing extremities, it may create shearing forces across the joint and will burden a portion of the surface as well as the investing ligaments of the joint with abnormally high stresses. Posttraumatic instability or arthritis may develop. In non-weight-bearing extremities the arc of motion may change. The shoulder joint can adjust to posttraumatic deformities of the humerus because of the wide range of motion and degrees of freedom within the joint. The elbow is less accommodating.

Translational displacement of fractures is relatively unacceptable when the expected remodeling is unlikely to restore a fairly normal appearance to a subcutaneous bone or when the degree of displacement is severe enough to impair bone healing. As a general rule, when translational displacement does not exceed half the width of the bone, the position is acceptable.

Growing bones can correct a significant degree of nonrotational displacement. Greater remodeling potential exists if the fracture is close to an epiphysis and if the angulation is in the plane of the adjacent joint. Rotational deformity does not remodel well in growing or mature bone and significant deformity should be corrected by reduction.

Because the criteria for "acceptable reduction" differs significantly with the patient and the injury, it is recommended that the reader consult the details for management of specific injuries in the appropriate chapters. A primary care physician who is not experienced in the management of these injuries should consult the orthopaedist for help in the evaluation and management of these patients.

DIRECTION OF FORCES OF REDUCTION

Most reductions are accomplished by manually applying a gentle, sustained traction force to the fragment that can be controlled. Apply the force in line with the long axis of the proximal part to gain the necessary length. Then, to achieve satisfactory anatomic alignment, apply appropriate angular and/or rotational forces to reduce the deformity. Traction forces sometimes must be strong and persistent (but always controlled and gradual in application) to overcome muscle spasm and friction forces that bind impacted fractures. Angular and rotational forces are applied gently and more briefly.

Traction is effective in gaining a reduction only if the bone ends are connected with sufficient soft tissues. These tissues usually survive the injury by their location in the concavity of the deformed bone or joint. By utilizing this natural tension band or hinge, the bone ends can be manipulated into a stable or relatively stable position (Fig. 10.1). If there is no soft tissue tension band, a stable reduction is more difficult to achieve by closed manipulation. While the length can be restored, displacement and angulation may persist.

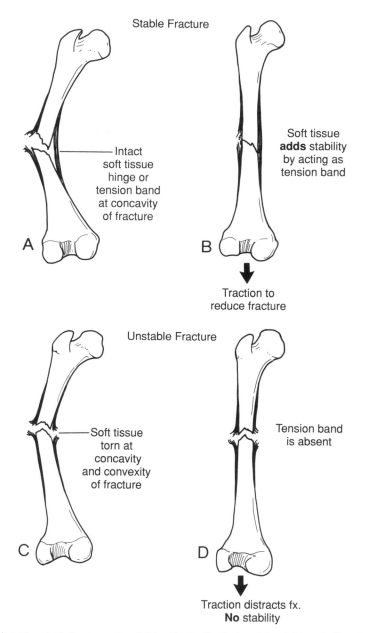

Stable Fracture

Intact
soft tissue
hinge or
tension band
at concavity
of fracture

A

Soft tissue
adds stability
by acting as
tension band

B

Traction to
reduce fracture

Unstable Fracture

Soft tissue
torn at
concavity
and convexity
of fracture

C

Tension band
is absent

D

Traction distracts fx.
No stability

Figure 10.1. Stable and unstable fractures. *A* and *B*, traction is effective in gaining stable reduction of a fracture when the soft tissue tension band or hinge is intact (shown at the concavity of the fracture). *C* and *D*, traction is ineffective in gaining stable reduction when the soft tissue is torn from the concavity and convexity of the fracture.

FORCES APPLIED TO DISLOCATIONS

Good analgesia and/or anesthesia will greatly diminish muscle resistance and often make the difference between success and failure when manipulating dislocations of the larger joints. The manipulator should await evidence that the patient is relaxed, then should begin with fairly gentle traction, e.g., merely the weight of the dependent arm when manipulating an anterior dislocation of the shoulder. Gentle rotational and angular forces are then applied, as described in the specific chapters, stopping when mechanical resistance is encountered. Forceful angular and rotational forces have caused fractures during efforts to reduce large joint dislocations. When these gentle maneuvers fail, stronger traction should be applied for many minutes before the appropriate rotational and angular forces are again gently applied.

At times, a dislocation will be "irreducible." In certain dislocations the bone end has "buttonholed" through the capsule and ligaments, and may be entrapped by these structures or adjacent tendons. In these circumstances, traction may not be beneficial and it is recommended that orthopaedic consultation be obtained. In addition, a dislocation may not be reducible because better muscle relaxation or pain relief is necessary. Caution should be exercised in the use of increasing doses of analgesics or relaxants. When one cannot gain a reduction under usual and customary doses of such medication, a regional anesthesia or general anesthesia under an anesthesiologist's direction should be considered.

FORCES APPLIED TO FRACTURES

Unless the operator is uncommonly strong, impacted and overriding fractures are more readily reduced by weighted traction. This can outlast the strongest muscular forces, is usually not very painful, and leaves the operator free to apply well-controlled angular and rotational forces to the fracture fragments. The angular and rotational forces needed rarely require more strength than abides in the hands and wrists of the operator. Various gripping forces that bridge the fracture site are typically all that are required to complete the reduction of most forearm, wrist, hand, and ankle fractures. Modest arm forces are required to complete the reduction of shaft fractures of the tibia and fibula, one hand gripping above and the other below the fracture site. Angular and rotational forces are initiated gently and increased smoothly until the desired position is achieved.

Having gained a satisfactory reduction, immobilization in a splint, a cast, or continuous traction is required. Radiographs should be taken to confirm maintenance of reduction. The injured extremity should be elevated and ice applied to the injury site. Appropriate neurovascular checks of the extremity are always mandatory.

Exceptions to the general principles of reduction as outlined above are considered in the specific chapters.

Principles of Immobilization

Immobilization techniques include casts, splints, and weighted traction. Two types of cast and splint materials will be discussed: plaster of Paris and fiberglass.

Plaster of Paris rolls are muslin-impregnated with starch and the hemihydrate of calcium sulfate. This material has a long, successful "track record" in that it is strong, rigid, moldable, porous (allows the skin to "breathe"), absorbent (absorbs any drainage from a wound), relatively inexpensive, and accessible. Its disadvantages include a prolonged curing (hardening) period, which delays weight bearing for 36 hours. Also, it is destroyed by moisture and is relatively radiopaque.

Fiberglass materials are available as an alternative. Fiberglass is durable, radiolucent, and light in weight, allows immediate weight bearing, and is stronger than plaster of Paris (less material required). It is, however, more expensive, less available, less moldable, and harder to cut and trim than plaster of Paris. Fiberglass occasionally causes skin irritation and is therefore less useful on fresh fractures. While fiberglass does provide an advantage because it tolerates wetness much better than plaster, this, in practice, is of limited benefit. A patient still must keep the underlying skin clean and dry. If a fiberglass-casted extremity is immersed in water, there is potential for skin maceration. Consequently, these extremities need to be protected from moisture in a fashion similar to extremities casted in plaster of Paris.

SPLINTING

Indications

A splint is usually chosen for temporary immobilization of an injury while awaiting definitive treatment, or for immobilization of an injury that needs protection but not great stability. In emergency situations, any material that can safely provide stability or protection to the injured part may be used, e.g., magazines, cardboard, padded wood, plastic, prefabricated air/plastic or metal splints, and traction splints for femur fractures. In the emergency or outpatient departments, however, plaster or fiberglass splints are preferred. Splints are useful for joints affected by acute arthritis and periarticular pain syndromes when rest to the painful structures is indicated, and when comfortable stability is needed in the context of the patient's expected activities.

Five splints are often used by primary clinicians for the upper extremities:

1. The volar forearm splint is used to temporarily immobilize distal forearm, wrist, and hand fractures, to protect wrist sprains and strains, and to rest an acutely arthritic wrist.

2. A volar splint with a thumb extension is useful to immobilize an ulnar collateral ligament tear at the first metacarpophalangeal joint.

3. An ulnar or radial gutter splint is useful for treatment of stable fractures and dislocations of the wrist and hand following reduction. For sprains and strains, the gutter splint protects involved metacarpals and phalanges, while freeing the uninvolved portions of the hand for function.

4. The dorsal forearm splint is used for protection of fractures at the base or shaft of metacarpals two through five, as an alternative to the ulnar or radial gutter splint. The dorsal splint is also used to rest inflamed flexor tendons associated with carpal tunnel syndrome.

5. The long-arm splint is used for temporary immobilization of fractures, dislocations, sprains, and strains of the forearm, elbow, and distal humerus. It is also used to protect contusions, infections, or inflammatory processes of the upper extremity.

Splints for the lower extremity include:

1. The short posterior leg splint, used for temporary immobilization of ankle and foot injuries until swelling subsides and proper evaluation for stability can be conducted. It is also used to rest an arthritic ankle or foot joint or to immobilize sprains, strains, and fractures of the foot or ankle.

2. The long posterior leg splint is used for temporary immobilization of injuries of the extensor apparatus, and potentially or obviously unstable injuries of the collateral or cruciate ligaments of the knee. It is used to immobilize fractures of the shaft and proximal condyles of the tibia, and if

a traction splint is not available, the condyles of the femur. The long posterior splint is also used to protect a stable knee sprain and/or fracture, and to rest the arthritic knee.

3. Femur fractures are better splinted with traction splints, i.e., the "Thomas" splint, one of the many modifications (Fig. 10.2). The traction splint's force is applied distally to the foot while proximally the padded ring, or half ring, is secured to the thigh and hip area. Wide, soft bandages are then tied at intervals along the splint to support the limb. Distal circulation and neural function should be monitored frequently before and after application of the splint. Femoral fractures should be referred to an orthopaedic surgeon for management following immobilization.

Splinting Technique (Fig. 10.3)

Depending on the mass of the extremity, the splint must be 8 (upper extremity) to 16 (lower extremity) plaster strips (or 6 to 8 fiberglass strips) in thickness. Such splints are made by stacking precut plaster splints on top of one another then cutting the whole to the desired length, or by rolling out strips of the desired length back and forth from a plaster roll. The width of the plaster is chosen so that approximately half the girth of the extremity will lie within the splint. The length varies: a short-arm splint to include finger fractures would extend from the fingertips to a point two finger breadths distal to the antecubital crease, or 2 cm from the biceps tendon in the antecubital space with the elbow at a right angle. Arm splints are shaped at one end to fit around the thenar eminence and to parallel the distal palmar crease. Other splints are left square at the ends. Where the plaster must round a flexed joint, slits are made in the sheets of plaster-impregnated muslin at right angles to the long axis of the splint to allow a smooth overlap at the turns or angles (Fig. 10.4, *A* and *B*), or careful tucks are taken to avoid skin pressure (Fig. 10.4*C*).

An alternative method would be to wrap a thick layer of cast padding to the extremity and apply the water-soaked splints directly to the cast padding, overwrapping with wet gauze or a layer of padding plus Ace bandage (Fig. 10.4, *D* and *E*). This often gives a better contouring than the "complete splint application" method.

The plaster is immersed in warm water until thoroughly wet, stripped of excess water, and laid on three or four layers of cast padding. It is covered with an additional strip or two of padding to prevent the Ace bandage or gauze (that will be applied over the plaster to hold the material in place) from sticking to the surface of the plaster. This would interfere with rewrapping. The splint then is applied to the extremity, and firmly wrapped and molded into place using wet Kling or gauze. As the plaster or fiberglass

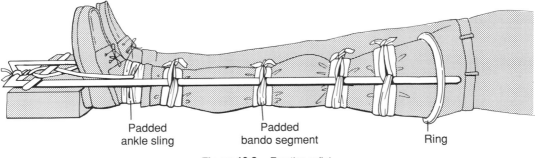

Padded   Padded
ankle sling   bando segment   Ring

Figure 10.2. Traction splint.

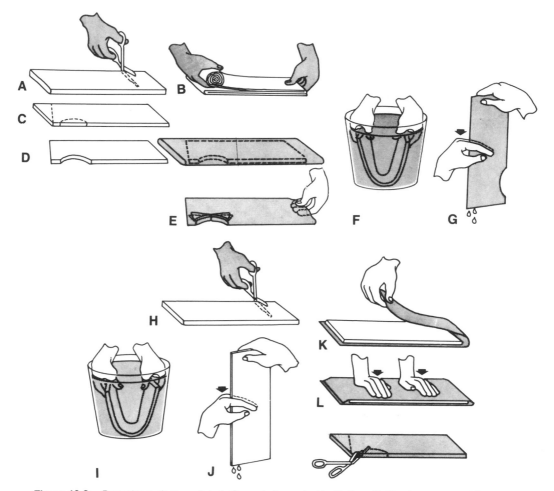

Figure 10.3. Preparing a plaster splint. *A–G*, employing a stockinette liner. *H–M*, using a cast-padding liner.

hardens, the extremity is held in the desired position while the splint is molded to the contours of the extremity. Direct pressure over bony prominences should be avoided. When the plaster is hardened, the circulation is evaluated. If it is normal, the Kling, along the margins of the splint, is cut through to prevent a tourniquet effect on the extremity should further swelling occur. The Kling is cut about 2 to 2½ inches at a time, beginning distally and working proximally, while an assistant begins distally to roll an Ace bandage without added tension to maintain the splints in place. Care must be taken not to lose the position of reduction while rewrap-

ping the splints. Always check neurovascular status after rewrapping and elevate the extremity to lessen swelling.

CAST IMMOBILIZATION
Indications

Casts immobilize by rigidly enveloping the unstable injured extremity and effectively producing soft tissue compression (a positive hydraulic force) that maintains apposition and alignment of the bone ends. In addition, a cast can provide a three-point force to maintain the position of a fracture, as seen in Figure 10.5. Avoid excessive point

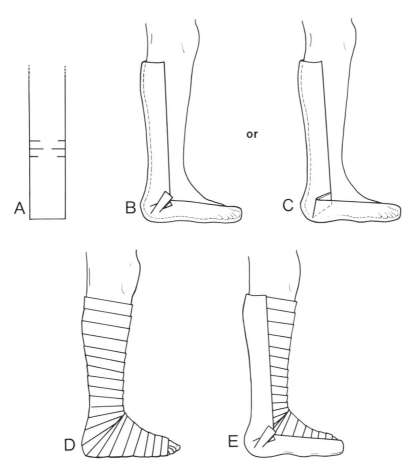

Figure 10.4. Application of plaster splints around a flexed joint. *A* and *B*, slits are made at right angles to the long axis of the splint and overlapped smoothly; or *C*, the redundant material is tucked and smoothed at the angles. *D* and *E*, a thick layer of cast padding is wrapped on the extremity and a posterior splint is applied over the padding.

pressure over bony prominences, especially the fracture site, as this could cause skin necrosis. Rather, disperse the force over a larger surface area.

In certain circumstances, the cast also must maintain a distracting force necessary to prevent overriding or angulation of the fracture fragments. Casts are less efficient in maintaining distraction, however. With the elbow flexed to 90° and with snug molding of the hand and wrist, a long-arm cast may maintain the necessary distraction force on oblique and spiral fractures of the forearm. With the knee in 90° of flexion, a long-leg cast may maintain the necessary distraction

force on oblique and spiral fractures of the tibia. A similar effect can be achieved using gravity, so that a long-arm "hanging cast" applies a gentle distracting force to an overridden fracture of the humerus. It must be emphasized that casts alone can rarely safely maintain strong distractive forces without skin problems. They consequently should not be used in that application.

Six basic casts are often used by primary care clinicians:

1. The short-arm cast is used in appropriate forms for stabilization of finger splints, and for immobilization of metacarpal fractures, carpal fractures, reduced carpal

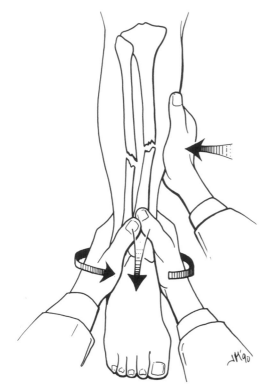

Figure 10.5. Three-point force applied while molding the cast to hold the position of a fracture with an intact soft tissue tension band.

dislocations, and fractures of the distal third of the forearm.

2. The long-arm cast is used in appropriate forms for immobilization of upper and middle-third forearm fractures. It is used for immobilization of reduced elbow dislocations and condylar and supracondylar fractures of the humerus after the circulatory response to injury has stabilized and swelling has subsided. The long-arm cast is also used for carpal and distal-third forearm fractures when swelling, muscle mass, or obesity prevent the well-molded short-arm cast from adequately limiting rotation.

3. The hanging arm cast provides traction immobilization of humeral shaft and humeral neck fractures. The cast is suspended by a strap connecting a collar about the neck and a cuff about the wrist.

4. The short-leg cast is used in appropriate forms for immobilization of unstable ankle sprains, stable ankle fractures, fractures of the proximal phalanges of the great toes, metatarsal fractures, minimally displaced fractures of the tarsus and calcaneus, and subluxations of the peroneal tendons.

5. The long-leg cast is used for immobilization of fractures of the ankle, fractures of the shaft of the distal femur, tibia, or fibula, undisplaced fractures of the tibial condyles, injury to the extensor apparatus of the knee, unstable ligament injuries of the knee, and for treatment of Achilles tendon ruptures.

6. The patellar tendon weight-bearing cast is preferred to the long-leg cast for immobilization of stable reduced transverse fractures of the lower extremity when weight bearing is to begin. This cast prevents rotation while allowing knee motion.

Techniques of Cast Application

Position the extremity with the fracture reduced as much as possible. Final adjustment is made as the cast is setting up (hardening). The practitioner usually needs assistance to control the limb. The position of the extremity and the areas of the cast that require special molding are unique to each injury and cast and are described in the specific chapters. Small wads of padding may be placed between the toes or fingers to provide adequate space in the cast for these members. The stockinette may be applied in stable injuries to cover the upper and lower ends of the cast. These should be of an approximate size to fit firmly without wrinkles (Fig. 10.6). In unstable injuries, the additional manipulation required for placement of the stockinette is not worth the extra step.

Cotton padding is then applied as

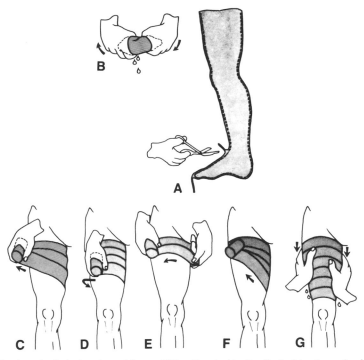

Figure 10.6. Application of roll plaster. *A*, applying and fitting the stockinette. *B*, pinching the ends of the wet plaster roll. *C* and *D*, plaster must not be pulled on as in *C*, but rolled on as in *D*. *E* and *F*, directing the lie of the plaster. *F*, the contour of the extremity guides the plaster in a wrong direction. *E*, by pleating, the plaster can be guided as desired. *G*, stroking the plaster to fuse the layers and to smooth the surface.

smoothly as possible from the distal to the proximal end of the limb. Each layer is overlapped about 60% to achieve a uniform two-layer padding (minimal padding feasible). The roll is held a few inches from the limb and pulled slightly as one circles the limb in a direction oblique to the long axis of the limb. There will be slight bagging of the lower edge of the cotton padding as one proceeds from distal to proximal. These areas are simply torn away and the remaining edges smoothed into place. The cotton padding surfaces must be wrinkle-free to avoid wrinkles in the plaster that can cause skin irritation or breakdown. The layers of padding vary. If considerable swelling is expected, an extra layer or two should be added. Also, extra layers should be added over and about bony prominences. Excessive padding

should not be used, however, because it lessens control of the fracture fragments.

The width of the plaster roll depends on the size of the extremity. Five- to six-inch rolls can be used for the adult thigh, 4- to 5-inch rolls for the lower leg, and 2- to 4-inch rolls for the wrist and forearm. The widest rolls that can be conveniently controlled allow the most rapid delivery of plaster to immobilize the part, giving the physician more time to mold and manipulate the fracture. The roll of plaster is thoroughly immersed in water with the end free so that it can be easily identified after soaking. Wearing gloves is optional when working with plaster of Paris, but mandatory for fiberglass. The water temperature should be as cool as possible to retard the setting time and allow more time to apply, mold, and manipulate. In addition, as casts set, they give off heat; using warm water can increase the overall temperature and lead to superficial burns. The plaster should be left in water until all of the bubbles stop rising. The ends of the roll are squeezed to force plaster into the body of the roll (Fig. 10.6B).

Plaster should be applied wet. The plaster is rolled obliquely onto the limb, in the same direction as the cotton padding, keeping the roll on the surface and using the fingertips to control the unrolling of the plaster (Fig. 10.6, D–F). The roll should be kept moving at all times, and should not be lifted off the extremity or pulled. The loose lower border is controlled by taking tucks and smoothing them into position to avoid wrinkles in the plaster. When using fiberglass, use slightly narrower rolls to offset the stiffer and thicker material. This prevents ridges in the cast when taking tucks around prominences or changes in diameter of the extremity. Each turn should be overlapped by 50% to ensure a uniform thickness. (Uneven application creates stress risers in the finished product, which cause breakage.) A second pass with additional rolls of plaster will result in a uniform four-layer cast about ⅛-inch thick, which is adequate for the upper extremity. A ³⁄₁₆-inch cast is adequate for most lower extremity fractures. These casts can be reinforced with additional longitudinal splints across the concavity of the elbow, wrist, knee, or ankle joints to lessen the overall weight of additional rolls of plaster. Avoid reinforcing splints over the convexity of joints because they are mechanically less effective.

The plaster is rubbed and smoothed constantly, adding water as necessary, to mold the cast to the contours of the limb. This avoids irregular ribs and depressions that cause skin damage, and also prevents air and water from being trapped between the layers of plaster, which creates weak spots that can cause early breakage. This rubbing motion is done with the entire palm for large surfaces, and the thenar and hypothenar eminences and the fingertips for smaller surfaces. Direct point pressure is never applied over a bony prominence. Instead, the plaster is shaped around the prominence. Avoid manipulation of the cast during the late stages of hardening. Motion at this stage will cause cracks and subsequent weakening of the cast. If this occurs, additional plaster must be added.

With experience, casts can often be made to the appropriate length and require little trimming. Before a practitioner becomes experienced, however, casts should usually be made longer than necessary and trimmed after they harden. This is most easily and safely done using a cast saw once the cast is hardened. A cast knife or scalpel can be used prior to full hardening of the cast. The handle of the knife or scalpel is gripped with all four fingers and steady counterpressure maintained on the cast with the thumb. Pull the margin of the cast to be trimmed up into the knife blade with the opposite hand, rather than incising downward into the plaster surface and risk cutting the patient. A special hardened saw blade is necessary to trim or cut fiberglass.

In routine long- or short-leg casts, the plantar aspect of the cast may be extended beyond the toe tips to protect them from injury. The metatarsophalangeal joint is kept at neutral by molding with the fingertips along the plantar aspect of the foot piece at the metatarsophalangeal joint level, while the toes are molded down into a neutral position. Hyperextension of these joints must be avoided. The extra padding previously placed between the toes is removed to afford adequate toe space for active motion. (This also applies for hand casts: removal of the padding in the web space allows the fingers to be comfortable and not compressed.) A walking plaster cast cannot support weight bearing until the cast has completely dried, usually 24 to 36 hours.

IMMOBILIZATION BY CONTINUOUS TRACTION
Weighted Traction while at Bed Rest

Indications. Weighted traction in bed is a distracting force exerted parallel to the axis of the extremity or trunk. It maintains the length and alignment and stability of a fractured extremity, or stability of the axial skeleton. It is especially effective if the soft tissue tension band is intact. It allows joint motion while maintaining length, alignment, and control of the extremity. With the patient at bed rest, it supplements immobilization of a painful joint while lessening the protective muscle spasm, providing relief of pain and swelling, and allowing minimal motion of the affected joint. The primary care physician will be involved in the use of skin traction techniques. Traction techniques using transcutaneously placed skeletal pins are also widely used by orthopaedic surgeons when larger forces must be exerted.

Technique. Commercial skin traction boots and sleeves, when available, or moleskin traction tapes backed with sponge rubber are applied over an unshaved lower extremity, with appropriate felt or cotton padding to prevent pressure over bony prominences or on superficial nerves. The straps are held in place by elastic bandages that are wrapped distally to proximally. Do not apply the bandages too tightly. They are rolled on—not pulled under tension. The proximal end of the straps must be well anchored. A distal-to-proximal pressure gradient is produced to prevent a tourniquet effect on the limb. This is done by wrapping the distal extremity slightly tighter than the proximal extremity. Distally, each turn is overlapped by three-fourths of the width of the bandage. The overlap is gradually lessened proximally, so that the proximal wrap overlaps one-third of the width. Moleskin traction tapes are attached to a spreader, and through this to a rope, which passes through pulleys to an attached weight. The amount of traction that can be applied is a function of the surface area of skin. In a child, usually 4 pounds of traction can be applied to the lower extremity, while an adult can tolerate approximately 8 pounds. The traction straps must be rewrapped at least 3 times a day. The skin must be inspected and wiped with alcohol to cleanse and toughen before rewrapping.

Types of Skin Traction

Buck's Traction (Fig. 10.7). This type of traction is used to relieve pain, inflammation, and muscle spasm about the knee and hip. Traction tapes (as described above) are applied to the lower legs, from immediately proximal to the malleoli to below the knee. Pads are placed over the malleoli and about the proximal fibula over the peroneal nerve. This prevents skin breakdown over the malleoli or damage to the peroneal nerve, which runs subcutaneously two finger breadths distal to the head of the fibula. For comfort, pillows may be placed under the knees, and the head of the bed may be raised. An example of the use of Buck's traction is for toxic synovitis of the hip in a child. Four to five pounds of weight are required, and intermittent heat to the involved hip is used 3 to 4 times a day. The child is removed from traction for gentle active-assistive range of motion exercises 3 to 4 times a day.

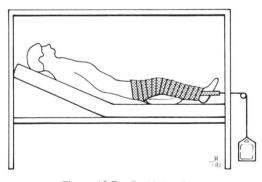

Figure 10.7. Buck's traction.

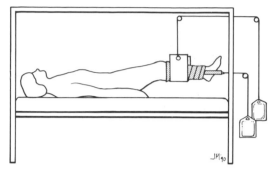

Figure 10.8.   Split Russell traction.

Split Russell Traction (Fig. 10.8). This type of traction is used for the same conditions as Buck's traction, but allows better control of rotation and some active motion of the knee and hip. Traction straps are applied as for Buck's traction. A soft felt sling is placed under the knee. This attaches to a spreader, then by a rope to an overhead pulley placed over the knee, and finally over the foot of the bed, through a second pulley, to a weight at the end of the bed. Weight is selected according to the patient's age and size. Typically, the axial traction is 3 to 5 pounds, and 3 to 5 pounds is used for the knee sling. This usually provides comfort and support to an acutely inflamed hip or knee. Traction could be coupled with ice massage or moist hot packs and gentle active-assistive range of motion as tolerated.

Pelvic Traction (Fig. 10.9). A corset-like lined canvas is wrapped about the waist.

Straps with rope extension extend from the corset at its midlateral points, through pulleys, to the bottom of the bed, and to weights. Adults can tolerate 20 to 30 pounds of weight. The foot of the bed is elevated, and body weight acts as countertraction. Traction is applied for 1 to 3 hours, 4 to 6 times per day, with intermittent heat for 20 minutes, 3 times per day. This amount of weight is really not enough to cause any significant distraction through the lumbar or lumbosacral spine. Much larger forces are necessary to provide true distraction but these cannot be tolerated in any type of corset or skin traction arrangement.

Cervical Traction (Fig. 10.10). A head halter or a soft head harness is commercially available to apply traction to the mandible and occiput. Avoid excessive pressure on the mandible by positioning the occipital strap to accept most of the load, or use a bite plate or mouthpiece to minimize the pressure on the temporomandibular joint, which can precipitate the temporomandibular (joint) syndrome. The halter is attached to a spreader bar above the head. A rope is attached to the spreader and is carried through a pulley at the head of the bed to a weight. The patient is usually positioned comfortably with the neck in slight flexion.

Cervical traction can also be effectively performed with the patient sitting using an over-the-door arrangement, demonstrated in Figure 10.11. Treatment begins with

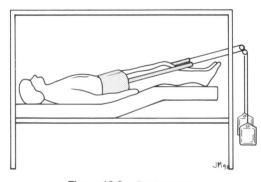

Figure 10.9.   Pelvic traction.

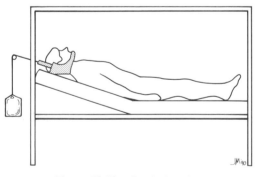

Figure 10.10.   Cervical traction.

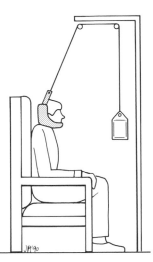

Figure 10.11. Over-the-door arrangement for cervical traction.

about 5 pounds of weight, which is gradually increased to 10 to 15 pounds as tolerated. The patient's comfort is used as a guide. The traction is used intermittently for 20 minutes to 1 hour, 4 to 6 times per day. Cervical traction requires appropriate skin care to avoid skin breakdown over the chin or occiput. This therapy is useful for neck pain associated with degenerative conditions and secondary to muscular strain or cervical sprains without instability.

COMPLICATIONS

Complications of immobilization techniques include tight cast, cast sores or burns, joint stiffness, thrombophlebitis, compartment (cast) syndrome, soft tissue contracture, allergic reaction to fiberglass, pressure ulcers, and nerve palsies secondary to traction apparatus. Three of the most common cast complications—compartment (cast) syndrome, skin necrosis, and joint stiffness—will be discussed.

Compartment (Cast) Syndrome

The extremities are comprised of soft tissue compartments bounded by rigid fascial envelopes oriented along the long axis of the extremity. The muscles, nerves, and vessels of the extremity traverse these compartments. The fascial envelopes have little compliance and are anchored to the supporting bone (Fig. 10.12). Injury to the contained bone or associated soft tissues that traverse the compartment results in bleeding or swelling in the compartment, which may increase intracompartment pressure. If the acutely injured extremity has been wrapped in a rigid cast, the compliance of the leg is further reduced, and this in turn may further increase the compartment pressure. If the compartment pressures exceed the venous pressure, the venous system collapses. There is secondary failure of the capillary circulation and then subsequent collapse of the arteriole circulation. This results in ischemia of the soft tissues in the compartment. This ischemia in turn causes more edema. This further increases the fluid and consequently pressure within the compartment, further worsening the syndrome. Thus, a vicious cycle is triggered that unless treated, will continue until it effectively strangles the soft parts.

The key to prevention or successful treatment is early recognition. The earliest sign of an impending compartment syndrome is severe pain that is of greater magnitude than one would ordinarily expect in an extremity that is well supported subsequent to an injury. One of the earliest signs is increased pain on passive stretching of the muscles within the affected compartment. Paresthesia and paralysis are later findings. It should be noted that the distal pulses are usually present.

The first step in treating compartment syndrome is to split the cast medially and laterally along the midlateral and midmedial lines, respectively (Fig. 10.13). All wrappings should be cut down to the skin so that the limb can be fully decompressed. Compartment pressures diminish 65% after bivalving and spreading the cast. Cutting the padding and removing the cast further de-

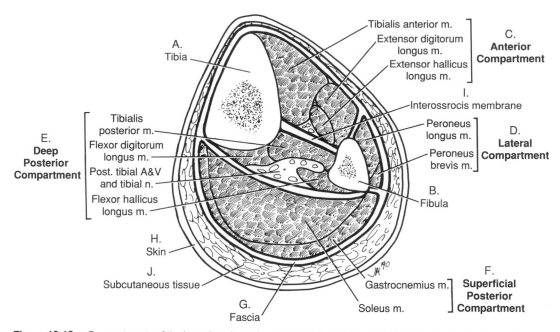

Figure 10.12. Compartments of the lower leg shown in a cross-section of the midcalf. *A*, tibia. *B*, fibula. *C*, anterior compartment. *D*, lateral compartment. *E*, deep posterior compartment. *F*, superficial posterior compartment. *G*, fascia. *H*, skin. *I*, interosseous membrane. *J*, subcutaneous tissue.

creases the compartment pressure by a small amount. The extremity should be elevated a few inches above the heart. Avoid excessive elevation as this might impair arterial circulation. Following this, the patient should be observed closely for signs of improvement.

If the syndrome persists, that is, the signs and symptoms do not return to normal, one assumes that the findings are related not only to the tight cast, but to a developing compartment syndrome. At this point, an emergency orthopaedic referral should be

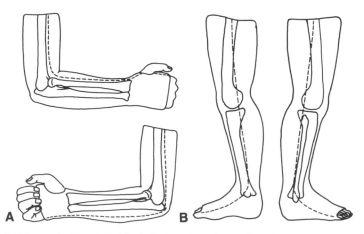

Figure 10.13. Splitting casts. The *dotted line* indicates where the cast is split. *A*, long-arm cast. *B*, long-leg cast.

made. Time is of the essence; any delay in this communication could be disastrous. Prolonged ischemia, greater than 6 hours, may result in irreversible tissue injury and significant sequelae.

If there is an obvious compartment syndrome, the orthopaedist may proceed directly with fasciotomy of the extremity. If there is any question, direct measurement of the compartment pressure can be performed. This is often the only means of making the diagnosis in an equivocal situation. Patients with fractures frequently have severe pain and, because of the damage to muscular tissue or slight movement of the fracture, may have increased pain with passive stretching. It is often difficult to assess these patients clinically and it becomes very difficult if the patient is heavily medicated. In the unconscious patient, only direct inspection of the involved compartment and compartment pressure measurement can be used to detect an early compartment syndrome.

Measurement of compartment pressure is a fairly simple procedure that the orthopaedist can perform using commercial kits or with a large-bore needle, intravenous tubing, three-way stopcock, and manometer. When the compartment pressure is measured to be above 30 mm Hg in a normotensive patient, the diagnosis of compartment syndrome is confirmed. Once this diagnosis is made, a fasciotomy is indicated on an emergency basis.

Because of the potential for increased swelling in an injured extremity that has been immobilized in a circumferential cast, patients must be carefully instructed and observed following cast application. Individuals who are stable and deemed at low risk for such complications may be treated on an ambulatory basis but must be instructed to be aware and observe their extremity for signs of circulatory or neurologic impairment. The following should be explained as

possible danger signs: coolness or sluggishness of capillary refill in the fingers or toes, cyanosis or pallor of the fingers or toes, tingling of the fingers or toes, and increasing pain, particularly with passive stretching. The patient is instructed to return promptly if these conditions develop. Patients who are judged to be at high risk for compartment syndrome should be hospitalized and observed for at least 24 to 48 hours until their condition stabilizes.

Skin Necrosis

A constant point of pressure will cause local cutaneous ischemia, and slight axial movement occurring under a cast will in time cause erosions over bony prominences and beneath the irregularities on the undersurface of the cast. To avoid these problems, the padding must fit snugly without wrinkles. The plaster must be applied smoothly over the padding, and must be separated from the skin over bony protrusions by padding and careful molding.

In addition to the circulatory precautions taught to patients, the following skin precautions are also taught. Patients are to return immediately if they experience burning pain inside a cast, or any other sensation which they interpret to feel like an abrasion or a boil. When faced with any such complaints, the primary care clinician is obliged to window the cast over the area of concern or split the cast and remove one-half of the cast at a time to better examine the extremity.

If a cutaneous injury is evident, the injured area is cleansed and dressed with a nonadherent dressing. Several layers of padding are applied over the dressing, the window of the cast is replaced and held in place with tape, or the bivalve is reapplied and held in position with cast straps. If the window is left open, tissue will swell up through the window, causing erosions at the margin of the window or possibly impairing circulation to the skin of that area (window edema).

Joint Stiffness

The stiffness that results following immobilization is proportional to the length of time immobilized. The main factor in the production of this contracture is shortening of the surrounding musculature; changes in the joint capsule contribute to a lesser degree. During immobilization, the normal pumping action that is generated by motion and produces the flow of tissue fluids out of an extremity is prevented. Tissue capillaries congest, and the capsules, ligaments, and tendons they serve also congest, become thickened, and consequently shortened. (Forces that stretch a viscoelastic material in one dimension will at the same time shorten it in the perpendicular direction.) Intraarticular changes also occur which can result in thinning of the cartilage, fibrosis, or bony anklylosis.

It follows that no joint should be immobilized unnecessarily. Certain injuries do not require rigid immobilization. For example, fractures of the shaft of the femur can be managed in traction, which allows controlled knee motion as well as isometric and limited isotonic exercises. Salter introduced the concept of continuous passive motion, which utilizes an apparatus that supports the injured extremity while passively moving the joint through a carefully controlled arc of motion at a specific rate, to avoid pain. This alleviates pain, preserves joint range of motion, and may enhance healing in both articular and ligamentous injuries.

The benefits and hazards of prolonged immobilization must be weighed before initial treatment is chosen, and a regimen of mobilization as well as strengthening must follow the period of immobilization. Treatment with a cast and discharge before following the patient through a well-guided rehabilitation program is incomplete treatment. Each specific chapter in this book describes exercises used to mobilize and recondition stiffened extremities.

RADIOGRAPHIC MONITORING

At least two views at right angles to one another should be taken of any suspected fracture. At times special views, such as obliques, spot views, stress films, tomograms, or computed tomography scans, are required to adequately visualize the injury. These have been discussed appropriately in other chapters.

Once the diagnosis is made and treatment accomplished, an x-ray should be obtained after manipulation and casting or splint to assess the accuracy of reduction and the maintenance of position. The extremity should then have repeat x-rays at 5 to 7 days to detect any change in position of unstable injuries. This should be repeated at an interval of another 5 to 7 days. In fractures that heal rapidly, another x-ray is appropriate in 2 to 4 weeks, when the fracture should be assessed clinically and radiographically for progress in healing. An x-ray should also always be taken when it is felt that the fracture is clinically stable and immobilization is going to be discontinued. This provides information about the degree of healing and, consequently, the degree of further protection necessary. Another x-ray should be obtained when it is thought that remodeling of the fracture is fairly mature to assess the integrity and form of the final structure. X-rays should be taken during treatment if there is further injury to the extremity, if the cast becomes grossly loose or breaks, or if there is increased pain at the fracture site at a time remote from injury.

The exact timing of x-ray examination depends on many variables, including the nature and location of the fracture as well as the age of the patient. For example, the time course of fracture healing of the femur can be 3 to 5 weeks in a 3-year-old patient, 8 to 10 weeks in an 8-year-old patient, 12 to 14 weeks in a 12-year-old patient, and 20 to 24 weeks in an adult patient. A developing deformity in an unstable fracture must be recognized before healing becomes too advanced for remanipulation to correct the malposition. The practitioner consequently must be aware which fractures heal rapidly, and carefully follow unstable injuries in the initial phase. For example, a metaphyseal fracture of the distal radius in a 6-year-old patient will be quite stable by 2 weeks and there is little chance of progressive deformity. Recurrent deformity must be recognized before 2 weeks postinjury to correct the deformity by remanipulation. Fractures that heal more slowly must have a longer period of close follow-up. A midshaft tibial fracture in an adult can change position 2 to 4 weeks after reduction.

Rehabilitation following Musculoskeletal Injuries

Rehabilitation efforts begin in the emergency department when the patient is admitted. The goals for the patient's recovery include regaining full range of motion of the involved joints, regaining full strength, endurance, and power in the affected motor groups in the extremity, gradually increasing functional activity of the injured parts to promote healing, and returning to as near a normal state as possible. The specific rehabilitative regimens are outlined in the specific chapters. It is best to utilize the resources of the acute physical rehabilitation services at the hospital or in the community to ensure optimal recovery.

BASIC PRINCIPLES

Muscle strengthens in proportion to load moved. It is usually safe and effective to choose a resistance that will fatigue the muscles, but not precipitate pain, within 20 repetitions. To increase muscle strength, it is necessary to make a muscle contract with maximum power every day without overloading. To increase its endurance, utilize repetitions of lighter loads, stopping short of fatigue. Strength of a muscle contraction is proportional to the starting length of the muscle. Therefore, fully extend the muscle prior to exercising. Avoid overstretching of muscles, as this retards healing. Weak or partially innervated muscles should be protected from overstretching.

There are three basic types of exercise routines: isometric, isotonic, and isokinetic. The routines are prescribed by the physician in specific situations. Warm towels should be placed on the muscle group for 5 to 10 minutes prior to the workout to promote relaxation and warm-up.

Isometric exercises strengthen muscle groups by contracting the muscle (producing tension) but not moving the affected joint or changing the length of the muscle. This is the best way to develop strength if joint motion is painful and there is secondary muscle inhibition. For example, quadriceps isometrics or "setting" involves maintaining the knee in a fixed position and contracting the muscle in rhythmic, gentle, gradual fashion to avoid pain. The contraction is sustained for 5 to 10 seconds and then relaxed for an equal period. This is repeated 10 to 20 times per "set," followed by a 5-minute rest period. The sets are repeated 2 to 3 times to the patient's fatigue point tempered by pain. The routine may be repeated 2 to 3 times per day as tolerated. Again, pain and fatigue are the controlling end points.

In isotonic exercises, the joint and muscle group move an applied load through a range of motion. This is probably the best way to regain motion, strength, and endurance when the joint is not painful. A useful technique to enhance the effects of isometric and isotonic programs is progressive resistance exercises, in which the load is increased progressively as strength increases, thereby enhancing strength, power, and endurance.

Isokinetic exercises control the rate of joint motion while the resistance varies with the strength of the subject's muscular effort. For example, patients may push or pull as little or as much as they wish, but the cadence is unchanged. Therefore, muscle power, which is the amount of work accomplished over a unit of time, may be increased by exercising at a higher rate even if the loads are smaller. This also increases endurance. An isokinetic machine can also measure torque; thus, it is a simple matter to graph the actual motor strength and power generated. The physician, therapist, and patient can see the results and, hence, gauge progress or lack of progress in the therapy program. Joints begin to mobilize when moved regularly, barely through the point of pain. Active exercise is preferred to passive exercise because it is independent, strengthens while it mobilizes, and is less likely to do harm than passive movements. Gentle active-assistive exercise is necessitated by weakness, timidity, harmful incoordination, or a pain process that is worsened by active movement, e.g., traumatic hemarthrosis or acute arthritis. As discussed above under "Complications," congestion is relieved by movements that rhythmically compress the congested structures. Joint movement to the mechanical limit of motion or the onset of pain (whichever occurs first) will apply such compression. This technique can be useful at the outset of a rehabilitation program, when pain, stiffness, and patient reluctance are greatest. Often, after a single session, the patient is capable of performing a therapeutically beneficial range of motion.

Wet heat is more analgesic than dry heat. Heat can burn; hence, the heat source must be tested on the volar forearm of the therapist before applying to the patient. It must not be applied to insensitive or ischemic skin. If the skin is prevented from cooling by the patient's position or a covering, a continuous source of heat must not be applied. For example, a common and blistering error is to lie on a heating pad. Wet heat is best applied as a local bath but may be applied as a hot, wet towel kept hot with a heating pad that has been insulated in plastic. Note that local

heating, e.g., immersion of the injured part alone, is more effective than total heating, e.g., immersion of the whole body, as the part can be kept hotter longer without harm to the patient. Usually, heat applications are limited to 10 or 15 minutes, 3 or 4 times a day. If exceeded, this tends to produce a hyperemic state in the local area, which causes more local inflammation and congestion, and attendant pain and tenderness.

Cold is less likely to congest an area than is heat, and it can be analgesic. The analgesic benefit is more likely to be appreciated after, rather than during, the application. Cold is unequivocally preferred to heat during the first 36 to 72 hours after injury. After that initial period of cold applications, heat or cold may be applied symptomatically on a trial basis.

Cold can be effectively applied in several ways. Water can be frozen in a paper cup and the ice, held in the cup or a washcloth, massaged over the painful areas. To avoid thermocutaneous injury, the ice must be kept moving throughout the treatment. Five to 10 minutes of massage is usually effective. The patient will experience a burning sensation before the analgesic effect is achieved. Alternatively, a bath towel can be folded to the size of the area to be treated, dampened thoroughly but not dripping, and chilled. The chilled or "soft-frozen" towel may then be applied to the painful area for 5 or 10 minutes. To prevent an ice burn, a damp towel must be placed between the soft-frozen towel and the disordered part. For example, the individual with a painful disorder of the low back can lie with the back on a damp towel over a chilled towel. Finally, an ice bag or pack are effective means of cooling an injured part. To avoid injury, the skin must not be in direct contact with the ice. The application should be for 5 to 10 minutes and the part should be allowed to return to normal temperature before reapplying the cold application.

Painfully reactive muscle tone must be

kept at a minimum. Any manipulation or motion, active or passive, that is followed by an increase in painfully reactive muscle tone must be avoided, or its harmful influence on muscle tone somehow neutralized. Topical and systemic analgesics facilitate a decrease in painfully reactive muscle tone. Topical analgesics include heat, cold, and gentle massage. Systemic analgesics include medications such as salicylates and nonsteroidal anti-inflammatories. Fatigue must be recognized, relieved, and subsequently avoided when it appears to augment pain. Anxiety and depression must be recognized and relieved.

MEASUREMENT OF JOINT MOTION

While a qualitative sense of joint motion is often adequate for diagnostic and planning purposes, a quantitative measure provides a more objective assessment of the effect of therapy and a better-documented report of disability. Joint motion is most accurately measured with a goniometer. One limb, the static limb, of the goniometer is aligned with a reference axis along the body part just proximal to the joint, and the other limb, the dynamic limb, of the goniometer is aligned with the moving axis along the body part just distal to the joint. The joint motion is measured from a position as close in line with the reference axis as the moving axis can attain, to a position as far from the reference axis as the moving axis can attain, within the intended plane of motion. The reference axis is always designated 0°. With experience, the examiner can fairly accurately estimate the degrees of joint motion without a goniometer.

Figures 10.14 through 10.28 name the motion and the plane of its measurements, designate the reference axis, and show the proper alignment of the goniometer for each measurement.

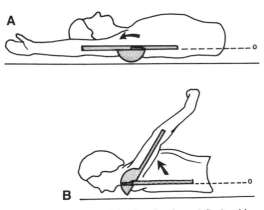

Figure 10.14. *A,* shoulder elevation through flexion. Measurement is made in the sagittal plane of the trunk. *B,* shoulder extension. Measurement is made in the sagittal plane of the trunk.

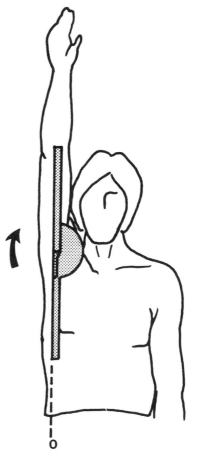

Figure 10.15. Shoulder elevation through abduction. Measurement is made in the frontal plane of the trunk.

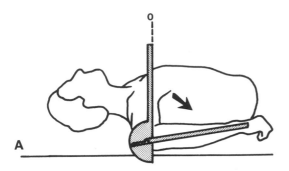

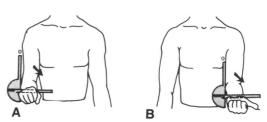

Figure 10.18. *A*, forearm pronation with the elbow at 90° of flexion, and the forearm in the sagittal plane of the trunk. Measurement is made in the frontal plane of the trunk. *B*, forearm supination with the elbow at 90° of flexion, and the forearm in the sagittal plane of the trunk. Measurement is made in the frontal plane of the trunk.

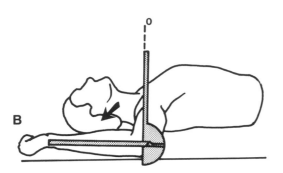

Figure 10.16. *A*, internal rotation of the shoulder at 90° abduction. Measurement is made in the sagittal plane of the trunk. *B*, external rotation of the shoulder at 90° abduction. Measurement is made in the sagittal plane of the trunk.

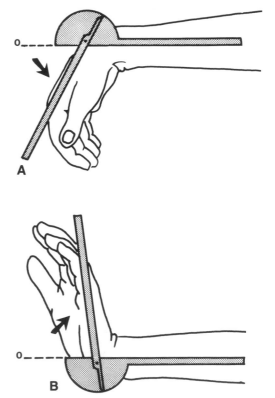

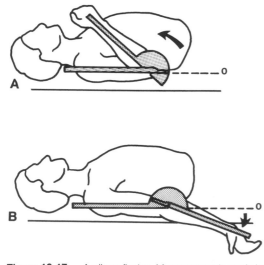

Figure 10.17. *A*, elbow flexion. Measurement is made in the sagittal plane of the arm. *B*, elbow extension. Measurement is made in the sagittal plane of the arm.

Figure 10.19. *A*, wrist flexion. Measurement is made in the sagittal plane of the forearm. *B*, wrist extension. Measurement is made in the sagittal plane of the forearm.

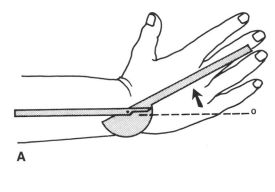

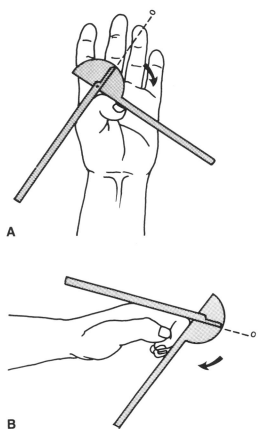

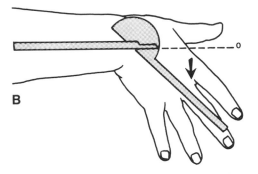

Figure 10.20. *A*, radial deviation of the wrist. Measurement is made in the frontal plane of the forearm. *B*, ulnar deviation of the wrist. Measurement is made in the frontal plane of the forearm.

Figure 10.22. *A*, flexion of the first interphalangeal joint. Measurement is made in the frontal plane of the hand. *B*, flexion of the second, third, fourth, and fifth interphalangeal joints. Measurement is made in the sagittal plane of the hand.

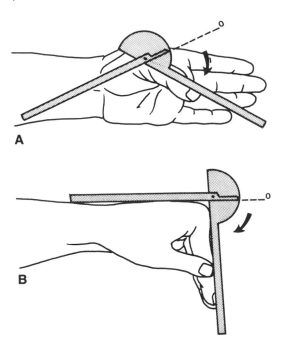

Figure 10.21. *A*, flexion of the first metacarpophalangeal joint. Measurement is made in the frontal plane of the forearm and hand. *B*, flexion of the second, third, fourth, and fifth metacarpophalangeal joints. Measurement is made in the sagittal plane of the forearm and hand.

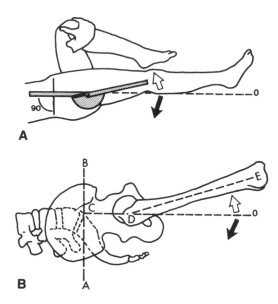

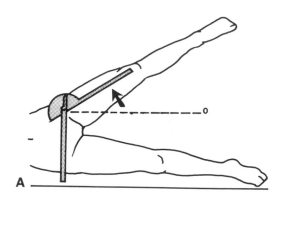

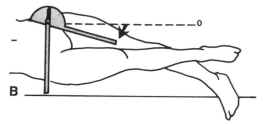

Figure 10.23. *A,* skeletal landmarks used to orient the goniometer when measuring hip extension and flexion. The 0° axis is perpendicular to a line connecting the point of the anterior-superior iliac spine with the point of the posterior iliac spine. *B,* hip extension. Measurement is made in the sagittal plane of the trunk. The example illustrates limitation of extension to a point short of the 0° axis (note the *open arrows*).

Figure 10.25. *A,* hip abduction. Measurement is made in the frontal plane of the trunk. *B,* hip adduction. Measurement is made in the frontal plane of the trunk.

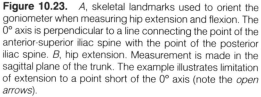

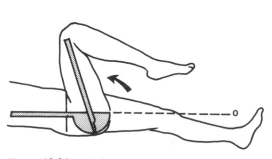

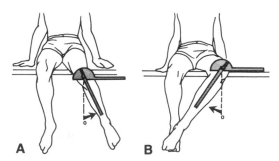

Figure 10.24. Hip flexion. Measurement is made in the sagittal plane of the trunk.

Figure 10.26. *A,* internal rotation of the hip. Measurement is made in the transverse plane of the thigh. *B,* external rotation of the hip. Measurement is made in the transverse plane of the thigh.

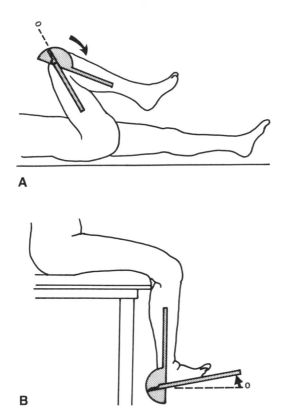

A

B

Figure 10.27. *A*, knee flexion. Measurement is made in the sagittal plane of the thigh. *B*, ankle dorsiflexion. Measurement is made in the sagittal plane of the leg.

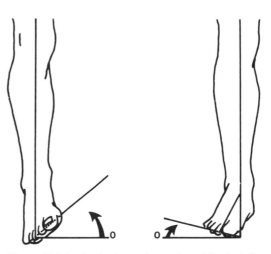

Figure 10.28. Supination and pronation of the foot. Supination is measured in the transverse plane of the foot. Pronation is measured in the transverse and frontal planes of the foot.

MUSCLE STRENGTH GRADING

The strength of individual muscles may be indicated by functional grades (Table 10.1).

AMBULATION AIDS AND GAIT TRAINING

Patients with injuries to the lower extremities usually require some form of ambulation aid (crutches, canes, walkers) to protect the injured parts. Prior to this, as soon as possible following injury and definitive care, prepare the patient for ambulation by regaining full range of motion, strength, endurance, balance, and control of the trunk and uninjured extremities. The most important muscles for assisted walking using aids are the abdominal and paraspinous muscles of the trunk; the shoulder abductors, depressors, adductors, flexors, and extensors; the elbow extensors; the forearm rotators, wrist extensors and finger flexors in the upper limbs; as well as the antigravity muscles of the uninjured lower extremity. Isometric exercises are utilized first, followed by isotonic and isokinetic exercises as described earlier. Patients must be taught a proper gait pattern utilizing support. They begin standing in the parallel bars with their feet slightly apart to get their balance. Next, they transfer their weight front-to-back and side-to-side to at-

Table 10.1.
Muscle Strength Grading

Grade	Characteristics
Normal (5)	Full active range of motion against gravity and normal resistance
Good (4)	Full active range of motion against gravity and good resistance
Fair (3)	Full active range of motion against gravity
Poor (2)	Full active range of motion with gravity eliminated
Trace (1)	Muscle contracts but no joint motion
None (0)	No muscle contraction

tain balance on each foot. They are then taught to use crutches, a cane, or a walker.

Crutches

Crutches should be adjusted for the patient so that there are three fingers between the "axillary" pad of the crutch and the axilla when the tip of the crutch is located slightly lateral and anterior to the tip of the shoe with the feet side by side. The axillary pad is designed to take pressure on the lateral side of the upper chest, and not in the axilla where the brachial plexus could be injured. The hand piece should be positioned so that the elbow is flexed comfortably (approximately 10° to 20°) while bearing weight. The tip of the crutch should be covered with a wide rubber crutch tip to add traction and stability.

Crutch Gaits. The simplest gait is the swing-through gait, in which both crutches are placed forward and the patient swings the body and both lower extremities through both crutches, so that the feet end up ahead of the crutch tips. Weight can be borne on both feet or on the well foot with the injured foot non-weight bearing. This is a non-physiologic gait, but it is quick and easy to learn.

The three-point gait is a smoother gait biomechanically. In this method, the two crutches are advanced and followed closely by the injured extremity, so that the crutch tips are firmly planted just before the injured extremity strikes the ground. The degree of weight bearing to the injured extremity is controlled by the weight borne on the upper extremities, and is expressed as a three-point, partial weight-bearing crutch gait. The desired weight (or none) to be borne on the injured extremity is specifically prescribed by the physician.

Canes

Canes are fitted by having the patient hold the cane in the hand opposite to the injured lower extremity. The length should be such that the elbow is flexed about 20° while the rubber cane tip rests on the ground 3 to 4 inches lateral to and slightly ahead of the tip of the ipsilateral shoe. Canes are less cumbersome and easier to use than crutches, but they are much less effective in unloading an extremity. Patients advance the cane with the normal alternating swing of the upper extremity, e.g., the right hand swings forward with the left foot. The cane and the heel of the injured limb should strike the ground simultaneously. At contact, the elbow should be flexed 10° to 20°, and the tip of the cane should be slightly outside the progression of the swing phase of the normal extremity, and opposite the midfoot of the injured extremity. The requirements for muscle strength are similar to those for crutches. The cane is a useful intermediate device when weaning a patient from crutches to full weight bearing.

Walkers

A walker is more stable than a cane or crutches, and offers an alternate device for protected weight bearing that is particularly useful for patients who do not have the strength, agility, or coordination to use crutches or a cane. Walkers are fitted to the patient while the patient stands with both hands on the handles of the walker and flexes the elbows 20° to 30° (handlebars approximately at the level of the greater trochanter). Patients should be instructed to stand in the embrace of the walker in a comfortable position with the necessary weight on the handles of the walker to protect the injured part. They then advance the walker for the length of their arms and set it firmly on the ground. Patients then shift their weight to the handles and walk into the bars of the walker. This provides a partial or non-weight-bearing gait, much like the three-point or four-point crutch gait. The walker is particularly useful for elderly patients following hip fracture.

SUGGESTED READINGS

Nickel VL, ed. Orthopedic rehabilitation. New York: Churchill Livingstone, 1982.

Rockwood CA Jr, Green DP, eds. Fractures in adults; Vols 1 and 2. 2nd ed. Philadelphia: JB Lippincott Co, 1984.

Rockwood CA Jr, Wilkins KE, King RE, eds. Fractures in children, Vol 3. Philadelphia: JB Lippincott Co, 1984.

Salter RB. Textbook of disorders and injuries of the musculoskeletal system: an introduction to orthopaedics, fractures and joint injuries, rheumatology, metabolic bone disease and rehabilitation. 2nd ed. Baltimore: Williams & Wilkins, 1983.

Southmayd W, Hoffman M. Sports health: the complete book of athletic injuries. New York: Quick Fox, 1981.

Staff, Prosthetics and Orthotics. Lower-limb orthotics. New York: New York University Postgraduate Medical School, 1986.

Staff, Prosthetics and Orthotics. Lower-limb prosthetics. 1990 revision. New York: New York University Postgraduate Medical School, 1990.

Staff, Prosthetics and Orthotics. Upper-limb prosthetics. New York: New York University Postgraduate Medical School, 1982.

Turek SL. Orthopaedics: principles and their application. 4th ed. Philadelphia: JB Lippincott Co, 1984.

CHAPTER 11

Aspiration and Injection Techniques: Joints, Bursae, and Local Anesthesia

Carlton M. Akins, M.D., and W. Thomas Edwards, Ph.D., M.D.

During the evaluation of orthopaedic disorders, the clinician may introduce a needle for a variety of reasons: (*a*) aspiration for diagnosis of joint or bursal effusion, (*b*) evacuation of painful hemarthrosis or other effusion, (*c*) injection of corticosteroid into the joint or bursa, or (*d*) local anesthesia. An understanding of both general and local principles is important in the safe and effective use of these techniques. These local principles are concerned with specific applications and are described and diagrammed later in this chapter.

Aspiration and Injection Techniques

GENERAL PRINCIPLES

Aspiration is performed as part of the evaluation of a joint or bursal effusion (see Chapter 12), and/or to relieve the painful pressure of a tense effusion. This also facilitates further clinical examination. Corticosteroids may be injected into an inflamed bursa or joint once it has been established that the inflammation is not secondary to an infection. The clinician is most likely to use these techniques in the following areas for the conditions listed: injuries with effusion—knee, elbow, ankle, shoulder; degenerative joint disease with synovitis—trapeziometacarpal joint of the thumb, knee, metatarsophalangeal joint of the great toe, ankle; rheumatoid arthritis—knee, metacarpophalangeal and interphalangeal finger joints, wrist, ankle; bursae—subacromial,

greater trochanteric, olecranon, prepatellar, and pes anserine.

The following general technique is recommended (Fig. 11.1):

1. Identify joint or bursal landmarks by fingertip palpation and define the site of needle insertion. (Specific sites are designated later in this section.)
2. Cleanse the area with povidone-iodine solution. Drape the site with sterile drapes.
3. Create a 1% lidocaine wheal at the site of needle entry using a small (25- to 27-gauge) needle and sterile gloves.
4. For joint or bursal aspiration, use an 18- or 19-gauge needle (smaller sizes are often ineffective) and syringe appropriate to the site. For the knee, ankle, shoulder, elbow, and wrist, use a 20-ml syringe; and for smaller joints and bursae, a 5- or 10-ml syringe.
5. For corticosteroid injection, after aspiration, use the same needle for both. For injection alone, use the narrowest gauge needle of appropriate length. For the shoulder, elbow, wrist, knee, and ankle, a 1½-inch 22-gauge needle usually suffices; finger and toe joints can usually be injected with a ¾-inch 25-gauge needle.
6. Draw the corticosteroid preparation from the vial into a small syringe, using an 18- or 20-gauge needle; then exchange the needle, using sterile technique, for the needle intended for the injection. The volume of corticosteroid to be injected

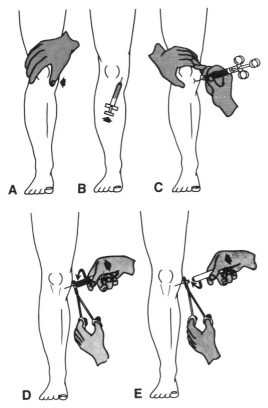

Figure 11.1.   Aspirating the knee. *A*, identifying the joint space. *B*, anesthetizing the skin. *C*, passing the needle. *D*, removing the filled syringe. *E*, replacing the emptied syringe.

depends on the size of the joint or bursa: finger and toe joints, 0.25 ml; elbow, wrist, and ankle, 0.5–1.0 ml; shoulder, hip, knee, and associated bursae, 1.0 ml.

7. Continue to use sterile technique for the process of needle insertion. Introduce the needle with a steady thrust, not an abrupt push. Hold the syringe like a pencil, and use only the force of the fingers and wrist to introduce the needle. The opposite hand may be used to steady the syringe hand, or to stabilize the area, or to compress the joint, if necessary.

8. When aspirating a joint or bursa, the syringe may have to be detached from the needle hub and emptied several times, leaving the needle inserted. Use a hemo-

stat to hold the needle back while twisting off the syringe, and when replacing it.

Specific Applications

Figures 11.2 through 11.12 identify the landmarks and proper site of needle insertion for aspiration and/or injection.

Local Anesthesia

GENERAL PRINCIPLES

It should be remembered that the most common cause of serious problems in the performance of any local anesthetic procedure is related to the toxic effects of local anesthetic agents. These toxic effects can occur because of accidental intravascular injection of the appropriate amount of the drug, injec-

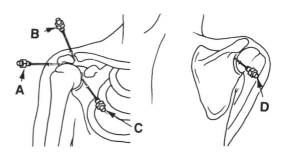

Figure 11.2.   Placing a needle into the shoulder joints. *A*, into the subacromial bursa. *B*, into the acromioclavicular joint. *C*, into the glenohumeral joint. Anterior approach. *D*, into the glenohumeral joint. Posterior approach.

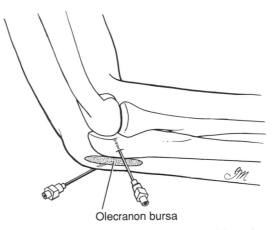

Olecranon bursa

Figure 11.3.   Placing a needle into the elbow joint or the olecranon bursa from the radial aspect.

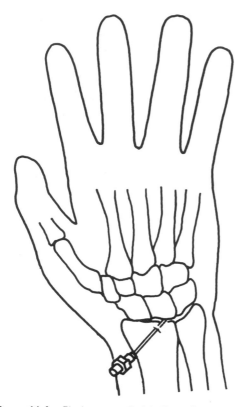

Figure 11.4. Placing a needle into the radiocarpal joint through the dorsal aspect of the wrist.

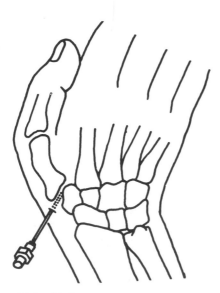

Figure 11.5. Placing a needle into the trapeziometacarpal joint.

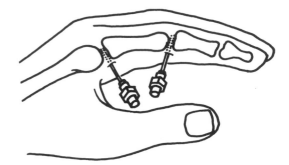

Figure 11.6. Placing a needle into the metacarpophalangeal and interphalangeal joints.

tion of an overdose of the drug into the appropriate tissue space, toxic reactions to drugs with which a local anesthetic agent is compounded, or allergic reaction to the local anesthetic drug or any substance with which it is prepared. Put simply, these can be remembered as: (*a*) right amount of drug in the wrong place; (*b*) wrong amount of drug in the right place; (*c*) right drug in the right place; wrong adjunct; (*d*) right drug, right place; unexpected reaction.

These problems can be avoided by taking some simple precautions in choosing drugs and dosages as well as being prepared to deal with unexpected outcomes. In general, every local anesthetic administration should follow these simple principles:

1. Always be familiar with the drugs you are administering, especially with the maximum safe dose of all drugs contained in the agent you are using.
2. Expect the unexpected and be prepared. Be sure your office is equipped to deal with the consequences of toxic and allergic reactions.
3. Have the necessary resuscitation equipment and drugs at hand when you administer local anesthetics. At the minimum, these include: equipment to establish intravenous line and intravenous fluids; oxygen and the appropriate equipment for its administration; appropriate airway support equipment includ-

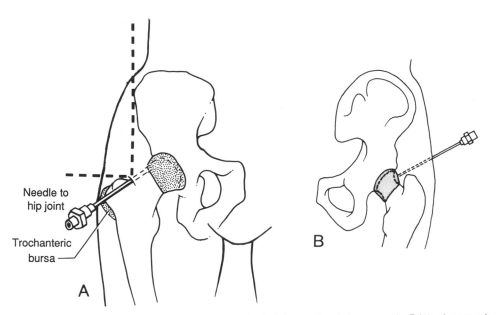

Figure 11.7. Passing a needle into the hip joint or trochanteric bursa. *A,* anterior approach. *B,* lateral approach.

ing suction, oral and nasal airways, endotracheal tube, laryngoscope, and hand resuscitator (Ambu bag); drugs for cardiovascular support in the event that advanced cardiac life support techniques need to be instituted.

LOCAL ANESTHETICS—DRUGS, AGENTS, ADJUNCTS

The author distinguishes the local anesthetic drug (such as lidocaine) from the agent used for local anesthesia. The agent includes the drug, its concentration, all adjunctive agents and their concentrations as well as the total volume of the solution administered to produce anesthesia. For example, the agent for a digital block might be 4 ml of 1% plain lidocaine (Xylocaine). A complete statement of the agent used can give an indication of why a problem has occurred.

A bewildering array of local anesthetics is commercially available. Five drugs are in

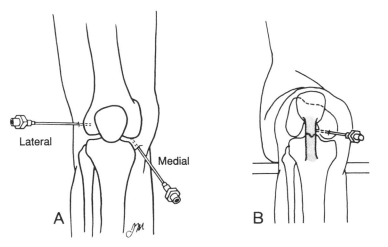

Figure 11.8. Passing a needle into the knee joint. *A,* medial or lateral. *B,* anterior approach, with the knee flexed to 90°.

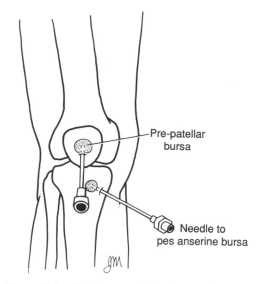

Figure 11.9. Passing a needle into bursae of the knee.

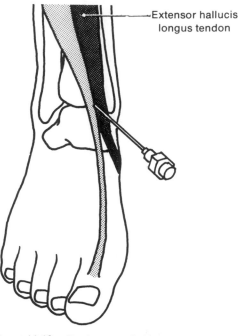

Figure 11.10. Passing a needle into the tibiotalar joint.

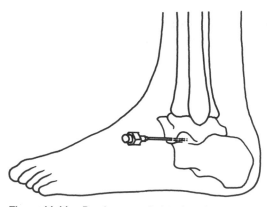

Figure 11.11. Passing a needle into the subtalar joint by way of the sinus tarsi. Note the position relative to the lateral malleolus. The depression of the sinus tarsi is palpable there, especially when the ankle is inverted.

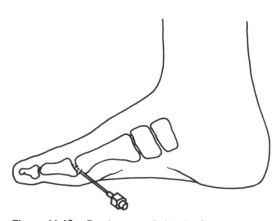

Figure 11.12. Passing a needle into the first metartarso-phalangeal joint.

common use today: cocaine, chloroprocaine, lidocaine, mepivacaine, and bupivacaine. For practical purposes, it is advisable that the physician become familiar with a limited number of drugs and use only these.

Cocaine is available in a 5% solution and is used only for application to mucosal surfaces of the upper airway to produce topical anesthesia. Higher concentrations are available but the toxicity can be profound. Chlo-

roprocaine is available in 1 to 3% solutions. The use of concentrations between 1 and 2% for routine office practice is recommended. This drug is the most rapidly acting of all injectable local anesthetics and generally has the lowest systemic toxicity. As with cocaine, chloroprocaine is a member of the group of ester local anesthetics that are hydrolyzed in the circulation by plasma pseudocholinesterase. Procaine and tetracaine are other available esters, but they are not particularly useful in the office setting. This group of local anesthetics has been associated with a measurable incidence of allergic phenomena.

Lidocaine (Xylocaine and others), mepivacaine (Carbocaine and others), and bupivacaine (Marcaine and others) are the three commonly used amide-type local anesthetics. All are metabolized in the liver and the degradation products are excreted in the urine. Speed of onset is roughly the same with all of these. Duration of action is in the following order: lidocaine *less than* mepivacaine *less than* bupivacaine, but this is dependent in part on the total dose administered. Amide-type local anesthetics have not been associated with true allergic phenomena. Recommended concentrations and maximum total doses are listed below.

1. Chloroprocaine (plain) 1–2% (10–20 mg/ml); not to exceed 10 mg/kg.
2. Lidocaine (plain) 0.5–1.5% (5–15 mg/ml); not to exceed 5 mg/kg.
3. Lidocaine (with epinephrine) 0.5–1.5% (5–15 mg/ml); not to exceed 7 mg/kg.
4. Mepivacaine (plain) (0.5–1.5%) (5–15 mg/ml); not to exceed 5 mg/kg.
5. Mepivacaine with epinephrine is not comercially available and not particularly useful.
6. Bupivacaine (plain) 0.25–0.5% (2.5–5 mg/ml); not to exceed 2.5 mg/kg.
7. Bupivacaine (with epinephrine) 0.25–0.5% (2.5–5 mg/ml); not to exceed 3.5 mg/kg.

Epinephrine (adrenaline) is commonly added to local anesthetics to extend the duration of action and to decrease blood flow in the region being blocked. Solutions containing epinephrine in a concentration greater than 1:200,000 (5 μg/ml) cannot be recommended. The commercial preparations of lidocaine containing 1:100,000 epinephrine do not offer any particular advantage to practitioners of office anesthesia. Other agents found in commercially prepared local anesthetic solutions include preservatives designed to retard growth of molds in multidose vials, and agents needed to adjust the pH in such a way as to keep the local anesthetic in solution. Since all local anesthetic agents are weak bases, the pH is adjusted to an amount below their pKa. Solutions of lidocaine and mepivacaine may have a pH as low as 2.5 to 3.0. This may explain in part why these drugs are painful to inject.

PREVENTION OF TOXIC REACTIONS

Before administering the medication, calculate the maximum allowable volume of the agent to be used. Remember to adjust downward the maximum allowable dose for elderly patients by 10 to 30%, depending on each patient's general state of health. If a field block with 1% lidocaine with 1:200,000 epinephrine is planned and the patient is a healthy 25-year-old person weighing 60 kg, 420 mg or 42 ml of this solution should not be exceeded. In addition, all resuscitation equipment should be immediately available (i.e., not in the next room). The following rules should also be observed:

1. Take a careful history. Patients who state that they are allergic to local anesthetics rarely are, but more likely they have had a toxic reaction. You may be able to identify the type of reaction from the history. Some of these reactions are simple "faints" or vasovagal reactions. Some are reactions to an overdose of a vasoconstrictor, usually epinephrine, and are characterized by a pounding sensation in the head followed by rapid heartbeat and sometimes by loss of consciousness. Occasionally these reactions are examples of intravascular injection of local anesthetic with vasoconstrictor and may have been followed by convulsion. These types of

problems are commonly seen during dental blocks. An episode that is characterized by the onset of buzzing in the ears, numb mouth or tongue, blurred vision, and loss of consciousness is probably an episode of an overdose of local anesthetic (wrong amount of drug, right place). A question should arise in the physician's mind if a patient has been told that he or she is allergic to lidocaine because of the low incidence of true allergy to amide local anesthetics.

2. Monitor carefully during injection. Pulse and blood pressure monitoring during the performance of a block may go far to prevent toxic reactions, as intravascular injection can usually be noted immediately, particularly if an epinephrine-containing solution is being used. It is heralded by rapid increase in heart rate followed quickly by increase in blood pressure. Monitor the patient's sense of well-being and frequently ask questions about "funny feelings in the head" or tingling around the mouth.

3. Perform all local anesthetic injections in a "fractionated" manner. Inject no more than 5 ml, wait one circulation time (15 to 30 seconds), inject another 5 ml, wait another 15 seconds, etc. It is rare to miss the onset of a toxic reaction from intravascular injection, although it will still be very mild if this technique is used regularly.

4. Recognize the early warning signs. Toxic reactions are described above. Be aware that if one stops injection at the earliest sign of toxicity and a fractionation technique has been used, it is unlikely that the worst will happen. This may not be true for bupivacaine, however, so this drug should be chosen with due appreciation for its tendency to produce high-grade ventricular arrhythmias as a first manifestation of toxicity. These can degenerate rapidly into ventricular tachycardia and fibrillation that may be refractory to treatment. With almost *all other drugs*, the usual progression of symptoms and signs when toxicity occurs is tinnitus > circumoral numbness > dizziness and excitation > unconsciousness and seizures > cardiovascular collapse > cardiopulmonary arrest. Each of these sets of events happens at definable blood levels of local anesthetic. Thus, with all commonly used local anesthetics (with the exception of bupivacaine), careful monitoring can identify the onset of a toxic reaction before it becomes serious.

What to do if the worst happens:

1. Stop the injection.
2. Administer oxygen.
3. Remember the "ABCs" of cardiopulmonary resuscitation:

   (*a*) open the airway;
   (*b*) breathe for the patient if spontaneous ventilation has stopped;
   (*c*) support circulation as indicated by external cardiac massage and principles of basic life support (and advanced cardiac life support if necessary).

4. Convulsions that follow toxic reactions to most local anesthetics are brief. Intubation of the trachea may not be needed and will only protect against aspiration if it is performed correctly. The airway must be kept open and oxygenation sustained by administration of oxygen by mask. Diazepam 5 mg or Midazolam 3 to 5 mg may help suppress a seizure but usually are not needed.

REGIONAL BLOCKS

The use of regional blocks is advantageous because relatively large areas of the body can be anesthetized (by the injection of local anesthetic agents) in specific areas close to an individual nerve, or where bundles of nerves are congregated. The disadvantage of this method is that if the nerves are damaged by the needle, there will likewise be a relatively large area subject to paresthesia or numbness; also, the nerves may lie deep and close to other vital structures (such as lungs or arteries), thus risking possible damage to these areas. Consequently, if local infiltration will do the job without having to use excessive volumes, it would be foolish for the occasional anesthetist to subject a patient to the potential hazards of these blocks. The goal of regional blocks is to deposit the anesthetic solution as close as possible to the nerve without actually penetrating it. For regional blocks requiring large volumes of solution, the simplest method is to draw up the maximum dose into a 30- to 50-ml syringe with an extension tube and needle attached, to inject the recommended amount after proper location of the needle, and to alternate small increments with repeated aspiration, as described previously. The needle should be a 1½-inch 22-gauge B-bevel needle.

Blocks of the Forearm and Hand

Elbow Block (Fig. 11.13). The radial, median, and ulnar nerves can be blocked independently at the elbow and will provide analgesia to their respective areas in the hand. However, this will not be adequate for operations on the forearm, unless a subcutaneous block of the area above the elbow is also administered to block the medial cutaneous nerve to the forearm. The arm is flexed 90° and a line is drawn along the crease of the elbow. The arm is then extended, and injections are made on this line.

Radial Nerve. The needle is inserted approximately 1 cm lateral (radial side) to the biceps tendon, and 5 ml are deposited in a fan-wise manner down to the bone, unless paresthesias are encountered. This generally blocks the musculocutaneous nerve as well, because the needle passes through the brachiolradialis.

Median Nerve

The needle is inserted medial to the brachial artery until paresthesias are elicited; 5 to 10 ml are injected.

Ulnar Nerve (Fig. 11.14). The nerve is rolled under the palpating finger proximal to the cubital tunnel behind the medial epicondyle. Two milliliters are injected on either side of the nerve. It is not wise to inject directly into the sulcus, as the nerve may be impaled against the bone and could possibly suffer from compression.

Medial Cutaneous of the Forearm. This can be accomplished by superficial injection of the medial half of the arm just above the elbow.

Wrist Blocks (Fig. 11.15). These blocks are indicated for specific areas in the palm or fingers. Each of the three blocks is made by injection into the volar aspect of the wrist at a level identified by a line drawn between the radial and ulnar styloid processes.

Ulnar. The needle is inserted perpendicular to the skin immediately radial to the flexor carpi ulnaris tendon and ulnar to the ulnar artery, at the level of the styloid pro-

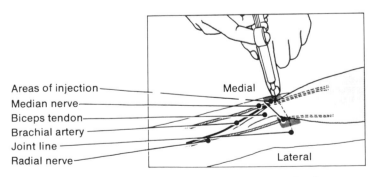

Areas of injection
Median nerve
Biceps tendon
Brachial artery
Joint line
Radial nerve

Medial

Lateral

Figure 11.13. Block of the radial and median nerves at the elbow.

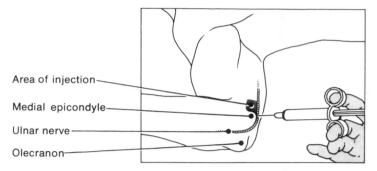

Area of injection

Medial epicondyle

Ulnar nerve

Olecranon

Figure 11.14. Block of the ulnar nerve at the elbow.

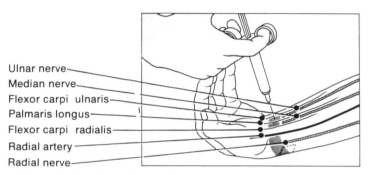

Ulnar nerve
Median nerve
Flexor carpi ulnaris
Palmaris longus
Flexor carpi radialis
Radial artery
Radial nerve

Figure 11.15. Block of the median, radial, and ulnar nerves at the wrist.

cess of the ulna. Four milliliters are injected, with or without paresthesias.

Median. The needle is inserted perpendicularly between the tendons of the palmaris longus and flexor carpi radialis through the flexor retinaculum. Five milliliters are injected at this site.

Radial. The needle is inserted perpendicularly over the radial artery, just proximal to the radial styloid, and directly dorsally, injecting 5 ml superficially around the radial aspect of the wrist. The needle must not enter the radial artery.

The specific danger with these blocks is nerve damage following needle penetration of a nerve. Intravascular injection is guarded against by repeated aspiration during the injection.

Metacarpal Blocks (Fig. 11.16). These blocks are useful for operations on the fingers, where digital injections are not suitable by reason of location of the operation, or

compromise of blood flow due to compression of finger vessels. The needle is inserted on either side of the adjoining metacarpal, proximal and close to the metacarpophalangeal joint. The solution is injected continuously as the needle is advanced until the tip of the needle can be felt in the palm. If an-

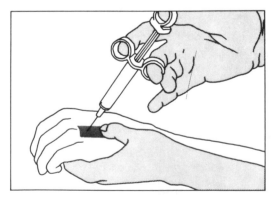

Figure 11.16. Metacarpal block.

esthesia is still inadequate after 5 minutes, the needle is reinserted through the same puncture site and advanced distally into each web, close to the designated digit, and 1 to 2 ml are injected at each site.

Intravascular injection is guarded against by repeated aspiration during the injection.

Digital Blocks (Fig. 11.17). These blocks are indicated for operations on the distal portion of the finger or nail. The needle is inserted from the dorsal aspect on each side of the finger, and 2 ml are injected at each site as the needle is advanced toward the volar surface.

A specific danger of digital blocks is the swelling of the proximal phalanx with solution which can result in impaired circulation to the remainder of the finger.

Epinephrine should not be used with either the metacarpal or the digital block.

Foot Blocks

The anterior tibial (deep peroneal) and posterior tibial nerves can be blocked individually, and the saphenous, sural, and terminal cutaneous branches of the superficial peroneal nerve may be blocked by circumferential subcutaneous infiltration proximal to the ankle joint. Metatarsal and digital blocks (Figs. 11.18 and 11.19) are performed as are the metacarpal and digital blocks of the hand.

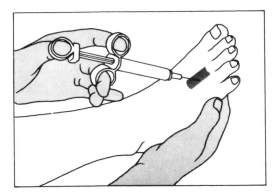

Figure 11.18. The metatarsal block.

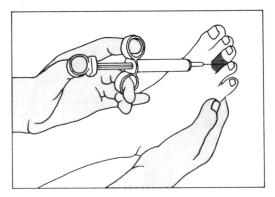

Figure 11.19. Digital block of the toe.

Anterior Tibial Block (Deep Peroneal Block, Fig. 11.20). A line is drawn across the front of the ankle, between the two malleoli. The needle is inserted lateral to the tendons of the tibialis anterior and extensor hallucis longus and advanced until a paresthesia is elicited, and 5 ml are then injected. Risk of injection into the anterior tibial artery which may lie on either side of the nerve can be minimized by intermittent aspiration during the injection.

Posterior Tibial Block (Fig. 11.21). The needle is inserted midway between the medial malleolus and the Achilles tendon. The nerve is posterior and lateral to the artery. The needle is advanced until a paresthesia is elicited, and 5 ml are then injected. If no paresthesia is elicited, the needle is withdrawn, and a fan-wise injection made.

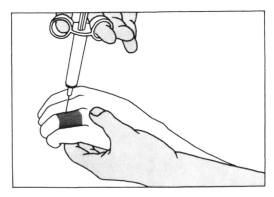

Figure 11.17. Digital block of the finger.

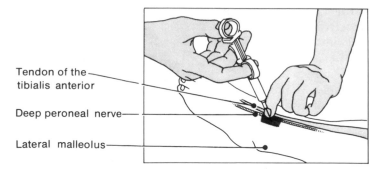

Tendon of the tibialis anterior

Deep peroneal nerve

Lateral malleolus

Figure 11.20. Block of the deep peroneal nerve at the ankle.

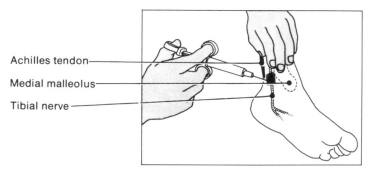

Achilles tendon

Medial malleolus

Tibial nerve

Figure 11.21. Block of the tibial nerve at the ankle.

Block of the Saphenous, Sural, and Terminal Branches of the Superficial Peroneal. This block is accomplished by circumferential posterior subcutaneous infiltration of 10 to 15 ml proximal to the ankle joint.

Intravenous Regional (Bier Block). This is suitable for most operations on the upper limb but has a limited application to the lower limb because of the huge volume of solution required. A double tourniquet is recommended. It should be reiterated that an intravenous infusion must be set up in the other arm and the patient's vital signs monitored. The double tourniquet is positioned in the upper arm and connected to the inflator, but not turned on. The pressure is set at approximately twice the systolic blood pressure, generally in the area of 300 mm Hg.

A small plastic cannula, 22-gauge, is inserted into a vein on the dorsum of the hand. Following aspiration of blood, it is flushed with 2 ml of saline, preferably with a heparin-type lock. The cannula is taped in position. The arm is then raised vertically and exsanguinated by means of an Esmarch's bandage. The distal cuff is inflated and then the proximal one; following satisfactory inflation of the latter, the distal cuff is then released. It is very important to check the tourniquet by palpation to see if it is inflated, and not simply rely on the pressure gauge. Forty milliliters of 0.5% lidocaine *without epinephrine* are now injected, making sure that the lidocaine is not infiltrating. The cannula is then withdrawn and pressure maintained over the puncture site for approximately 3 minutes. Anesthesia develops within approximately 5 minutes and will last for 60 to 70 minutes.

If the operation lasts over 15 minutes, and the patient is complaining of tourniquet pain, the distal tourniquet is then inflated, and after 1 minute, the proximal tourniquet released. By this time, the agent will have anesthetized the arm under the distal cuff. It is very important not to release the tourniquet completely until a minimum of ½ hour has elapsed following injection, as it takes that long for the bulk of the anesthetic to diffuse out of the vasculature into the tissue fluid. If the operation finishes before then, the tourniquet is kept inflated for the required time. If deflated sooner, the amount of anesthetic remaining in the vasculature can be enough to cause a toxic reaction. Following deflation, the patient should be carefully monitored for a further ½ hour, to make sure no toxic reaction develops.

Specific Dangers

1. Inadequate or noninflation of the tourniquet prior to administrating the agent will result in a failed anesthetic as well as a bolus dose injection of the local agent into the circulation.
2. Premature release of the tourniquet will result in a similar effect. Complications of local anesthetic toxicity are treated with administration of oxygen, up to 5 mg of intravenous diazepam, and intravenous fluids. If seizure occurs, follow the ABCs described earlier in this chapter.
3. Administration of an epinephrine-con-

taining solution will result in hypertension, arrhythmias, and possible cardiac arrest.

Local Infiltration of Fracture Sites

This is a relatively easy procedure and consists of the injection of approximately 10 ml of 1% lidocaine into the hematoma of the fracture site. An intradermal wheal is raised over the fracture site with a 1-inch 25-gauge needle and, following this, a 1½-inch 22-gauge needle is attached to the syringe and inserted into the fracture site. Following aspiration of blood, 10 ml are injected. This procedure has the theoretic disadvantage of converting a simple fracture into a compound one. Consequently, surgical preparation of the area is necessary. In addition, there are the dangers of intravascular absorption of the agent with its consequent effect. For a Colles' fracture, it will be necessary to inject not only the radial fracture site, but the styloid process of the ulna as well, in the event that this fractured.

SUGGESTED READINGS

Akins CM. Aspiration and injection of joints, bursae, and tendons. In: Vander Salm TJ, ed. Atlas of bedside procedures. Boston: Little, Brown and Co, 1988:451–464.

CHAPTER 12

Nontraumatic Arthropathies

David F. Giansiracusa, M.D., and Steven L. Strongwater, M.D.

Common nontraumatic disorders include osteoarthritis (OA), rheumatoid arthritis (RA), systemic lupus erythematosus (SLE), crystal-induced arthritis (gout, calcium pyrophosphate, and hydroxyapatite), the spondyloarthropathies (ankylosing spondylitis, psoriatic arthritis, Reiter's syndrome, and arthritis associated with inflammatory bowel disease), fibrositis, and Lyme disease.

Anatomy, Innervation, and Joint Function

Two types of joints are commonly affected by nontraumatic arthropathies: (*a*) diarthrodial or synovial joints, which move freely and are lined by a synovial membrane; and (*b*) amphiarthrotic or fibrocartilaginous joints, which have a more restricted range of motion. Diarthrodial joints (knee, wrist, shoulder, etc.) may be affected by a wide range of disorders, such as OA, RA, SLE, and crystal-induced arthritis. The fibrocartilaginous joints, including the pubic symphysis, sacroiliac joints, and intervertebral disks, are frequently involved in the spondyloarthropathies.

Diarthrodial joints consist of two or more bones or bone ends with opposing surfaces covered by extremely low-friction hyaline cartilage. The joint is lubricated by synovial fluid produced by the synovial membrane, and surrounded by capsule, ligaments, and often tendons adjacent to the capsule. The articular cartilage is composed of type II collagen fibers, which form the structural skeleton of the cartilage; between these fibers there is ground substance composed of aggregates of large proteoglycan molecules that contain negatively charged sulfate branches. These generate a strong osmotic force and facilitate the flow of nutrients from synovial fluid into the cartilage, and contribute to the expansile properties of cartilage. The collagen fibers and proteoglycans are synthesized by chondrocytes present in the cartilage. Cartilage is devoid of blood vessels and is dependent for its nutrition on diffusion of nutrients. This process is facilitated by the normal compression and decompression of the cartilage during joint use.

Articular cartilage is bathed in synovial fluid, which serves several functions: it nourishes cartilage; it helps maintain a low coefficient of friction as a result of a protein called lubricin; and it contains a number of proteins and other substances important in the regulation of inflammatory joint processes.

In contrast to articular cartilage, the synovium has a well-developed vascular, lymphatic, and nerve supply. Nerve fibers arise from roots supplying muscles that span the joint. Irritation of nerves in one joint may cause pain referred to surrounding muscle and adjacent joints. The synovium shares the same blood supply as the joint capsule and juxtaarticular bone. Fenestrations in the microvasculature allow diffusion of small solutes from the plasma and interstitial spaces into the joint. If, as in the case of chronic rheumatoid synovitis, the microcirculation is compromised, the delivery of nutrients (glucose and oxygen) may be significantly impaired.

The synovium is composed of two types of lining cells. Type A lining cells are derived from monocytes and resemble macrophages. Type B cells synthesize hyaluronic acid and other synovial fluid proteins. Other cellular components include antigen-presenting "dendritic" cells, mast cells, and white blood cells, important in regulating inflammatory conditions.

The composition of synovial fluid proteins is the result of diffusion from blood vessels, synthesis by synovium, articular consumption, and removal via lymphatic channels. Proteins passively diffuse from the microcirculation into the synovial interstitium and synovial fluid. The rate of diffusion is inversely proportional to the molecular size. Consequently, large molecules such as immunoglobin G are found in lower concentrations in synovial fluid than in plasma, while small proteins are more abundant. Hyaluronic acid, which gives synovial fluid its viscosity and lubricates the contact surface between the synovium and articular cartilage, is synthesized by the synovial membrane.

Several factors provide stability throughout a joint's range of motion. Joint shape enhances a close, congruous fit of the articular surfaces during weightbearing. Ligaments maintain the relationship of opposing articular surfaces and guide joints through normal range of motion, preventing excessive movement or movement into an unstable position. Muscles and tendons are particularly important in conferring dynamic stability while facilitating polyplanar motion, as in the shoulder where the rotator cuff muscles and tendons are essential. Synovial fluid facilitates the sliding motion of articular surfaces and resists distraction of the joint. This stability is lost when the normal film of synovial fluid is replaced by a "pathologic" joint effusion.

Any disorder that causes a joint effusion ultimately interferes with the normal synthetic activity or physical characteristics of synovial fluid, synovial lining cells, articular cartilage, ligaments, tendons, and/or subchondral bone. Reflex changes affect the function of the neuromuscular apparatus so that joint protection is limited. In the process, pain, joint instability, and functional impairment develop.

Osteoarthritis

Osteoarthritis is the most common nontraumatic arthropathy. Its prevalence increases with age, and it is present in almost everyone by the age of 65. Physical demands, anatomic abnormalities of joints, and genetic factors predispose to OA. It is characterized pathologically by progressive injury to and loss of articular cartilage, accompanied by reactive changes at joint margins and in subchondral bone; clinically, by slowly progressive pain, stiffness, loss of joint motion, and bony joint enlargement. An inflammatory process involving the synovium may occur, associated with flares of joint symptoms (inflammatory variant of OA).

PATHOGENESIS AND PATHOPHYSIOLOGY

Osteoarthritis is initiated by biomechanical, biochemical, inflammatory, or immunologic insults that stimulate chondrocytes to release enzymes that break down articular proteoglycans and collagen. Biomechanical factors potentiate disruption of collagen and cause microfractures into subchondral bone. Loss of the stress-absorbing properties of cartilage and subchondral bone leads to progressive joint injury, prompting reparative responses, which include bony proliferation (osteophyte formation), chondrocyte proliferation, and chondrocyte synthesis of smaller proteoglycan subunits that are less effective in supporting the normal function of cartilage. Locally produced prostaglandins augment the inflammatory response while immune complexes and T lymphocyte responses, directed against proteoglycan components, accelerate cartilage damage.

Pathologically, OA is characterized by thinning, fissures, and focal erosions of articular cartilage. As the disease progresses, the erosions become deeper and more confluent, leading to complete loss of cartilage in stress-bearing areas. Osteoarthritic spurs form at joint margins. Microfractures in subchondral bone lead to sclerosis and cyst formation. In advanced stages of the disease, inflammatory reactions may cause flares of pain and joint effusions.

CLINICAL CHARACTERISTICS

Early in the course of OA, pain is aggravated by weight bearing and relieved with rest; there may be transient morning stiffness. As the disease progresses, pain may occur even at rest. Nocturnal pain and prolonged morning stiffness may develop due to progressive irritation of nerves within subchondral bone, periosteum, joint capsules, ligaments, tendons, and muscles. Cracking, popping, or grinding with joint motion, called crepitus, often occurs due to joint destruction and intraarticular fragments of bone or cartilage. Joint motion becomes progressively restricted. An inflammatory synovitis may develop because of microcrystals of calcium pyrophosphate dihydrate, apatite, and/or monosodium urate. Cartilage fragments or minor trauma exacerbate this process.

Several clinical subsets of OA have been defined: (a) primary OA of weight-bearing joints (knee, hip, first metatarsophalangeal); (b) nodal OA of the distal and proximal interphalangeal (DIP and PIP) finger joints and thumb carpometacarpal joints; (c) erosive inflammatory OA; (d) ankylosing hyperostosis (also called Forestier's disease or diffuse idiopathic skeletal hyperostosis; and (e) secondary OA.

The various clinical presentations of OA of the weight-bearing joints will be found in the pertinent chapters of this text. They present with pain, swelling, stiffness, and crepitation. On examination tenderness, contracture, deformity, and swelling are demonstrable.

Primary OA of the hands, often referred to as nodal OA, is an autosomal dominant trait that tends to affect women. Distal interphalangeal and PIP joint involvement results in bony proliferation, termed Heberden's and Bouchard's nodes, respectively. The carpometacarpal joint of the thumb and the metatarsophalangeal joint of the great toe are commonly affected. In most patients, the disease begins insidiously and progresses slowly. Pain and erythema, if present, may be severe early in the course of the disease. Later, low-grade aching and stiffness, limited flexion, deviation of the fingers, and the nodular appearance of the joints predominate. Mucinous cysts resembling ganglions may develop over the Heberden's or Bouchard's nodes.

Inflammatory OA represents another OA subset and, like nodal OA of the hands, involves the interphalangeal joints of the fingers and can involve other joints as well, including the carpometacarpal joints of the thumbs, the first toe metatarsophalangeal, the hips, and the knees. It is characterized by acute bouts of inflammation leading to erosive joint disease. Radiographically, the margins and central aspect of the joint are destroyed, resulting in deformities and occasionally ankylosis of bone. This arthropathy may be confused with monoarticular or oligoarticular forms of arthritis, such as psoriatic arthritis, another form of erosive disease which affects the DIP joints.

The subset of OA termed ankylosing hyperostosis, also called diffuse idiopathic skeletal hyperostosis or Forestier's disease, may affect the spine. Manifestations include stiffness, loss of motion, and ossification of the anterolateral aspect of the vertebral bodies with preservation of intervertebral disk spaces (in contrast to primary OA in which disk height is reduced). Patients with diffuse idiopathic skeletal hyperostosis may also produce proliferative spurs at sites of tendon and ligament attachments and heterotopic bone following joint surgery.

Primary OA most often affects the knees, hips, and cervical and lumbar spine. It tends to spare the metacarpophalangeal (MCP), wrist, elbow, and shoulder joints. Osteoarthritic involvement at these sites should raise concern of some other joint insult. Secondary causes of OA include mechanical joint injury, following a treated inflammatory arthropathy, deformity from congenital or developmental disease (congenitally dislocated or dysplastic hip, slipped capital femoral epiphysis, Legg-Calvé-Perthes, etc.), metabolic abnormalities of cartilage (hemochromatosis and acromegaly), neurologic diseases causing neuropathic arthropathy (diabetes, tabes dorsalis), or repetitive bleeding within the joint (hemophilia).

Laboratory and Radiographic Features

Laboratory studies in OA are generally normal, including erythrocyte sedimentation rate (ESR), complete blood count, and other acute phase reactants. Synovial fluid, when present, is noninflammatory (Table 12.1). Synovial fluid may contain calcium pyrophosphate, monosodium urate, or hydroxyapatite crystals (see section on "Crystal-Induced Rheumatic Diseases"), and/or

cartilage fragments and have mildly inflammatory features.

X-rays reveal joint space narrowing (indicative of cartilage loss), which in the knees and hips is best demonstrated by weight-bearing views. Also seen are joint effusions, increased density of subchondral bone (termed sclerosis or eburnation), subchondral cysts, and osteophytes. Radionuclide bone scans reveal discrete areas of increased uptake and are more sensitive in detecting early disease than are x-rays.

TREATMENT

The patient should be instructed to minimize stress to the affected joints. This includes weight loss, avoidance of activities producing a high load across the joint, judicious rest, splinting, and the use of assistive devices such as a cane for patients with hip or knee disease. Other modalities include heat, ice, exercise, analgesic and anti-inflammatory agents (Table 12.2), along with selective use of injectable steroid preparations. When pain becomes severe, symptoms are unresponsive to conservative measures, and joint dysfunction leads to inability to perform activities of daily living, surgery should be considered.

Rheumatoid Arthritis

Rheumatoid arthritis is a chronic, inflammatory immunologic process that affects

---

Table 12.1.
Classification of Synovial Effusions

Characteristic	Normal	Noninflammatory (type I)	Inflammatory (type II)	Septic (type III)
Color	Clear, straw-colored	Straw to yellow	Yellow	Variable
Clarity	Transparent	Transparent	Translucent	Opaque
Viscosity	High	High	Low	Variable
WBC (mm³)	<200	200–2000	2000–75000	>100,000
Polys (%)	<25	<25	>50	>75+
Culture	Negative	Negative	Negative	Often positive
Mucin clot	Firm	Firm	Friable	Friable
Glucose	Near blood	Near blood	<25 mg/dL Lower than blood	>25 mg/dL Lower than blood

Table 12.2.
Nonsteroidal Anti-Inflammatory Drugs[a,b]

Class and Generic Name	Brand Name(s)	Tablet Size (mg)	Daily Dose
Salicylates			
Acetylsalicyclic acid (aspirin examples)	Anacin, Ascriptin, Bayer, Bufferin, Ecotrin, Empirin	325–500 mg	1000–6000 mg/day
	Easprin	975 mg	
	Zorprin	800 mg	
Diflunisal	Dolobid	250, 500	250–500 mg b.i.d.
Nonacetylated			
Choline salicylate	Arthropan	500 mg/tsp	1–2 tsp q.i.d.
Choline magnesium salicylate	Trilisate	500, 750, 1000	1000 mg t.i.d. 1500 mg b.i.d.
Salsalate	Disalcid	500, 750	1000 mg t.i.d. 1500 mg b.i.d.
Propionic Acids			
Ibuprofen	Advil, Nuprin	200	
	Motrin	400, 600, 800	400–800 mg t.i.d.
Naproxen	Naprosyn	250, 375, 500	250 mg b.i.d. to 500 mg t.i.d.
Fenoprofen	Nalfon	300, 600	300–600 mg q.i.d.
Ketoprofen	Orudis	50, 75	50–75 mg t.i.d.
Flurbiprofen	ANSAID	50, 100	100–150 mg b.i.d.
Indolacetic acids			
Indomethacin	Indocin	25, 50, 75 SR[c]	75–150 mg/day
Sulindac	Clinoril	150, 200	150 mg b.i.d. to 200 mg b.i.d.
Tolmetin sodium	Tolectin	200, 400, 600	1200–2000 mg in divided doses
Fenamic acid			
Mefenamic acid	Meclomen	50, 100	200–400 mg in 3–4 divided doses
Oxicam			
Piroxicam	Feldene	10, 20	10–20 mg/day
Phenylacetic acid			
Diclofenac sodium	Voltaren	25, 50, 75,	50–75 mg b.i.d.
Pyranocarboxylic acid			
Etodolac[d]	Lodine	200, 300	600–1200 mg/day in 2–4 divided doses

[a]Indications for use: see text.
[b]Common adverse side effects include: gastrointestinal intolerance (dyspepsia, nausea, vomiting, diarrhea, bleeding); impairment of renal function; inhibition of platelet function (minimal inhibition by nonacetylated salicylates); and central nervous system effects (headache, tinnitus, depersonalization).
[c]Sustained release.
[d]Approved only for osteoarthritis and general purpose analgesia.

joints and may also involve visceral structures (Table 12.3). The incidence of RA is highest in women (two to three times that of men) ages 30 to 50, with an overall incidence of 0.3% to 1.5%. The HLA-DR4 haplotype confers susceptibility in most ethnic groups; however, only a minority of individuals with this haplotype develop rheumatoid arthritis.

PATHOGENESIS

Although the etiology of rheumatoid arthritis is unknown, two immune mechanisms are important. (*a*) Within the synovial fluid, immune complexes form as a result of interaction of antibodies with self immunoglobulin (Ig) molecules. These Ig-anti-Ig complexes are called rheumatoid factors.

Table 12.3.
Extraarticular Manifestations of Rheumatoid Arthritis

Skin
  Subcutaneous nodules
  Vasculitic lesions (leg ulcers, medium vessel
    vasculitis)
  Ecchymoses and thin skin
Respiratory tract
  Lung (pleural effusions, pleural thickening;
    pneumonitis and interstitial lung disease;
    rheumatoid nodules; necrotizing bronchiolitis)
  Upper airway (dryness secondary to Sjögren's
    syndrome; laryngeal obstruction secondary to
    cricoarytenoid arthritis)
Cardiovascular
  Pericarditis
  Rheumatoid nodules of myocardium/valves
  conduction system
  Interstitial myocarditis
  Coronary arteritis
Nervous system
  Mononeuritis multiplex secondary to arteritis
  Peripheral nerve entrapment (carpal tunnel
    syndrome, ulnar nerve entrapment at the elbow
    (cubital fossa), tarsal tunnel syndrome, popliteal
    cyst compression of posterior tibial nerve)
  Compressive myelopathy, cervical subluxation
  Stroke
Eye
  Dryness due to keratoconjunctivitis sicca (Sjögren's
    syndrome)
  Episcleritis or scleritis

Antibodies are also generated to constituents of damaged articular cartilage. These immune complexes activate the complement cascade, producing an inflammatory reaction with attendant microvascular injury, increased vascular permeability, and formation of subsynovial edema. Polymorphonuclear leukocytes, which are chemotactically attracted, ingest immune complexes and in the process release injurious oxygen radicals, hydrolytic enzymes (collagenases, elastases), and arachidonic acid metabolites (prostaglandins). (*b*) Infiltrates of lymphocytes, macrophages, and dendritic cells liberate interleukin-1, which stimulates antibody production and proliferation of synovial lining cells, chondrocytes, and osteoclasts. Granulation tissue, termed pannus, is formed from synovial tissue and erodes bone and cartilage. Osteoclasts release destructive substances that erode cartilage and bone, and contribute to periarticular injury of ligaments, tendons, and joint capsules. Vascular engorgement, thrombosis, perivascular hemorrhage, proliferation of macrophage-like (synovial type A) and fibrocyte-like (synovial type B) cells can be seen. Collections of mononuclear cells, predominantly lymphocytes and plasma cells, locally produce rheumatoid factor and other antibodies.

CLINICAL CHARACTERISTICS

The severity of RA is variable. It may affect one or many joints for a few months, or may be widespread, symmetrical, and destructive, with associated extraarticular manifestations.

Rheumatoid arthritis characteristically begins insidiously over weeks to months. Prolonged morning stiffness (one or more hours), fatigue, malaise, and gelling (stiffness after immobility) may be prominent symptoms. Joint stiffness improves with activity but may be followed by afternoon fatigue and pain. Periarticular and diffuse muscle aching, low-grade fevers, malaise, weight loss, and depression are not infrequent symptoms. Although RA may remit (10% or less), the majority of patients have progressive disease. Joint involvement is typically symmetrical and involves the PIP and MCP joints of the hands, wrists, elbows, shoulders, cervical spine, hips, knees, ankles, subtalar, tarsal, and metatarsophalangeal joints. Less frequently, the temporomandibular, cricoarytenoid, and sternoclavicular joints are affected.

Synovitis of the hands results in symmetric fusiform swelling, most prominently affecting the second and third MCP and PIP, and wrist joints of the dominant side. With soft tissue injury to ligaments and tendons, the fingers deviate laterally at the MCP joints (so-called ulnar deviation). Soft tissue injury to the MCP and interphalangeal joints may cause a swan neck deformity, which is a flexion contracture of the MCP and DIP joints with hyperextension of the PIP joint. A boutonnière deformity may also develop as a result of a flexion contracture of the PIP and hyperextension of the DIP joints. For the details of finger and wrist involvement by rheumatoid arthritis, see Chapter 4.

Elbow involvement may lead to flexion contractures, occasionally in the absence of pain. Synovial proliferation and effusion may be palpated at the joint line between the lateral epicondyle and the tip of the olecranon process. Synovitis at the elbow in the ulnar (cubital) groove may cause a compressive neuropathy of the ulnar nerve.

Cervical spine disease causes pain, stiffness, and muscle spasm. Erosion of the transverse ligament of C-1 may allow the odontoid process to compress the spinal cord during neck flexion due to anterior subluxation of C-1 on C-2. Another cause of compressive cervical myelopathy is "staircase" subluxation of multiple cervical vertebral units.

Like OA, rheumatoid hip disease tends to be felt as pain in the groin, buttock, medial or anterior thigh, and/or knee. In contrast to OA, pain may be significant even with non-weight bearing. Motion of the hip is globally restricted.

Knee synovitis is readily apparent. Since the true knee joint is almost always continuous with the suprapatellar bursa, swelling is appreciated above, medial, and lateral to the patella. A firm or cystic swelling behind the knee in the medial popliteal space indicates the presence of a popliteal or Baker's cyst.

Foot and ankle involvement cause considerable morbidity due to difficulty standing and walking. Tibiotalar arthritis is manifest by swelling adjacent and anterior to the malleoli, with restricted dorsiflexion and plantar flexion. Tenderness anterior and inferior to the lateral malleolus and pain on inversion and eversion of the ankle are indicative of subtalar joint disease. With progression, the ankle develops a valgus deformity and the foot becomes flattened. Patients walk by rolling off the inner aspect of a flattened foot. Involvement of the metatarsophalangeal joints may also cause subluxation, forcing patients to walk on tender metatarsal heads. If the phalanges sublux superiorly, claw or hammer toe deformities develop.

Laboratory Features

Rheumatoid factor is present in 75 to 80% of patients. Normochromic, normocytic anemia develops as a result of chronic disease. Low-grade gastrointestinal bleeding caused by nonsteroidal anti-inflammatory medications may cause hypochromic anemia. White blood cell counts are generally normal unless the patient has either systemic-onset (Still's) disease, in which a marked leukocytosis may be evident, or Felty's syndrome, manifested by leukopenia (generally granulocytopenia) and splenomegaly. Nonspecific markers of inflammation, including thrombocytosis, and elevation of the ESR, reflect the degree of inflammatory activity. Synovial fluid is classified as type II, inflammatory (Table 12.1).

Radiographic Features

Early radiographic features of RA consist of fusiform soft tissue swelling, joint effusions, and periarticular demineralization. Ligamentous and tendon laxity result in joint subluxations, which on x-ray reflect the clinically apparent deformities previously described. With disease progression, erosions of articular cartilage and bone occur. Uniform joint space narrowing reflects irreversible and global injury to cartilage. Erosions occur earliest at the margins of subchondral bone, at so-called bare areas of bone where bone is not protected by articular cartilage. Erosions also occur at sites of ligamentous and tendinous attachments, and inflamed bursae. Large subchondral cysts are seen. An important abnormality that may lead to profound neurologic complications is the C-1, C-2 subluxation. Lateral flexion and extension radiographs of the cervical spine will demonstrate this finding.

TREATMENT

As a chronic systemic disease, RA is best managed by an interdisciplinary team consisting of the primary care physician, rheumatologist, orthopaedist, physical and occupational therapists, social worker, nurse, and vocational counsellor. Management of each patient must be individualized. Goals of therapy are to relieve pain, stiffness, and muscle spasm; to provide education regarding sexual, marital, and work-related problems; and to maintain or improve joint function, and thereby the quality of life. Adequate rest, including late morning or afternoon naps, may help counteract fatigue. Occupational therapists fashion splints, provide aids to assist with activities of daily living, and instruct patients in exercise to maintain and improve fine motor control.

The nonsteroidal anti-inflammatory medications are effective first-line agents in the treatment of RA (Table 12.2). When synovitis is not well-controlled by these medications or bony erosions appear, slow-acting disease-modifying drugs should be added. These include antimalarial drugs, gold salts, penicillamine, azathioprine, methotrexate, and sulfasalazine. All of these second-line agents have the potential for causing serious adverse reactions, and regular clinical and laboratory monitoring is necessary.

Periarticular (bursal and tendon sheath) and intraarticular corticosteroid injections may be helpful in suppressing inflammation in one or two particularly painful joints while waiting for a second-line agent to work.

Due to the toxicity of systemic corticosteroids, use of these agents should be restricted. When used, they should be prescribed only in low doses (equivalent to 2.5 to 10 mg of prednisone per day) while waiting for disease-modifying agents to become effective. Higher steroid doses may be required for extraarticular manifestations, such as pericarditis, pleuritis, rheumatoid vasculitis, and rheumatoid pneumonitis.

Once the diagnosis of RA has been made, consultation is appropriate if questions arise about the diagnosis, if synovitis is not controlled by conservative measures, if joint damage is evident radiographically or by clinical examination, or if serious extraarticular problems become evident.

Systemic Lupus Erythematosus

Systemic lupus erythematosus is a multisystem, chronic inflammatory disease. While the etiology is unknown, it appears to develop as a result of the interaction of genetic, environmental, and hormonal factors. Like RA, SLE most frequently affects women during their childbearing years. Underlying abnormalities of immune regulation result in the production of autoantibodies, proliferation and alteration of lymphocyte subsets, and activation of the complement system. Autoantibodies to cell membranes cause immune thrombocytopenia, hemolytic anemia, leukopenia, lymphopenia, and some forms of lupus cerebritis; immune complex formation leads to vasculitis, pleuritis, rashes, and glomerulonephritis.

CLINICAL CHARACTERISTICS

Musculoskeletal manifestations of SLE include arthralgias and arthritis (synovitis). Involvement of wrists, finger joints, elbows, and knees in a symmetrical distribution (similar to RA) with morning stiffness, joint pain, and swelling are common. Inflammatory disease of soft tissues, specifically joint capsules, tendons, and ligaments, may cause joint malalignment and subluxation. Although erosive arthritis is rare, reversible ulnar deviation of the fingers, deviation of the toes, and tendon rupture may occur.

Other musculoskeletal manifestations include myalgias and, less commonly, inflammatory muscle disease (myositis) and osteonecrosis. Myalgias are characterized by aching and occasionally muscle tenderness with maintenance of strength. In contrast, myositis causes weakness, particularly of the shoulder and hip musculature, and is associated with elevated muscle enzymes (creatine kinase, aldolase, aspartate aminotransferase) and electromyographic abnormalities.

Osteonecrosis, also termed avascular necrosis or ischemic necrosis of bone, may develop spontaneously in patients with SLE. Predisposing factors are vasculitis, Raynaud's phenomenon (digital vasospasm), and systemic corticosteroid therapy. The femoral head is most often affected, but numerous other bones, including the humeral head, talus, and bones of the knees and wrist, may be affected. Symptoms of osteonecrosis include pain, often sudden in onset, aggravated by weight bearing and use. The diagnosis is made on the basis of symptoms and findings on plain radiographs, bone scans, and/or magnetic resonance imaging studies.

The diagnosis of SLE requires a constellation of clinical and laboratory abnormalities, which might include malar rash, arthralgias/arthritis, polyserositis, oral ulcerations, photosensitivity, glomerulonephritis, seizures or psychoses, vasculitis, leukopenia, thrombocytopenia, hemolytic anemia, positive antinuclear antibodies, antibodies to double-stranded DNA, to the Sm antigen, and to cardiolipin.

Radiographic Features

Skeletal radiographic abnormalities in SLE are those that develop as a result of ligamentous instability, osteonecrosis, or osteoporosis.

TREATMENT

Lupus tends to have a fluctuating clinical course requiring ongoing monitoring and adjustments in therapy. Polyarthralgias, myalgias, and arthritis are treated with nonsteroidal anti-inflammatory medications (Table 12.2), splints, and physical therapy. Resistant joint or skin disease is treated with antimalarials, generally in the form of hydroxychloroquine (Plaquenil). Severe systemic manifestations, such as pleuritis, pericarditis, lupus pneumonitis, hemolytic anemia, immune thrombocytopenia, cerebritis, transverse myelitis, glomerulonephritis, vasculitis, and severe rash, are generally treated with high-dose glucocorticosteroids (1 mg/kg methylprednisolone a day or its equivalent). Consultation with a rheumatologist for management of such serious disease manifestations is recommended. To avoid the toxicities associated with long-term, high-dose steroid therapy, a number of alternative therapeutic regimens employing cytotoxic agents (cyclophosphamide), antimetabolites (azathioprine), and pheresis (plasmapheresis, lymphopheresis) have been developed.

Spondyloarthropathies

The spondyloarthropathies are a group of rheumatic diseases that includes ankylosing spondylitis (AS), psoriatic arthritis (PA), Reiter's syndrome (RS), and the arthritis associated with inflammatory bowel disease. Inflammation at sites of ligament or tendon insertion is common. All have a predilection for the sacroiliac joints (sacroiliitis), longitudinal ligaments of the spine (spondylitis), facet joints, peripheral diarthrodial joints, ligaments, tendons, and fascia. Additionally, all share a strong association with the class I histocompatibility antigen, HLA-B27.

ANKYLOSING SPONDYLITIS

Ankylosing spondylitis is regarded as the prototype of the spondyloarthropathies. It occurs most frequently in men 20 to 30 years old (threefold male predominance), with an overall prevalence of 0.1 to 0.2%. Ankylosing spondylitis affects the sacroiliac joints symmetrically and the spine in a progressive ascending fashion.

Clinical Characteristics

The earliest manifestations of AS are back discomfort and stiffness that are most severe in the morning and improve over the course of 1 or 2 hours. Stiffness may return after periods of immobility associated with late afternoon or early evening fatigue. Sacroiliac joint discomfort is felt in the region of the posterior iliac crest, but may be interpreted as occurring in the hip or down the back of the legs. Occasionally, a peripheral tendinitis, such as Achilles or supraspinatus tendinitis, or plantar fasciitis occurs. In women, bouts of tendinitis and/or plantar fasciitis may predominate, or they may present with a peripheral arthritis (wrist and hand or ankle arthritis, cervical spine disease, or both, with a paucity of sacroiliac or lumbar involvement.

The physical examination of patients with AS characteristically reveals tenderness of the sacroiliac joints on direct palpation and pain with stress of the sacroiliac joints. Lumbar motion is restricted, and the reduction may be documented by the Schober index. A mark is made on the skin between the posterior iliac crests and a second mark 10 cm cephalad. The patient is asked to touch his or her toes (maximally flex the back with knees extended) and the distance between the two skin marks is remeasured. Normally, the distance in flexion (the numerator) is more than 5 cm greater than the initial 10 cm (the denominator). Therefore, a normal Schober index is greater than 15/10. Chest expansion at the nipple line during full inspiration compared with full expiration may also indicate spondylitis: expansion of less that 3 cm may indicate arthritis of the costovertebral and/ or costochondral joints. Other physical findings include limited motion of the shoulders and hips, synovitis of the knees, plantar fasciitis, and supraspinatus and Achilles tendinitis.

Extraarticular manifestations of AS consist of anterior uveitis (photophobia, difficulty with accommodation, eye redness and soreness, and headache), cardiac abnormalities (aortic insufficiency due to valvular disease, aortic dissection, and heart block as a result of atrioventricular nodal disease), and fracture of the fused osteopenic spine (most commonly involving the cervical area, which may result in quadriplegia or death). Inflammation of the arachnoid of the lower spine may cause intermittent sciatica and, rarely, a cauda equina syndrome. In less than 1% of patients, interstitial lung disease develops in the upper lobes.

Laboratory Features. Normochromic, normocytic anemia and elevation of the ESR are common in AS. The HLA-B27 antigen can be detected in approximately 80 to 90% of Caucasians with this disease, compared to an incidence of 4 to 8% in the general population.

Radiographic Features. Radiographic features of AS include bilaterally symmetrical sacroiliitis. As the disease progresses, fibrous union followed by eventual ankylosis may occur. Early changes of spondylitis include a "squared" appearance of the lumbar vertebral bodies as a result of erosion of the anterosuperior and inferior margins of the vertebral bodies and deposition of bone in the concave aspect of the vertebral body. Ossification of paraspinal ligaments creates a "bamboo" appearance, often accompanied by ankylosis of the facet joints. Generalized osteopenia of the spine is common.

REITER'S SYNDROME

The triad of conjunctivitis and/or uveitis, arthritis, and urethritis represent the classical features of Reiter's syndrome. Sacroiliitis, spondylitis, tendinitis, bursitis, and mucocutaneous disease also occur commonly. Like AS, this disease is most common in young men with the HLA-B27 haplotype. Reiter's syndrome has also been referred to as a form of "reactive arthritis" because it often occurs after venereal infection or after an epidemic of dysentery caused by *Yersinia, Shigella, Salmonella,* or *Campylobacter* species. Infectious agents are regarded as possible triggers of the disease in a genetically predisposed individual.

Clinical Characteristics

Urethritis, manifested by dysuria or a urethral discharge or both may develop several weeks after venereal exposure or a diarrheal illness. Other genitourinary manifestations include acute and chronic prostatitis, cervicitis, and vaginitis. Development of conjunctivitis or anterior uveitis or both may follow.

The arthritis of RS typically affects less than four peripheral joints in the lower extremities, most commonly the knees and foot joints. Involvement of the periosteum of the phalanges and tendon mechanisms may result in a diffusely erythematous and swollen digit, referred to as a "sausage" digit. Tendinitis, particularly of the Achilles tendon, and plantar fasciitis often occur as isolated musculoskeletal manifestations of RS.

Axial joint disease includes sacroiliitis (unilateral or bilateral) and spondylitis. The latter may involve the cervical spine with sparing of the lower spine.

Mucocutaneous manifestations of RS include a hyperkeratotic rash termed keratoderma blennorrhagica, painless oral mucosal ulcers, circinate balanitis, and nail ridging and pitting. Keratoderma blennorrhagica may be clinically and pathologically indistinguishable from psoriasis. Other extraarticular manifestations of RS include intermittent fever, weight loss, heart block, aortitis, and amyloidosis.

Laboratory Features. Laboratory abnormalities in RS are similar to those in AS. Joint effusions, when present, tend to have inflammatory characteristics (Table 12.1).

PSORIATIC ARTHRITIS

Approximately 5% of patients with psoriasis develop arthritis that affects the back or peripheral joints. Typically, joints of the upper extremities are involved. Psoriatic arthritis resembles RS clinically and radiographically. Approximately 20% of individuals with PA have sacroiliitis and spondylitis, and half of these have the HLA-B27 haplotype.

Clinical Characteristics

Psoriatic arthritis affects men and women with equal frequency in their young adult years. Usually, the rash precedes the arthritis, but not infrequently the joint disease precedes or accompanies the onset of psoriasis. In a small number of individuals, the arthritis may be present with only subtle evidence of skin disease, such as nail pitting or excessive dandruff.

Psoriatic arthritis affects the joints in five distinct patterns. The most common is a peripheral, asymmetric arthritis involving four or fewer joints of the hands. A second subset consists of DIP arthritis involving the fingers or toes, often associated with severe psoriatic nail disease of the same digit. The third form is a symmetric polyarthritis resembling RA but without subcutaneous nodules and rheumatoid factor in the blood. A fourth form, a severe, destructive arthritis termed arthritis mutilans, results in joint erosions and resorption of bone to the degree that the affected fingers and toes become shortened and markedly unstable. A fifth form is sacroiliitis with or without spondylitis, similar to that of RS.

A characteristic pattern of peripheral psoriatic arthritis is the so-called "ray" distribution, in which all of the joints of a given digit are inflamed, resulting in the appearance of a sausage digit. These findings are similar to the toes of patients with RS.

Laboratory Features. The ESR is frequently elevated. Rheumatoid factor is characteristically absent. Approximately 50% of individuals with psoriatic spondylitis possess the HLA-B27 haplotype.

Radiographic Features. The sacroiliitis of psoriatic arthritis may be unilateral or asymmetric, as in RS. Spondylitic involvement may proceed in a progressive, ascending manner as in AS, but may also skip areas of the spine. Syndesmophytes in psoriatic and Reiter's spondylitis may be nonmarginal (originate and join adjacent vertebral bodies some distance from the inferior and superior end plates), in contrast to the marginal syndesmophytes seen in AS or spondylitis of inflammatory bowel disease.

ARTHROPATHIES OF INFLAMMATORY BOWEL DISEASES

Approximately 5 to 10% of individuals with ulcerative colitis and regional enteritis (Crohn's disease) develop either sacroiliitis and spondylitis and/or peripheral arthritis affecting the large joints of the lower extremities. These forms of spondyloarthropathy have been termed enteropathic or colitic arthritis. The peripheral arthritis may be associated with skin lesions, including erythema nodosum, pyoderma gangrenosum, oral mucosal ulcers, and/or uveitis. The activity of the peripheral arthritis tends to correlate with that of the bowel disease, while the axial arthritis may progress independently.

The laboratory and radiographic features of the spine resemble those of AS, while the peripheral arthritis is generally not erosive.

TREATMENT OF THE SPONDYLOARTHROPATHIES

The major treatment goals for the spondyloarthropathies are to suppress inflammation (Table 12.2), relieve discomfort, and facilitate physical therapy to maintain maximal function. Physical therapy is crucial to minimize joint contractures, maintain optimal posture, and improve joint motion. Exercises as well as participation in sports that emphasize back extension and deep breathing are valuable. Patients should sleep on firm mattresses and use thin pillows, and sleep or lie prone to minimize the development of flexion contractures of the back.

Referral to a rheumatologist is indicated for the patient with erosive peripheral arthritis associated with psoriasis or RS. The rheumatologist will consider treatment with slow-acting drugs, analogous to the treatment of erosive rheumatoid arthritis with gold compounds, methotrexate, sulfasalazine, or azathioprine.

Local injections of depot corticosteroid preparations are helpful. Systemic corticosteroids aggravate the accelerated osteoporosis associated with these arthropathies and do not improve inflammatory back disease, and therefore should not be prescribed. Appropriate footwear and orthotic devices are often prescribed for pain caused by infracalcaneal bursitis or plantar fasciitis.

Extraarticular manifestations of the spondyloarthropathies may require specialized care. This would be necessary for uveitis, cardiac conduction defects, inflammatory bowel disease, and cutaneous manifestations. Nongonococcal urethritis should be treated with a 14-day course of tetracycline, as often the infecting agent is *Chlamydia trachomatis.*

Crystal-induced Arthropathies

GOUTY ARTHRITIS

Gout occurs as a result of sustained hyperuricemia secondary to uric acid overproduction (defined as a urinary excretion of more than 600 mg of uric acid per day on a purine-restricted diet, or more than 800 mg/day on a regular diet), or excessive intake, and/or diminished urinary excretion of uric acid. Hyperuricemia most commonly occurs because (*a*) diminished renal clearance of uric acid, (*b*) disease states that increase purine turnover, such as psoriasis, sarcoidosis, myeloproliferative and lymphoproliferative diseases, multiple myeloma, and hemolytic anemia, or (*c*) acquired renal disease or drug ingestion that impairs excretion. Clinically, gouty arthritis manifests as recurrent acute attacks of arthritis and/or a chronic erosive deforming arthritis (tophaceous gout).

Pathogenesis

During the initial phase of a gouty attack, monosodium urate crystals are shed into the synovial fluid. This initiates an inflammatory process leading to formation of a painful swollen joint. Gout characteristically affects "cooler" joints, such as the feet, ankles, knees, hands, and elbows; tophi deposit in the cartilaginous helix of the external ear and the olecranon bursa because of the cooler temperature. Stresses such as twisting an ankle or stubbing the great toe may dislodge urate crystals from otherwise stable sites. Crystal shedding, leading to acute gouty arthritis, can also occur because of rapid changes in urate concentration, such as institution of uric acid-lowering therapy or ingestion of alcohol or salicylates.

Clinical Characteristics

Acute gouty arthritis is characterized by the abrupt onset of exquisite pain, tenderness, swelling, and erythema most commonly affecting a single joint, generally after 10 or more years of asymptomatic hyperuricemia. It most frequently affects men in their fourth through sixth decades of life and, less commonly, postmenopausal women. Approximately 50% of patients experience their first attack in the metatarsophalangeal joint of the great toe (podagra). Other peripheral joints are involved in a monoarticular or migratory fashion. Approximately 10 to 15% of patients present with polyarticular gout. Even if untreated, acute attacks are usually self-limited, lasting 3 to 7 days, after which the patient becomes asymptomatic, referred to as the intercritical period. With the passage of time, attacks become more frequent and prolonged, eventually resulting in chronic persistent gout with tophi palpable on examination or erosions visible on radiographs.

Radiographic and Synovial Fluid Features. Radiographically, acute gout is manifest as soft tissue swelling and joint effusions. In chronic or tophaceous gout, cortical erosions that have sharply defined sclerotic margins as a result of tophaceous deposits in the periosteum of cortical bone

may be seen, as well as oval-shaped cysts with sclerotic margins in periarticular medullary bone. Joint space preservation, absence of profound periarticular demineralization, and the eccentric location of soft tissue swelling are characteristic of gout.

The diagnosis of gouty arthritis is established by demonstration of needle-shaped monosodium urate crystals within polymorphonuclear leukocytes in synovial fluid aspirated from affected joints. The monosodium urate crystals are readily visualized by polarizing microscopy.

Treatment of Hyperuricemia and Gouty Arthritis

The goals of treatment of gouty arthritis are (a) to terminate the acute attack, (b) to prevent recurrent attacks, and (c) to prevent or resorb tophi. Agents employed are either antiinflammatory, prophylactic, or urate- (and uric acid-) lowering drugs.

The earlier an acute attack of gouty arthritis is treated, the more rapidly the inflamed joints respond. Nonsteroidal anti-inflammatory medications are generally given in high doses for the first 2 to 3 days (Table 12.2), then tapered to lower doses. If treatment is begun within several hours of onset, 0.6 mg of oral colchicine given every hour for a maximum of eight tablets or until gastrointestinal side effects develop, followed by maintenance therapy of 0.6 mg twice daily may be effective. Colchicine may also be given intravenously. Initial infusion is 2.0 to 3.0 mg, followed by 0.5 to 1.0 mg 8 to 12 hours later, not to exceed a total dose of 4.0 mg in 48 hours. Colchicine is extremely irritating to soft tissues and should be diluted in 20 ml of normal saline and infused over 10 to 20 minutes in a well-running intravenous line, with care taken to prevent extravasation. Colchicine is particularly useful in patients requiring oral anticoagulation, or who have gastrointestinal bleeding or heart failure, but it should not be used in patients with significant liver or renal disease.

Corticosteroids may be required to treat acute gouty arthritis if contraindications exist to the use of other agents. Systemic or intraarticular administration may be given once joint sepsis has been excluded.

After an acute attack of gout has subsided, chronic maintenance therapy with colchicine (0.6 mg twice daily) or low doses of nonsteroidal anti-inflammatory medications can be used to prevent subsequent attacks.

Indications for chronic uric acid-lowering therapy are (*a*) repeated attacks of disabling arthritis, (*b*) presence of tophaceous deposits, (*c*) clinical or radiographic signs of chronic gouty joint disease, (*d*) progressive renal impairment, (*e*) recurrent urolithiasis, and (*f*) gross overproduction of uric acid (urinary uric acid excretion more than 1000 mg/day). Uric acid-lowering therapy is also used in patients with lymphoproliferative and myeloproliferative disease prior to cytotoxic therapy to prevent hyperuricemic nephropathy.

Two types of uric acid-lowering agents are available, uricosuric drugs, which increase urate clearance, and xanthine oxidase inhibitors (allopurinol), which block uric acid production. Uricosuric agents are given to patients with near-normal renal function who excrete less than 700 mg of uric acid per day. Probenecid is given initially in a dose of 250 to 500 mg twice daily and increased to 1.5 g twice daily; alternatively, sulfinpyrazone 100 mg to 400 mg twice daily may be used. An agent to prevent acute gouty arthritis (prophylactic colchicine or a nonsteroidal anti-inflammatory medication) should be administered and continued for at least 6 months after the serum urate level is below 6 mg/dL, or 6 months after resolution of tophi. Side effects of probenecid include headache, nausea, anorexia, skin rash, and (rarely) nephrotic syndrome, hepatic necrosis, and aplastic anemia. Sulfinpyrazone may cause gastrointestinal irritation and bone marrow suppression.

Allopurinol is used with excessive uric acid excretion (over 1 g in 24 hours), with urolithiasis or tophaceous gout, and in patients with renal insufficiency who require uric acid-lowering therapy. Allopurinol should only be instituted after resolution of an acute attack of gout and with the concurrent prophylactic administration of either nonsteroidal antiinflammatory medications or colchicine 0.6 mg once or twice daily. The initial dose is 100 mg/day; this is increased by 100 mg every 2 to 4 weeks to the dose required to depress the serum urate level below 6 to 7 mg/dL, up to a maximum of 300 mg/day. In renal insufficiency, the dose must be reduced considerably (100 mg/day or less). Allopurinol reduces the metabolism of warfarin, 6-mercaptopurine, and azathioprine, and therefore the dose of these medications must be appropriately reduced. Potential toxicities of allopurinol include a severe allergic reaction, nausea, diarrhea, drug fever, leukopenia, hepatotoxicity, interstitial nephritis, vasculitis, and a rash that may evolve into exfoliative dermatitis or toxic epidermal necrolysis. Serious side effects most commonly occur when allopurinol is prescribed in renal insufficiency, particularly in the setting of concomitant thiazide administration.

If gouty arthritis develops in a patient taking allopurinol or a uricosuric agent, the dose of the uric acid-lowering agent should not be changed until after resolution of the attack.

CALCIUM PYROPHOSPHATE DEPOSITION DISEASE

Calcium pyrophosphate dihydrate (CPPD) crystal deposition disease (pyrophosphate arthropathy) is a crystal-induced disease associated with the deposition of CPPD crystals in and around joints. The deposits may be found in the fibrocartilage, articular hyaline cartilage, and intervertebral disks as well as in tendons, ligaments, synovial membranes, and joint capsules.

Calcium pyrophosphate deposition disease is seen in disorders associated with elevated calcium levels, such as hyperparathyroidism, metabolic disorders characterized by diminished activity of pyrophosphatases (familial hypophosphatasia and hypomagnesemia), familial hypocalciuric hypercalcemia, hemochromatosis, and hypothyroidism. The degeneration of tissue seen with normal aging and osteoarthritic degeneration of cartilage also facilitate CPPD deposition.

Clinical Characteristics

Calcium pyrophosphate deposition disease commonly affects the knees and wrists and, less often, the MCP, ankle, shoulder, and elbow joints. Calcium pyrophosphate deposition is best known for causing "pseudogout." Pseudogout, which mimics gout, most commonly affects elderly women. The joint most often affected is the knee, in contrast to gout which most commonly affects the first metatarsophalangeal joint.

Calcium pyrophosphate deposition may also be associated with a more subacute, polyarticular presentation similar to RA ("pseudorheumatoid" form), a "pseudoosteoarthritis" form, and a destructive ("pseudoneuropathic") form. Calcium pyrophosphate dihydrate crystals may be asymptomatic and identified radiographically as articular chondrocalcinosis.

Workup of the patient with CPPD should include evaluation for underlying medical disorders; screening laboratory studies should include calcium, phosphorus, albumin, magnesium, thyroid function studies, alkaline phosphatase, iron and total iron binding capacity, and ferritin levels.

Diagnosis

The diagnosis of CPPD deposition disease is suggested by acute arthritis with radiographic articular chondrocalcinosis, and is confirmed by joint aspiration and visualization by compensated polarized microscopy of the rhomboid or square-shaped, positively birefringent CPPD crystals within synovial fluid leukocytes (blue crystals when parallel to the axis of light with the red compensator). Synovial fluid should also be cultured and evaluated by Gram stain to exclude bacterial infection.

Treatment

Like OA, CPPD deposition disease is managed with nonsteroidal anti-inflammatory medications (Table 12.2), non-narcotic analgesics, joint splinting as appropriate, and range of motion and strengthening exercises. Joint lavage and arthroscopic irrigation may be beneficial. In severe destructive cases of CPPD arthropathy, particularly involving the hips and knees, joint replacement is indicated. Management of CPPD should include treatment of underlying medical disorders.

HYDROXYAPATITE ARTHROPATHY

Calcium hydroxyapatite deposition, now a well-recognized entity, causes an acute or chronic arthropathy, as well as periarthritis (formerly termed degenerative calcific tendinitis and bursitis). These disorders range in severity from asymptomatic to severe and cause pain, tenderness, localized edema, and restricted motion. Conditions that may predispose to calcific periarthritis include excessive repetitive motion, diabetes mellitus, thyroid disorders, and chronic renal failure (particularly in patients on chronic hemodialysis). The most familiar form of hydroxyapatite-induced disease is supraspinatus tendinitis and/or calcific subacromial bursitis.

Synovial fluid is characterized by a paucity of white cells; crystals cannot be easily detected by polarized microscopic examination, but can be detected by alizarin red or von Kossa's stains.

Treatment includes analgesics, nonsteroidal anti-inflammatory medications (Table 12.2), aspiration, local injection of corticosteroids, and physical therapy (application of heat or cold, diathermy, and ultrasound). In recurrent and refractory cases, surgical removal of calcium deposits may be necessary.

Hydroxyapatite crystals may cause acute flares of arthritis in patients with OA in knee and finger joints. Hydroxyapatite crystals also cause a destructive form of arthritis of the shoulders (called Milwaukee shoulder or rotator cuff arthropathy), knees, and hips.

Lyme Disease

Lyme disease is a tick-borne disorder caused by the spirochete *Borrelia burgdorferi.* It closely simulates other rheumatic disorders in causing arthritis, systemic manifestations, and a tendency for remissions and exacerbations.

The vector carrying *B. burgdorferi* is a tick, typically *Ixodes dammini,* although other strains may carry the spirochete. After inoculation, a rash may develop 3 to 32 days later. The Lyme spirochete invades regional lymph nodes, and in some patients, spreads hematogenously to the eye, heart, joints, central or peripheral nervous system, resulting in clinical symptoms. The spirochete may also remain dormant, particularly in the central nervous system, and later cause organic brain or multiple sclerosis-like syndromes.

CLINICAL CHARACTERISTICS

Common complaints include the development of rash (erythema chronicum migrans), neurologic symptoms (Bell's palsy, meningoencephalitis), carditis, and arthritis. Rash is the earliest manifestation of Lyme disease, while other organ system involvement occurs 3 or more weeks after inoculation.

Arthritis affects approximately 60% of patients. In the early phase, joint involvement is generally asymmetric, affecting large joints (e.g., knees) in a migratory fashion. Months later, a destructive, erosive form of arthritis may develop that must be distin-guished from the spondyloarthropathies, RA, and crystalline arthritis.

Laboratory Features

The diagnosis of Lyme disease is confirmed by serologic tests (finding of specific IgM and IgG antibodies against the Lyme spirochete) or by the direct identification of a spirochete in tissue samples. IgM antibody titers peak between 3 to 6 weeks after inoculation of the organism. Specific IgG titers rise more slowly and are detectable for months to years thereafter. Culture is usually unsuccessful. Radiographic findings are nonspecific and depend on the extent of joint destruction.

TREATMENT

Therapeutic decisions are largely based on the extent of organ system involvement. For early disease, doxycycline is the drug of choice. During the latter phases, in the presence of significant joint, cardiac, or neurologic involvement, high-dose parenteral penicillin or ceftriaxone are preferred.

Fibrositis

Fibrositis, referred to also as myofascial pain syndrome, fibromyalgia, or simply a form of nonarticular rheumatism, is a chronic pain amplification syndrome. It is characterized by diffuse musculoskeletal aching of 3 or more months, localized muscle tenderness (trigger points), a sleep disorder characterized by interrupted and nonrestorative sleep, and morning stiffness. Other somatic complaints and stress-related disorders such as tension headaches, irritable bowel syndrome, primary dysmenorrhea, premenstrual syndrome, and depression are commonly associated.

PATHOPHYSIOLOGY

The etiology of fibrositis is unknown. The possibility of a primary sleep disorder playing a pathophysiologic role is suggested by three observations: (*a*) disrupted stage IV delta wave sleep in some individuals with fibrositis, (*b*) development of fibrositic symptoms in healthy subjects deprived of stage IV nonrapid eye movement sleep, and (*c*) improvement of sleep and musculoskeletal symptoms with therapy such as amitriptyline, which raises intracerebral serotonin levels that modulate stage IV nonrapid eye movement sleep.

CLINICAL CHARACTERISTICS

Pain, stiffness, and easy fatigability are the three most common presenting complaints in primary fibrositis. Perceived but unverifiable joint pain and swelling, muscle weakness, paresthesia, or burning are com-

mon symptoms, as is digital vasospasm (Raynaud's phenomenon). A disturbed sleep history may be reflected by not awakening refreshed and by excessive fatigue despite many hours of sleep. This cadre of complaints is often exacerbated by cold damp weather, excessive stress or anxiety, and exercise. Young, healthy, "driven" women are most often affected, comprising nearly 90% of those with the disorder. Men and children may also develop this syndrome.

Physical examination is normal except for the presence of tender points in characteristic locations (Fig. 12.1). Dermatographia and exquisite tenderness to rolling the skin between the thumb and index finger (positive skin rolling tenderness) may be demonstrated over tender points, particularly the

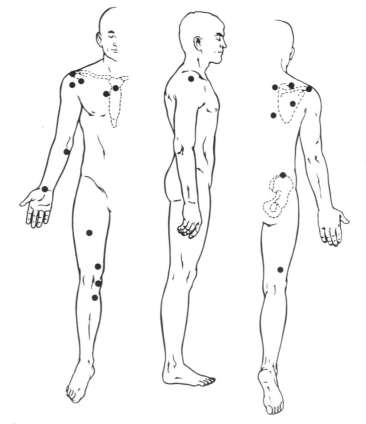

Figure 12.1. Sites of common tender points in primary fibromyalgia. (From Simms RW, Goldenberg DL, Felson DT, Mason JH. Tenderness in 75 anatomic sites. Arthritis Rheum 1988; 31:182–187. Reprinted with permission.)

upper back. Neurologic and musculoskeletal examinations are otherwise normal.

Laboratory and Radiographic Features

The absence of any radiographic or significant laboratory findings typifies patients with fibrositis. Erythrocyte sedimentation rate is normal. Psychometric testing may, however, be abnormal.

TREATMENT

Fibrositis does not cause weakness or joint destruction and is not progressive, despite the many significant problems it causes for the patient. Treatment is symptomatic and begins with patient education. Aerobic training is beneficial despite the initial discomfort that must be endured. Stress-reduction programs, mild analgesics or nonsteroidal anti-inflammatory medications (Table 12.2), massage, applications of moist heat, transcutaneous electrical nerve stimulation, and medication to restore sleep (amitriptyline or cyclobenzaprine) may be of benefit. Prognosis for the motivated and cooperative patient is excellent despite some episodic exacerbations.

SUGGESTED READINGS

Katz WA, ed. Diagnosis and management of rheumatic diseases. 2nd ed. Philadelphia: JB Lippincott, 1988.

Kelley WN, Harris ED Jr, Ruddy S, et al, eds. Textbook of rheumatology. 3rd ed. Philadelphia: WB Saunders Co, 1989.

McCarty DJ, ed. Arthritis and allied conditions. 11th ed. Philadelphia: Lea & Febiger, 1989.

Schumacher, HR Jr, ed. Primer on the rheumatic diseases. 9th ed. Atlanta: The Arthritis Foundation, 1988.

Sheon RP, Moskowitz RW, Goldberg VM. Soft tissue rheumatic pain. 2nd ed. Philadelphia: Lea & Febiger, 1987.

CHAPTER 13

Osteomyelitis and Septic Arthritis

Anna M. Korkis, M.D., and Nelson M. Gantz, M.D., F.A.C.P.

Acute Osteomyelitis

Acute osteomyelitis can be divided into three types: (*a*) hematogenous osteomyelitis, (*b*) osteomyelitis secondary to a contiguous focus of infection, and (*c*) osteomyelitis associated with diabetes and peripheral vascular disease. In addition, two specific forms of acute osteomyelitis will be discussed in detail at the end of this section: "Vertebral Osteomyelitis" and "Osteomyelitis in Sickle Cell Disease."

HEMATOGENOUS OSTEOMYELITIS

This disease has typically been described in children, but is being reported with increasing frequency in adults. While the femur and tibia are most frequently involved in childhood cases, the vertebrae are the more common site for adults. Multiple bone involvement may occur in up to 15% of patients. *Staphylococcus aureus* is the causative agent in approximately 50% of patients with hematogenous osteomyelitis. Recently, however, there has been a rise in the incidence of Gram-negative bacilli as the infective agent. Though staphylococcal osteomyelitis is frequently secondary to hematogenous spread of postoperative or soft tissue infection, osteomyelitis secondary to Gram-negative organisms is often attributable to diseases of the gastrointestinal or genitourinary tract.

Clinical Characteristics

The clinical features of presentation vary in children and adults. The classic presenta-tion in children consists of the sudden onset of high fever, systemic toxicity, and restricted, painful motion of the involved extremity. Pain and tenderness usually involve a bony metaphysis and, as infection progresses, the region may become erythematous, indurated, and swollen. Should the bony infection erode into the overlying soft tissue, an abscess may form. An inflammatory synovitis of an adjacent joint may develop or, in more severe cases, a septic arthritis occurs as the result of extension of the infection through an intraarticular portion of the bone metaphysis. Although infants may have the classic presentation of the older child, they can at times appear less ill. In addition to a motionless extremity, the child may develop lethargy, restlessness, decrease in appetite, and a variable fever. Adults may also present variably. Approximately 50% of patients will have symptoms of pain, swelling, fever, chills, or malaise for 3 weeks or less. Alternatively, they may present with vague symptoms of 1 to 2 months' duration, with the major complaint being that of pain in the involved bone.

OSTEOMYELITIS SECONDARY TO A CONTIGUOUS FOCUS OF INFECTION

This form of osteomyelitis may be secondary to a direct wound, an infection in an adjacent soft tissue focus, or a compound fracture or an open reduction of a closed fracture. Human and animal bites are common causes. While puncture wounds frequently involve the hands and feet, human and animal bites predominantly involve the hands. Postoperative infections may affect any bone, depending upon the site of surgery.

This form of osteomyelitis, unlike hematogenous osteomyelitis, is often associated with more than one organism. The causative organism varies with the bones involved. *S. aureus* is still the most common infective agent, but is often part of a mixed infection. While *S. aureus* is frequently associated with infections of the hip, long bones, and calvaria, Gram-negative organisms are more commonly associated with osteomyelitis of the mandible, pelvis, and small bones of the feet.

Clinical Characteristics

Presenting signs and symptoms with this form of osteomyelitis include fever, pain, swelling, and erythema, frequently accompanied by drainage.

OSTEOMYELITIS ASSOCIATED WITH DIABETES AND VASCULAR INSUFFICIENCY

Patients with severe atherosclerosis or diabetes have a predilection for the development of osteomyelitis. The toes or other small bones of the feet are most typically involved. While *S. aureus* is the most common pathogen, Gram-negative aerobic and Gram-positive and Gram-negative anaerobic bacteria may also be isolated.

Clinical Characteristics

The majority of patients lack systemic manifestations and present either with local symptoms of cellulitis, including pain, swelling, and erythema, or with indolent ulcers.

DIAGNOSIS AND TREATMENT OF ACUTE OSTEOMYELITIS

Diagnosis

The diagnosis and treatment of osteomyelitis hinges on the recovery of the infective organism, making immediate needle aspiration a procedure of paramount importance (see Chapter 11). If purulent fluid cannot be aspirated from the soft tissue or periosteum, the needle must be inserted into the underlying bone. If pus is obtained, the patient must undergo surgical drainage and will thus require orthopaedic referral.

Roentgenographic diagnosis is often difficult in the early stages of acute osteomyelitis. Deep soft tissue swelling and obliteration of the intermuscular planes occur early on and may provide the first clues. Bony changes, however, may not appear for 10 to 14 days after the onset of infection, and consequently are not helpful in early diagnosis. The changes include areas of destruction with cortical irregularity and lucency as well as regions of new bone formation and periosteal reaction.

Radioactive scans incorporating technetium or gallium may be positive as early as 3 days after the onset of symptoms. However, these radionuclide tests are nonspecific, and this makes them less useful since inflammatory processes, tumor, trauma, synovitis, and arthritis can all result in positive scans. The reading must be carefully correlated with the clinical presentation.

Ewing's tumor may mimic osteomyelitis because of the similarity of clinical and roentgenographic findings in these two processes. Thus, whenever the diagnosis is in question, a bone biopsy should be performed.

Laboratory data is frequently not diagnostic. Erythrocyte sedimentation rate and white blood cell count are often elevated, although the latter rarely exceeds 16,000/mm³. Calcium, phosphorus, and alkaline phosphatase are typically normal. In general, laboratory values are nonspecific and are not predictive for outcome of disease.

Treatment

Antibiotic therapy for acute osteomyelitis should be determined by the findings on Gram stain and culture. A 4- to 6-week course of high-dose parenteral antibiotic therapy is required, with no need for subsequent oral antibiotic administration. Serum drug levels must be carefully followed for selected agents such as aminoglycosides and vancomycin, and the patient monitored for toxic side effects. If acute osteomyelitis is strongly suspected but Gram stain is nonrevealing and needle aspirate unobtainable, antibiotics should be instituted to cover the most likely causative organism. If more than one organism is suspected or likely, broad-spectrum therapy is indicated.

Therapy for osteomyelitis often involves both antibiotics and surgery. In acute hematogenous osteomyelitis, surgery is indicated to drain an abscess, or if there is no response after 72 hours of appropriate antibiotic therapy. In osteomyelitis secondary to a contiguous focus of infection, surgery is indicated to drain pus and excise tissue that has an inadequate blood supply (sequestra). Indications for the removal of foreign material, such as internal fixation or prosthetic devices, are difficult to establish and require a combined approach by the orthopaedic surgeon and infectious disease specialist.

Prognosis in acute osteomyelitis is very good. The two major determinants of outcome are (a) duration of symptoms prior to onset of antimicrobial therapy, and (b) duration of the antibiotic course. If treated within 3 to 5 days of symptom onset with adequate dosing for more than 3 weeks, the incidence of recurrent or chronic disease is extremely low. However, once chronic osteomyelitis supervenes, the prognosis is much poorer.

VERTEBRAL OSTEOMYELITIS

Pyogenic infection of the spine most frequently involves the body of the vertebra. Infections may spread to adjacent soft tissue and vertebral bodies, and into the spinal canal. Once in the spinal canal, pus may collect to form an epidural abscess. This condition is seen more commonly in drug addicts, the immunocompromised, and those patients who have a remote site of infection and develop spinal involvement on a hematogenous basis. This latter presentation is particularly common with infections involving the genitourinary tract.

Staphylococci are the predominant causative organisms. While Gram-negative enteric rods (usually from the urinary tract) have been found with increasing frequency, tuberculosis of the spine has become a rarity. Blood cultures or aspirates from the vertebral body, disk space, or adjacent area should identify the organism.

Clinical Characteristics

Vertebral osteomyelitis is most commonly seen in children up to 15 years of age and in adults beyond 50 years of age. Back pain is the most common presenting symptom and varies in location according to the region of spinal involvement. The pain may be severe and acute in onset, or dull and of many months' duration. There may be referred pain to the lower hip or abdomen. Fever may be low-grade or absent. Paralysis may occur in the case of epidural abscess formation, which is more common in fungal and tuberculous infections and in the elderly.

Physical examination reveals tenderness to palpation of the involved vertebra. Muscle spasm and restricted motion of the spine and sometimes of the hip are present. The erythrocyte sedimentation rate is usually elevated, so that this, associated with back pain, with or without fever, should make one consider the diagnosis of vertebral osteomyelitis.

Neurologic impairment is common in advanced disease involving epidural or paravertebral abscesses or vertebral collapse. In addition to parenteral antibiotic therapy, orthopaedic or neurosurgical referral for surgical drainage and possible stabilization is mandatory. For the uncomplicated form, antibiotic therapy, bed rest, and spinal support are usually sufficient.

OSTEOMYELITIS IN SICKLE CELL DISEASE

Diagnosis of osteomyelitis in the presence of a sickle cell crisis can be difficult as the two may present with virtually the same clinical and radiologic signs. Early cultures of blood and stool are paramount to the detection of a septic process. The organism is usually a Gram-negative rod, with *Salmonella* species accounting for the majority of these. The sites of bone involvement are multiple. Clinically, the child may present with bone pain and fever, with development of the fever only after the 5th to 14th day. Thus, the diagnosis may be missed unless cultures are taken early. Antibiotic therapy should consist of agents effective against *Salmonella*, such as ampicillin, trimethoprim-sulfamethoxazole, or chloramphenicol, depending on the results of culture and sensitivity testing of the aspirate or surgical specimen.

Chronic Osteomyelitis

Chronic osteomyelitis is the recurrence of infection after treatment of the initial osteomyelitis. While drainage from a sinus tract is often the sign indicating an exacerbation, recurrent infection may present as pain without drainage. With chronic osteomyelitis, toxicity and high fever are uncommon and local tenderness, swelling, and erythema occur less frequently than in the acute form. There is often a history of preexisting fracture, injury, or surgery. In the absence of such a history, the diagnosis is more difficult and inflammatory soft tissue problems, stress fracture, and bone tumor must be included in the differential diagnosis. When the process is long-standing, active chronic septic osteomyelitis may be associated with loss of appetite and weight.

Diagnosis of chronic osteomyelitis is aided by the use of roentgenographic studies. Findings may include bony deformity consequent to previous infection or fracture, subperiosteal new bone formation, or a "sequestrum," an area of sclerotic avascular bone surrounded by radiolucency.

As with acute osteomyelitis, therapy depends on the identification of an infecting organism. While there is frequently a draining sinus tract, culture of this is inadequate because it often does not contain the infecting pathogen. While isolation of *S. aureus* from sinus tracts often correlates with its isolation in bone at surgery, isolation of bacteria other than *S. aureus* correlates poorly with the bone pathogen. Thus, it is important to obtain operative specimens for culture and pathology in chronic osteomyelitis.

When the diagnosis of chronic osteomyelitis is suspected or made, orthopaedic as well as infectious disease referrals are indicated as therapeutic recommendations may be complex, depending on the site, the infecting organism, and the extent and chronicity of infection. These factors determine whether aggressive therapy with surgical debridement and antibiotics is indicated. Surgical debridement is generally required to remove necrotic bone.

Potential complications of chronic osteomyelitis include, though rarely, epidermoid carcinoma and secondary amyloidosis.

Septic Arthritis

Septic arthritis may be mimicked by many other processes, and thus becomes a diagnostic challenge. It is a medical emergency, and failure to make an early diagnosis may lead to joint destruction and severe systemic toxicity.

The infection may develop via one of three routes: direct introduction, extension from a contiguous focus, or hematogenous spread. Hematogenous seeding of the synovium occurs most often. Multiple factors may predispose a host to septic arthritis. These include diabetes mellitus, neoplasia, immunosuppressive therapy, extraarticular foci of infection, and damaged joints from either rheumatoid arthritis or osteoarthritis.

The causative agents of septic arthritis are multiple and include bacteria, mycobacteria, viruses, and fungi. The frequency with which these causative agents occur varies with the age of the patient. *Haemophilus influenzae* type B is the most common causative agent in children under 2 years of age. In children over the age of 2, *S. aureus* becomes the most common bacterial cause. For adults under the age of 30, *Neisseria gonorrhoeae* is the predominant organism.

Infectious arthritides are commonly classified as either gonococcal or nongonococcal. Of the nongonococcal causes, *S. aureus* occurs with the greatest frequency, accounting for 30 to 50% of cases. Varying species of streptococci (including groups A, B, and G) comprise 25% of cases. In recent years, Gram-negative bacilli have emerged as important causative agents, especially in intravenous drug abusers and immunosuppressed patients, accounting for approximately 20% of nongonococcal cases. *Pseudomonas aeruginosa* is the frequent culprit among drug abusers, and has a predilection for the sternoclavicular joint. *Streptococcus pneumoniae* accounts for 5% of cases. While *H. influenzae* is a common cause of septic arthritis in infants and young children, it produces disease in less than 1% of cases in adults.

Viruses associated with arthritis include hepatitis B, rubella, mumps, and arbovirus. Fungal and tuberculous causes are rare. Other infectious causes of arthritis include Lyme disease, rheumatic fever, subacute bacterial endocarditis, and Whipple's disease.

A postinfectious arthritis may develop in patients following a *Salmonella*, *Shigella*, *Campylobacter*, or *Yersinia* enteritis. It is postulated to occur as an immune response because these pateints frequertly carry the specific histocompatibility antigen HLA-B27.

Bacterial or suppurative arthritis is monarticular in 90% of children and adults, the knee being the most commonly affected joint in both of these populations. This site is followed in frequency by the hip joint, with less common involvement of other joints. While adults tend to have involvement of the shoulder, sternoclavicular, and sacroiliac joints, children more frequently manifest infection of the ankle and elbow. The wrist and interphalangeal joints of the hands are more commonly involved when *N. gonorrhoeae* or *Mycobacterium tuberculosis* are the culprits. When viral induced, septic arthritis tends to involve multiple joints, especially the interphalangeal joints of the hands, and the wrists, knees, ankles, and elbows.

CLINICAL CHARACTERISTICS

Patients with bacterial arthritis usually present abruptly with fever, chills, and monarthritis manifested by warmth, erythema, swelling, and tenderness. Polyarthritis, however, may occur in 10% of patients.

Noninfectious inflammatory disorders involving joints may mimic septic arthritis and, therefore, should always be considered in the differential diagnosis of a warm, swollen joint or joints. These include gout, pseudogout, rheumatoid arthritis, psoriatic arthritis, Reiter's syndrome, collagen disease, and the arthritides of ulcerative colitis or regional enteritis. Hemarthrosis secondary to any hemorrhagic disorder or trauma should also be considered.

The gonococcus is the most common cause of septic arthritis in adults. This process usually occurs in young, healthy women, most commonly during the menses, pregnancy, or early postpartum period. The source may usually be traced to an asymptomatic genital, pharyngeal, or rectal infection. The disease may occur in two forms. Patients with one form of gonococcal arthritis present with fever, chills, and migratory polyarthritis with skin lesions and tenosynovitis. Little synovial fluid is present in the joint, joint cultures are often negative, and blood cultures are positive in only 20% of cases. In contrast, the second form manifests as a monarthritis with gonococcus frequently isolated from the joint fluid.

DIAGNOSIS

Synovial fluid analysis is the procedure critical to establishing the cause of the arthritis. Aspiration of a suspected septic joint is, therefore, mandatory. Fluid from a joint with pyogenic infection is characterized by a white blood cell count of 50,000 to 100,000 cells/ml with 90% neutrophils, a poor mucin clot, and glucose of at least 50 mg/dL less than the simultaneously obtained serum glucose. Gram stain (as well as other stains) and culture of the fluid for both aerobes and anaerobes are essential. In the case of suspected gonococcal infection, cultures of the throat, cervix, and skin pustules may be revealing. Synovial fluid from any adult with monarticular arthritis should also always be examined for crystals (uric acid and calcium pyrophosphate) to rule out a noninfectious origin.

Other helpful laboratory tests may include an elevated erythrocyte sedimentation rate, especially in those with bacterial infection or infection of long duration. Children tend to have an elevated white blood cell count with a predominance of neutrophils, while adults often do not manifest such an elevation.

The most frequent roentgenographic abnormality in bacterial arthritis is distention of the joint capsule and soft tissue swelling. Destructive changes are usually not noted until late in the course of the infection, often not until the 2nd week.

TREATMENT

Treatment consists of drainage and administration of antibiotics directed toward the specific organism. Splinting of the in-fected joint and avoidance of weight bearing are important until the signs of inflammation and pain have disappeared. The initial antibiotic therapy should be guided by the synovial fluid and Gram stain results, as well as the patient's age and underlying disease. Initial therapy should consist of parenteral antibiotics. Most antimicrobial agents reach therapeutic levels in the infected joint equal to or higher than serum levels. Oral antibiotics may be used later, but adequacy of serum levels must be monitored. The standard length of therapy for suppurative arthritis is 2 to 3 weeks. Intraarticular antibiotic regimens are unnecessary and may result in chemical synovitis.

Needle aspirations must be repeated whenever effusions reaccumulate to prevent cartilage destruction by leukocytic enzymes and debris. Open drainage is indicated for all hip joints, and often for the shoulder joint, when repeated aspiration does not succeed in preventing the reaccumulation of fluid, and whenever adhesions or loculations prevent adequate closed drainage of fluid. In such situations, orthopaedic referral is necessary.

Joint fluid cultures are usually negative within 7 days of initiation of antibiotic therapy. Effectiveness of therapy can be determined by clinical response and serial synovial fluid analyses. In the meantime, physical therapy should be instituted once pain and inflammation have subsided. Prognosis depends on the duration of symptoms prior to treatment, the organism, and any underlying illness. Prognosis is poorest in patients with symptoms for more than 5 days prior to initiation of antibiotic therapy and in patients infected with staphylococci or Gram-negative bacilli. Thus, recognition of a septic joint is of utmost importance in the prevention of a potentially fatal disease.

INFECTIONS OF PROSTHETIC JOINTS

Arthroplasty is a commonly performed procedure in the United States and carries with it a 0.5 to 2% infection rate. The immunocompromised patient or the patient with diabetes mellitus, rheumatoid arthritis, or previous joint surgery is at increased risk of developing infections. Prosthetic joint infections fall into three categories: early (within the first 3 months after replacement), delayed (within the first 2 years), and late (after 2 years). Two-thirds of these infections are discovered within the first 2 years, and many are probably a result of contamination at the time of surgery. In contrast, those that occur after 2 years are probably the result of hematogenous seeding from either an infected focus, such as a cellulitis, or a transient bacteremia. The hallmark of joint infection is pain, especially with motion. Fever and wound drainage are more commonly noted in the "early" infections; both are usually absent in the "late" cases.

Staphylococci are the most common cause of prosthetic joint infections, accounting for 30 to 40% of all infections (*Staphylococcus epidermidis* being more frequent than *S. aureus*). Gram-negative bacilli comprise 20 to 30% of infections, more commonly occurring in the earlier onset group. Anaerobes account for approximately 16% of cases. Ten percent of patients may be culture-negative despite clinical evidence of infection. Other organisms are implicated less frequently and polymicrobial infections may occur.

Aspiration of the joint is the most reliable test for diagnosis. An erythrocyte sedimentation rate greater than 20 mm/hr suggests infection, in the absence of other etiologic factors. The white blood cell count may vary. Plain radiographs, arthrogram, or bone scan may aid in the diagnosis.

If a prosthetic joint infection is suspected, an orthopaedic referral is necessary. Treatment of these infections, particularly the late or delayed type, may be complex and often requires removal of the prosthetic components and cement, as well as a prolonged course of antibiotics.

Prosthetic joint infections that occur at a time remote from surgery are often the result of a transient bacteremia. It is therefore recommended, although this is controversial, that the patient undergoing a procedure with this associated risk, e.g., cystoscopy or dental work, receive antibiotic prophylaxis immediately before and shortly after the manipulation.

SUGGESTED READINGS

Bayer AS, Guze LB. Fungal arthritis. I. Candida arthritis: diagnostic and prognostic implications and therapeutic considerations. Semin Arthritis Rheum 1978;8:142–150.

Buchholz HW, Elson RA, Engelbrecht E, et al. Management of deep infection of total hip replacement. J Bone Joint Surg 1981;63B:342–353.

Fitzgerald RH Jr, Nolan DR, Ilstrup DM, et al. Deep wound sepsis following total hip arthroplasty. J Bone Joint Surg 1977;59A:847–855.

Goldenberg DL, Cohen AS. Acute infectious arthritis. A review of patients with nongonococcal joint infections (with emphasis on therapy and prognosis). Am J Med 1976;60:369–377.

Goldenberg DL, Reed JI. Bacterial arthritis. N Engl J Med 1985;312:764–771.

Goldenberg DL, Brandt KD, Cohen AS, et al. Treatment of septic arthritis. Comparison of needle aspiration and surgery as initial modes of joint drainage. Arthritis Rheum 1975;18:83–90.

Ho G Jr, Gadbow JJ, Glickstein SL. *Hemophilus influenzae* septic arthritis in adults. Semin Arthritis Rheum 1983;12:314–321.

Hollander JL, Reginato A, Torralba TP. Examination of synovial fluid as a diagnostic aid in arthritis. Med Clin North Am 1966;50:1281–1293.

Kelly PJ. Bacterial arthritis in the adult. Orthop Clin North Am 1975;6:973–981.

Krey PR, Bailen DA. Synovial fluid leukocytosis: a study of extremes. Am J Med 1979;67:436–442.

Mackowiak PA, Jones SR, Smith JW. Diagnostic value of sinus-tract cultures in chronic osteomyelitis. JAMA 1978;239:2772–2775.

Nelson JD. Antibiotic concentrations in septic joint effusions. N Engl J Med 1971;284:349–353.

Nelson JD, Koontz WC. Septic arthritis in infants and children: a review of 117 cases. Pediatrics 1966;38:966–971.

Newman JH. Review of septic arthritis throughout the antibiotic era. Ann Rheum Dis 1976;35:198–205.

O'Brien JP, Goldenberg DL, Rice PA. Disseminated gonococcal infection: a prospective analysis of 49 patients and a review of pathophysiology and immune mechanisms. Medicine 1983;62:395–406.

Parker RH, Schmid FR. Antibacterial activity of synovial fluid during therapy of septic arthritis. Arthritis Rheum 1971;14:96–104.

Rosenthal J, Bole GG, Robinson WD. Acute nongonococcal infectious arthritis. Arthritis Rheum 1980;23:889–897.

Rotbart HA, Glode MP. *Haemophilus influenzae* type b septic arthritis in children: report of 23 cases. Pediatrics 1985;75:254–259.

Wallace R, Cohen AS. Tuberculosis arthritis. A report of two cases with review of biopsy and synovial fluid findings. Am J Med 1976;61:277–282.

CHAPTER 14

Diseases of Bone

Daniel T. Baran, M.D.

The skeleton is the major reservoir of calcium in the body. Diseases of bone affect the strength of the bony skeleton as well as calcium homeostasis. Likewise, hormones or drugs that affect calcium homeostasis also alter skeletal integrity. Thus, the patient with Paget's disease of bone may present with hypercalcemia or hypercalciuria following immobilization. Similarly, the patient with primary hyperparathyroidism may present with osteopenia and fracture prior to the discovery of hypercalcemia and elevated parathyroid hormone levels.

This chapter will review the clinical characteristics, pathophysiology, and differential diagnosis of the metabolic bone diseases encountered by the primary care physician: osteoporosis, Paget's disease of bone, and metastases to bone.

Osteoporosis

Osteoporosis is characterized by a decrease in bone mass. Both the organic matrix (collagen) and mineral component (hydroxyapatite crystal) are diminished in the osteoporotic patient. Osteoporosis is a major health problem in the United States. Approximately 15 to 20 million women over the age of 45 have osteoporosis. Each year, 1.2 million fractures are attributed to osteoporosis, resulting in health expenditures of 7 to 10 billion dollars annually.

CLINICAL CHARACTERISTICS

The woman at greatest risk for developing the disease is of northern European heritage, petite, a smoker, and sedentary, has a family history of osteoporosis (particularly in her mother), has a lifelong history of low dietary calcium intake, and has undergone an early menopause or an oophorectomy. Men are less likely to develop osteoporosis because of greater initial bone mass and slower rate of bone loss than women.

Osteoporosis is manifested by a decrease in bone substance and strength. The resulting diminution of bone tissue is expressed as a reduced bone mineral density. In the earliest stage, the patient is asymptomatic. However, as bone density decreases, spontaneous fractures occur, most commonly involving the spine, hip, or radius. The morbidity and mortality associated with osteoporosis are most evident in relation to hip fractures, which occur in 160,000 women each year and in one-third of women who live to age 90. Women who suffer hip fractures have a 12 to 20% greater risk of dying within the first year after the fracture. Vertebral fractures occur in 400,000 women each year causing loss of height, pain, and, if recurrent, deformity (dowager's hump).

PATHOPHYSIOLOGY OF OSTEOPOROSIS

Two general factors determine whether an individual will eventually develop osteoporosis: one is the peak bone mass attained at maturity and the other is the rate of bone loss as a function of age. Assume that two women lose bone density at the same yearly rate beginning at age 20. The individual with the lower initial bone density will cross the threshold of abnormally low density at an earlier age and be more prone to fracture.

The peak bone density reached in young adulthood is thought to depend on physical activity and calcium intake. Physical activity appears to be effective in maintaining and increasing normal bone mass. The exercise modality that optimally maintains or increases axial bone density has yet to be determined. However, positive correlations have been reported between bone mass and a variety of fitness and physical activity measurements, including maximal oxygen uptake, muscular strength, and lifetime physical activity. Similarly, a positive correlation between calcium intake and bone density has been noted in young women. This correlation is independent of physical activity. Likewise, calcium intake (1 to 1.5 g of elemental calcium per day) in premenopausal women appears to reduce the rate of age-related bone loss. Thus, prior to menopause, physical activity and diet are important determinants of bone health.

Loss of ovarian function, whether due to menopause or oophorectomy, is associated with an increase in the rate of bone loss for the ensuing 3 to 4 years. The premenopausal woman with low normal bone mass is therefore at greatest risk for the development of osteoporosis during the perimenopausal years. The mechanism(s) by which estrogen promotes bone health is unclear. Recently, estrogen receptors have been demonstrated in osteoblasts isolated from human bone, suggesting that the steroid may have direct effects on the cells to promote bone formation. The presence of estrogen is also associated with increased blood levels of the active vitamin D metabolite 1,25-dihydroxyvitamin D_3 and enhanced intestinal calcium absorption. Therefore, loss of estrogen due to either menopause or oophorectomy results in decreased intestinal calcium absorption, increased bone resorption to compensate for the decrease in calcium obtained

from the diet, and decreases in direct stimulation of osteoblastic activity.

Inactivity also augments the osteoporotic condition. The osteoporotic patient who fractures often immobilizes herself to reduce discomfort and the risk of additional fractures. Immobilization and the lack of weight bearing decrease bone formation, resulting in greater bone loss.

DIAGNOSIS OF OSTEOPOROSIS

The osteoporotic skeleton is quantitatively diminished but histologically normal. The diagnosis of advanced or severe osteoporosis can usually be made by routine x-rays of the spine (Fig. 14.1) or femur. Characteristic x-ray features of the osteoporotic skeleton prior to fracture include codfish vertebrae, accentuation of the vertebral end

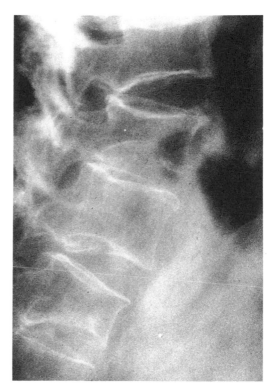

Figure 14.1. Lateral radiograph of the lumbar spine of an osteoporotic patient, demonstrating anterior and central vertebral compression fractures and accentuation of the endplates.

plates, and accentuation of the vertical trabecular pattern in the vertebral bodies and the trabecular pattern in the femoral neck. It must be remembered, however, that a 30% loss of bone mineral is required before one can appreciate these changes. Consequently, only the patient with severe osteoporosis can be diagnosed by these routine measures.

Awareness of osteoporosis has improved because of noninvasive techniques that quantify bone mass in vivo. Rather than relying on qualitative x-ray images of the axial skeleton, the physician can now obtain numerical values for bone mass in the spine and hip. Bone mass has been shown to be an important predictor of fracture risk: as bone mass decreases, the incidence of vertebral and hip fractures increases. Techniques to measure bone mass of the spine and hip include dual photon absorptiometry, dual energy x-ray absorptiometry (DXA), and single and dual energy computed tomography. The newest technique, DXA, has the advantage of speed (5 minutes for each scan), low radiation exposure (1 to 1.5 mrem), and reproducibility (a coefficient of variation of 1%) (Fig. 14.2). Other techniques are available to measure bone mass in the extremities. Both single photon absorptiometry and ultrasound (the attenuation of the sound wave as it passes through bone) have been used to measure bone mass in the forearm, the patella, and the calcaneus. Measurements of bone mass at these peripheral sites have now been shown to be excellent predictors of fracture at all sites.

These techniques now offer the physician the opportunity to quantitatively assess both the patient at greatest risk of fracture and the efficacy of treatment in patients with this common and disabling disease, thus improving the quality of care. The physician no longer needs to depend on a reduction in fracture rate to assess therapeutic effectiveness, but may assess increments in bone mineral density within 6 to 12 months of initiating therapy. About 95% of spine fractures occur in the 50% of elderly women with lumbar density levels below 1.0 g/cm^2 (by dual photon absorptiometry). Similarly, 95% of hip fractures occur in patients with a femoral density below 0.7 g/cm^2. Thus, these noninvasive procedures offer the opportunity of early detection of osteoporosis and fracture prevention.

DIFFERENTIAL DIAGNOSIS AND CLASSIFICATION

Idiopathic, postmenopausal osteoporosis is a diagnosis of exclusion. Osteomalacia, multiple myeloma, hyperparathyroidism, hyperthyroidism, carcinoma, and hypercortisolism must be considered. In the male, osteoporosis may be a manifestation of testicular failure, and in the young female, a presenting sign of Turner's syndrome.

Osteomalacia is a defect in collagen matrix mineralization. Because milk is supplemented with vitamin D in the United States, nutritional deficiency of the vitamin is rare in this country. Osteomalacia due to abnormality in vitamin D metabolism may occur in renal failure (decreased 1,25-dihydroxyvitamin D production in the kidney), steatorrhea (loss of fat-soluble vitamins through the intestinal tract), or vitamin D-resistant rickets (decreased 1α-hydroxylase activity in renal mitochondria). Abnormalities in bone mineralization also occur in the severely hypophosphatemic patient (typically the result of excess ingestion of phosphate-binding antacid or phosphate diabetes).

Multiple myeloma, hyperthyroidism, hyperparathyroidism, and carcinoma can all present as osteopenia. Plasma cells are capable of producing a variety of substances termed osteoclast-activating factors or transforming growth factors that induce bone resorption. Similarly, excessive parathyroid hormone and thyroid hormone induce bone resorption. Recent studies suggest that chronic administration of suppressive doses of thyroid hormone is associated with decreased bone mass. Finally, certain tumors

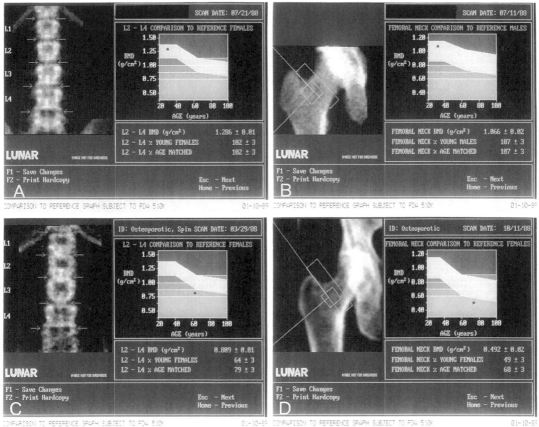

Figure 14.2. *A,* bone mineral density (BMD) of a normal lumbar spine determined by digital radiography. The lumbar vertebrae of this 29-year-old woman are visualized to the left and the bone mineral density plotted in comparison to normal reference females at the upper right. The numerical value is provided at the bottom right. *B,* bone mineral density of a normal femur determined by digital radiography. The right proximal femur of this 28-year-old man is visualized at the left and the bone mineral density plotted in comparison to reference males at the upper right. The numerical value is provided at the lower right. *C,* bone mineral density of osteoporotic lumbar vertebrae determined by digital radiography. The lumbar vertebrae of this 61-year-old woman are visualized at the left and the bone mineral density plotted in comparison to reference females at the upper right. The numerical value is provided at the lower right. *D,* bone mineral density of an osteoporotic femur determined by digital radiography. The right proximal femur of this 76-year-old woman is visualized at the left and plotted in comparison to reference females at the upper right. The numerical value is provided at the lower right. (From LUNAR Corp., Madison, WI.)

are capable of inducing bone resorption resulting in hypercalcemia. The typical tumors that secrete these humoral factors are squamous, renal, bladder, and ovarian carcinomas.

Glucocorticoid excess, either intrinsic or iatrogenic, causes osteoporosis. The glucocorticoids inhibit intestinal calcium absorption and bone formation. Bone resorption is often increased to compensate for the decreased intestinal calcium absorption. Therapy for osteoporosis requires treatment of glucocorticoid overproduction or reduction of steroid dose to the lowest effective level, preferably steroid treatment every other day.

Therefore, although idiopathic postmenopausal osteoporosis is the most common form of the disease that will be encountered by the practitioner, these other causes of diminished bone density need to be considered. Consequently, evaluation of these patients should include serum calcium, phosphorus, and alkaline phosphatase levels, a complete blood count, either serum or urine protein electrophoresis, thyroid function tests, parathyroid hormone and serum cortisol levels, and 24-hour urinary calcium excretion. With the exception of osteoporosis caused by humoral mechanisms associated with cancer and multiple myeloma, these entities may be treated by the practitioner with consultation from an endocrinologist.

TREATMENT OF POSTMENOPAUSAL OSTEOPOROSIS

The drugs currently available to treat the condition include estrogen, bisphosphonates, calcitonin, the coherence (ADFR) therapies, 1,25-dihydroxyvitamin D, and fluoride. These drugs affect bone mass and also decrease fracture rate.

Estrogen

The main effect of estrogen is the prevention of further bone loss, rather than the augmentation of bone mass. Therefore, it is indicated in women who have undergone oophorectomy. It can be used in the perimenopausal woman to prevent further bone loss. Estrogen is usually not indicated in the woman with established osteoporosis and fractures. Since estrogen does not appear to augment bone mass, its use in such a woman will prevent further bone loss but will not increase bone density, and thus will not reduce the established fracture risk. Estrogen therapy prevents axial bone loss when administered either orally or transdermally. The use of calcium supplements (1000 mg of elemental calcium per day) along with estrogen appears to be synergistic, allowing the oral estrogen dose to be decreased to 0.3 mg/day.

Candidates for estrogen therapy include women with a history of oophorectomy, women undergoing early menopause, or women who are perimenopausal with a slight build and a family history of osteoporosis. Since physical activity in postmenopausal women appears to increase bone mass, the combination of estrogen and weight-bearing exercises may prove to be the optimal regimen in the treatment of the perimenopausal woman.

Bisphosphonates

The bisphosphonates possess a strong affinity for the hydroxyapatite crystal and inhibit both bone formation and resorption. The latter effect is greater and occurs at lower concentrations, so the major effect of the drug at standard doses is the inhibition of bone resorption. The brief half-life of the compounds in the circulation plus their long half-life in bone explains their low toxicity and the restriction of their effects to the skeleton.

Cyclical therapy of osteoporosis with etidronate (Didronel) has been shown to increase bone density, decrease fracture rate, and reduce the loss of height that accompanies vertebral fractures. The bisphosphonates also prevent the bone loss that occurs shortly after menopause, and appear to reduce the loss of vertebral bone mass in 1- and 2-year follow-ups of steroid-treated patients. The low cost of these compounds, their ease of administration, their lack of side effects, and their efficacy in the prevention and therapy of osteoporosis may make them the ideal treatment for the average patient.

Calcitonin

Both salmon (Calcimar) and human (Cibacalcin) calcitonin are now available for the treatment of osteoporosis. The drug is a potent inhibitor of osteoclastic bone resorption, appears to increase bone mass by 20% per year in women with high turnover osteoporosis, and possesses analgesic properties. Its major disadvantages are cost (approximately $150 per month) and route of administration (subcutaneous). However, trials are now underway to assess the efficacy of alternate routes of administration. The intranasal route has been shown to be effective in the prevention of bone loss at menopause. The major advantage of the drug is its lack of significant side effects. Nausea is the main complication. The usual dose is 100 IU of Calcimar or 0.5 mg of Cibacalcin administered 3 times a week.

Coherence (ADFR) Therapies

These new treatments are based on the biology of osteoclasts and osteoblasts. Current evidence indicates that bone formation is in some way "coupled" to bone resorption. Increasing resorption increases formation, and decreasing resorption decreases formation. These treatments employ parathyroid hormone, phosphorus, or growth hormone to *Activate* the osteoclasts and thereby induce osteoblastic activity by the coupling phenomenon. 1,25-Dihydroxyvitamin D, etidronate disodium (Didronel), or calcitonin are then employed to *Depress* bone resorption; however, the osteoblastic activity (bone formation) proceeds. Calcium supplements are frequently used during the drug-*Free* period. This cycle is then *Repeated*. Marked increments in axial bone mass have been reported. Since these therapies are new, it is suggested that the practitioner refer these patients to an endocrinologist before beginning coherence therapy.

1,25-Dihydroxyvitamin D$_3$

1,25-Dihydroxyvitamin D$_3$ (Rocaltrol) is the most potent vitamin D metabolite. It augments intestinal absorption of both calcium and phosphorus and has been shown to prevent vertebral bone loss at an average dose of 0.6 μg/day. Its major side effects are the risk of hypercalciuria and hypercalcemia and, therefore, its administration requires constant monitoring. In one study the vitamin D metabolite increased bone density,

but all of the patients developed hypercalciuria, and 89% manifested a serum calcium greater than 11 mg/dL at one time during the study. Reduction in the dose of 1,25-dihydroxyvitamin D$_3$ lessens the risk of hypercalcemia and hypercalciuria but does not appear to prevent bone loss. It appears that the therapeutic window between efficacy of the drug and side effects is very narrow, making routine treatment difficult.

Fluoride

Sodium fluoride, 40 to 60 mg/day, increases vertebral bone density in approximately 70% of women. The new bone that is formed contains the fluorapatite crystal rather than hydroxyapatite. In a recent 3-year prospective study, sodium fluoride treatment of women with postmenopausal osteoporosis was associated with significant increments in vertebral bone density, but no reduction in fracture rate. Thus, at present, sodium fluoride is not indicated for the treatment of postmenopausal osteoporosis.

Paget's Disease of Bone

Paget's disease is characterized by increased bone resorption and resultant increments in bone formation. The "turnover" of bone is increased greatly and results in a "mosaic" pattern of bone formation.

CLINICAL CHARACTERISTICS

Paget's disease occurs in 0.1 to 1% of elderly hospitalized patients in the United States, with equal frequency in men and women. The bones most commonly affected by Paget's disease, in order of decreasing frequency, are sacrum, spine, femur, skull, sternum, and pelvis. The bones of the axial skeleton are most frequently involved, but the disease may occur at any skeletal site, and may involve one or many bones.

Pain is a common manifestation of Paget's disease, with some studies suggesting that prostaglandins may be the responsible agents. The skin over the affected bone is often warm. This is thought to reflect the increased vascularity of the bone with resultant increased blood flow. Because of the chaotic turnover of bone, the size and shape of the bones often change, with the skull enlarging and long bones becoming deformed. Although the bone in Paget's disease may increase in size, the mosaic pattern of deposited lamellar bone makes it weaker. Hence, "bowing" deformities of the lower extremities and fractures are common occurrences.

The treatment of fractures associated with Paget's disease is similar to treatment of fractures of normal bone; however, the practitioner must be aware that these bones are more vascular. Less than 1% of patients with Paget's disease progress to develop osteogenic sarcoma. This is heralded by increasing pain in a previously well-controlled patient, or rapidly increasing serum alkaline phosphatase.

The major complications of Paget's disease are spinal stenosis, degenerative arthritis, and nerve impingement caused by increasing bone size. Deafness is a common sequela of Paget's disease involving the skull. It may result from damage to the auditory nerve as it passes through the auditory canal, or from involvement of the bones of the inner ear with Paget's disease. Degenerative arthritis is a commonly associated finding when Paget's disease bridges a joint, e.g., pelvis and femur, femur and tibia.

PATHOPHYSIOLOGY OF PAGET'S DISEASE

The etiology of the disease remains unclear. Viral inclusion bodies have been reported in biopsies of bone with Paget's disease, but it is not certain that they are the causative agents. The observation that Paget's disease often occurs in several members of a family has led to speculation regarding genetic transmission. However, based on the known incidence of Paget's disease and the

incidence of identical twin births, the paucity of Paget's disease in twin pairs makes genetic transmission unlikely.

DIAGNOSIS OF PAGET'S DISEASE

Paget's disease is characterized by increased bone resorption and, frequently, increased bone formation. The stages of Paget's disease may thus involve (*a*) increased resorption, (*b*) resorption plus formation, or (*c*) a sclerotic quiescent phase. The practitioner is referred to a textbook of radiology for a thorough description of the radiographic changes in bones affected by Paget's disease. A bone scan can differentiate between active and quiescent Paget's disease, and serum alkaline phosphatase is a marker for the activity of the disease. Although alkaline phosphatase is produced by osteoblasts, increased alkaline phosphatase may also reflect liver disease, ectopic pregnancy, a healing fracture, or any osteoblastic process in bone. Alkaline phosphatase from bone can be distinguished by fractionating the total alkaline phosphatase. The bone fraction is heat-labile. Urinary hydroxyproline is increased in Paget's disease, reflecting increased collagen degradation. Although this is also an excellent marker for disease activity, the procedure requires the collection of a 24-hour urine sample, and the results may be affected by diet, e.g., gelatin, or skin disease, e.g., psoriasis. Acid phosphatase, most frequently thought of as a marker for prostatic malignancy, is also produced by bone cells and may be elevated in active Paget's disease. Since metastatic osteoblastic prostate malignancy is in the differential diagnosis of Paget's disease, increases in serum acid phosphatase must be further evaluated by measures of the prostatic fraction of acid phosphatase.

DIFFERENTIAL DIAGNOSIS

Any osteoblastic process, e.g., metastatic prostate cancer, may resemble Paget's disease roentgenographically, but appropriate testing should differentiate the conditions. Hereditary hyperphosphatasia may be similar to Paget's disease, but the age of the patient and the involvement of the entire skeleton should easily differentiate the two.

TREATMENT OF PAGET'S DISEASE

The drugs most commonly used to treat Paget's disease are etidronate disodium (Didronel) or calcitonin (Calcimar or Cibacalcin). Indications for treatment are increasing severity of symptoms (see above) and an elevated alkaline phosphatase (>300 IU).

Etidronate Disodium

Etidronate disodium (Didronel) is an oral medication effective in approximately 85% of patients with Paget's disease, decreasing both symptoms and activity of the disease as measured by alkaline phosphatase. The usual dosage is 5 mg/kg body weight per day in two divided doses for 6 months. Since food affects absorption of the drug, it should be given between meals. Sodium etidronate is an inhibitor of bone resorption and bone formation. At doses of 10 to 20 mg/kg body weight per day, the drug has been associated with increased incidence of fractures and the development of osteomalacia (impaired mineralization of the collagen matrix). Sodium etidronate may also cause a mild phosphaturia, and it is suggested that serum phosphorus as well as alkaline phosphatase be measured at 3-month intervals. In the patient on a normal diet, this mild phosphaturia is of no clinical significance. In the patient without skull involvement, this is the first drug of choice.

Calcitonin

Calcitonin is a polypeptide hormone produced by the C cells of the thyroid. Increasing serum calcium, or a pentagastrin infusion, stimulates calcitonin release. Its major action is inhibition of osteoclastic bone re-sorption. Since bone resorption and formation appear to be coupled, inhibition of bone resorption will ultimately inhibit bone formation. These effects result in decreased urinary hydroxyproline excretion and decreased serum alkaline phosphatase levels. Although the drug is effective in the treatment of hypercalcemia associated with malignancy (see below), calcitonin treatment does not cause hypocalcemia in patients with Paget's disease.

Calcitonin is administered subcutaneously, usually 3 times a week. The dose of salmon calcitonin is 100 IU, while that of human calcitonin is 0.5 mg. The response rate ranges between 95 and 100%. The most common side effect is transient nausea. This can be minimized by administration of the calcitonin at bedtime. Initial studies have demonstrated nasal calcitonin to be an effective treatment of Paget's disease. If substantiated, this will eliminate the need for subcutaneous injections.

Mithramycin

Mithramycin is a cytotoxic antibiotic that induces a hypocalcemic response similar to calcitonin. The drug is administered intravenously over 4 hours at a dose of 10 μg/kg body weight. Its side effects include liver and marrow toxicity. Baseline liver function tests, prothrombin time, complete blood count, and platelet count are necessary prior to its administration. Because of its side effects, the use of this drug should only be considered in the patient who is symptomatic and has failed treatment with sodium etidronate, salmon calcitonin, and human calcitonin. The practitioner is urged to consult an endocrinologist prior to its use.

Nonsteroidal Anti-inflammatory Agents

Although these drugs do not specifically treat Paget's disease, they may be useful in the patient with arthritic changes associated with Paget's disease.

Bone Metastasis

Tumors metastatic to bone may cause pain, hypercalcemia, and fractures. Osteolytic hypercalcemia results from bone resorption caused by tumors in direct contact with the bone cells. The tumors most likely to cause osteolytic hypercalcemia are breast cancers, multiple myelomas, and hematologic malignancies. In contrast, humoral hypercalcemia of malignancy in the absence of bone metastases is caused by osteoclastic resorption mediated by parathyroid hormone-like peptides. Tumors most commonly associated with humoral hypercalcemia are renal, squamous, bladder, and ovarian carcinomas. Although fractures occur in patients with hyperparathyroidism, the presence of hypercalcemia in a patient with a fracture should immediately raise concern regarding the possibility of a malignancy. A bone scan should be obtained to investigate potential skeletal involvement at other sites, and orthopaedic consultation should be requested. The bone scan may not show increased activity in patients with osteolytic tumor, e.g., myeloma, who have not yet developed a pathologic fracture.

TREATMENT

The practitioner should consult an oncologist prior to treatment of the underlying tumor. Often, however, the patient with hypercalcemia presents as a medical emergency with altered mental status and electrocardiographic changes, i.e., shortened QT interval. The goal of therapy is the rapid reduction in serum calcium to avoid cardiovascular and central nervous system complications. In the acute situation, this is initially accomplished by rehydrating the patient, thereby increasing renal calcium excretion. Intravenous fluids can be started quickly and can rapidly increase calcium excretion. The goal is to achieve a urine output of 3 to 5 liters every 24 hours. If the patient's cardio-vascular system is compromised, care must be used to prevent congestive heart failure. Concomitant use of loop diuretics can help achieve the desired urinary output while minimizing the risk of fluid overload. Calcitonin is effective in the treatment of hypercalcemia. Up to 80% of hypercalcemic patients will respond to calcitonin with a decrease in serum calcium levels within 4 to 6 hours. Unfortunately, tolerance to the calcitonin may develop within 6 to 10 days. Intravenous etidronate disodium may be a useful form of therapy. When administered along with intravenous fluids, calcium levels are normalized in 90% of patients. Glucocorticoids may also be beneficial in the treatment of hypercalcemia of malignancy caused by myeloma and other hematologic malignancies. Because a response to glucocorticoids is usually not seen for 7 to 10 days, they cannot be used to acutely lower serum calcium.

While the patient's serum calcium is being treated, the practitioner is urged to consult an oncologist so that diagnosis and therapy for the underlying malignancy may be initiated.

SUGGESTED READINGS

Barzel US. Estrogens in the prevention and treatment of postmenopausal osteoporosis—a review. Am J Med 1988;85:847.

Canalis E, McCarthy TL, Centrella M. The Role of growth factors in skeletal remodeling. Endocrinol Metab Clin North Am 1989;18:903–918.

Civitelli R, Gonnelli S, Zacchei F, et al. Bone turnover in postmenopausal osteoporosis: effect of calcitonin treatment. J Clin Invest 1988;82:1268–1274.

Cummings SR, Kelsey JL, Nevitt MC, et al. Epidemiology of osteoporosis and osteoporotic fractures. Epidemiol Rev 1985;7:178–208.

Cummings SR, Black DM, Nevitt MC, et al. Appendicular bone density and age predict hip fracture in women. JAMA 1990;263:665–668.

Favas MJ, ed. Primer on the metabolic bone diseases and disorders of mineral metabolism. Kelseyville, CA: American Society for Bone and Mineral Research Society, 1990.

Gallagher JC, Goldgar D. Treatment of postmenopausal

osteoporosis with high doses of synthetic calcitriol. Ann Int Med 1990;113:649–655.

Hui SL, Slemenda CW, Johnston CC, Jr. Age and bone mass as predictors of fracture in a prospective study. J Clin Invest 1988;81:1804–1809.

Riggs BL, Hodgson SF, O'Fallon, WM, et al. Effect of flu-oride treatment on the fracture rate in postmeno-pausal women with osteoporosis. N Engl J Med 1990;322:802–809.

Watts NB, Harris ST, Genant HK, et al. Intermittent cy-clical etidronate treatment of postmenopausal osteo-porosis. N Engl J Med 1990;323:73–79.

CHAPTER 15

Orthopedic Problems in the Pediatric Patient

M. Timothy Hresko, M.D., and Yvonne A. Shelton, M.D.

Nontraumatic Disorders of Childhood

While the nontraumatic disorders of adulthood are typically degenerative, the nontraumatic disorders of childhood are typically developmental. Therapy for adult disorders usually focuses on restoration of function and retardation of degeneration, while therapy for childhood disorders usually focuses on correction of distorted anatomy and prevention of a propensity to accelerated degeneration.

The following are the developmental anatomic abnormalities presented in this text:

Anatomic abnormalities recognized within the first 3 months of life: (*a*) congenital dysplasia of the hip, under "Nontraumatic Conditions of Childhood" in Chapter 6; (*b*) metatarsus adductus, under this heading in Chapter 9; (*c*) metatarsus primus varus, under "Hallux Valgus" in Chapter 9; and (*d*) talipes equinovarus, under "Newborn Foot Deformities" in Chapter 9.

Anatomic abnormalities recognized at the onset of standing and walking, about the end of the 1st year: (*a*) *pronated feet*—flexible flatfeet and rigid flatfeet, under "Flatfeet" in Chapter 9; (*b*) *pigeon-toed stance*—femoral anteversion, under this heading in Chapter 9, and internal tibial torsion, under this heading in Chapter 9.

Metatarsus varus will occasionally not be recognized until the end of the 1st year.

The osteochondroses cause various pain syndromes unique to children. Table 15.1 lists the osteochondroses presented in this text. In general, the etiology of the pain in these conditions is either (*a*) shear fractures through epiphyseal growth plates or (*b*) fractures through avascular necrotic bone. The treatment regimen for these conditions emphasizes restriction of activities, nonsteroidal anti-inflammatory medications, functional bracing, and physiotherapy to maintain joint range of motion and prevent muscular atrophy.

Certain acquired inflammations and structural displacements are also unique to childhood. Four have been presented in this text (Table 15.2).

Traumatic Disorders of Childhood

Developing bones and joints respond to injuries differently in several respects from fully developed and deteriorating bones and joints. The greater remodeling potential of growing bones and its effect on treatment plans was summarized under "General Principles of Treatment of Forearm Fractures" in Chapter 3. This principle allows acceptance of positions that would not be acceptable in adult injuries. Growing joint capsules, ligaments, and muscles are more tolerant to prolonged immobilization than mature joint capsules, ligaments, and muscles. Thus, the need for prolonged immobilization does not commonly contraindicate closed methods of treatment in children as it does in adults. This is often important in the

Table 15.1.
Osteochondroses Presented in the Text

Presentation	Disorder
Dorsal back pain	Adolescent kyphosis (Scheuermann's disease), under "Adolescent Kyphosis (Scheuermann's Disease)" in Chapter 5.
Hip and knee pain	Aseptic necrosis with stress fracture in the capital femoral epiphysis (Legg-Calvé-Perthes disease), under "Avascular Necrosis of the Femoral Head" in Chapter 6.
	Aseptic necrosis with stress fracture of the femoral condyles (osteochondritis dissecans), under "Necrosis within the Condylar Epiphyses of the Femur (Osteochondritis Dissecans)" in Chapter 7.
	Apophysitis of the tibial tubercle, under "Tibial Apophysitis (Osgood-Schlatter Disease)" in Chapter 7.
	Necrosis within the poles of the patella (Larsen-Johansson's disease), under this heading in Chapter 7.
Foot and ankle pain	Apophysitis of the calcaneal physis (Sever's disease), under "Calcaneal Apophysitis (Sever's Disease)" in Chapter 8.
	Aseptic necrosis with stress fracture of the talar navicular (Köhler's disease), under "Aseptic Necrosis of the Navicular (Köhler's Disease)" in Chapter 9.
	Aseptic necrosis of the head of the 2nd metatarsal (Frieberg's disease), under "Aseptic Necrosis of the Second Metatarsal Head (Freiberg's Disease)" in Chapter 9.

Table 15.2.
Acquired Inflammations and Structural Displacements Presented in the Text

Presentation	Disorder
Wry neck	Atlantoaxial subluxation, under "Acute Cervical Myalgia" in Chapter 1.
Hip and knee pain	Pyogenic arthritis of the hip, in Chapter 6.
	Nonspecific synovitis of the hip, under "Nonspecific or Transient Synovitis" in Chapter 6.
	Slipped capital femoral epiphysis, under this heading in Chapter 6.

treatment of fractures of the radius, ulna, femur, and tibia in a child. Unfortunately, application of these principles is difficult to teach in a text. Consequently, until experience is gained it is recommended that orthopaedic consultation be obtained when questions of this sort are problematic in the care of a specific injury.

Fracture patterns that involve the articular surface of a joint are much less common in children than they are in adults. Fractures in children that do involve the articular surface share the same risk involved in articular fractures in adults. Any fracture involving the articular surface in either a child or an adult should be referred to an orthopedist.

PHYSEAL FRACTURES

Physeal fractures of the long bones usually do not interfere with the growth of the injured bone. These fractures occur through the zone of provisional calcification in the physis. The growth potential of the physis usually is not disturbed. However, if the fracture extends through the zone of proliferation into the epiphysis, there is a significant risk of interfering with the growth of the injured bone (Fig. 15.1). Epiphyseal fractures have been classified into five groups, each of which presents different diagnostic and prognostic characteristics.

Salter I fractures are transverse fractures of the growth plate without injury to the bony metaphysis or epiphysis. When these fractures are undisplaced, they are not radiologically evident at the time of injury. Tenderness at the level of the growth plate of a long bone and a normal x-ray imply a Salter I fracture until developments prove otherwise. Stress views may be diagnostic. Repeat x-rays after 2 weeks will usually show bone

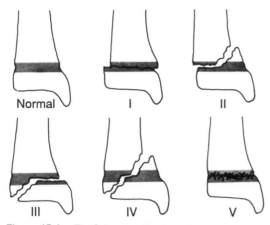

Figure 15.1.   The Salter classifications of epiphyseal fractures.

response characteristic of fracture healing, if the Salter I fracture has actually occurred. Salter I fractures must be reduced and immobilized until clinical union is evident. In the upper extremity this usually requires 3 to 4 weeks of immobilization, while in the lower extremity clinical union is usually present by 6 weeks after the injury. In most cases, nondisplaced Salter I fractures do not interfere with growth (see the discussion of Salter V fractures).

Salter II fractures are transverse fractures of the growth plate that extend obliquely into the bony metaphysis. This fracture and the Salter I fracture are by far the most common physeal fractures. The fracture separation of the distal radial epiphysis discussed in Chapter 3 under ''Fractures of Both Bones of the Forearm'' is an example. Since the fracture into the metaphysis is radiologically evident, a Salter II fracture is rarely missed at the time of injury. Treatment and prognosis are identical to those of the Salter I fracture. Special attention must be paid to injuries in the distal femoral physis. Growth inhibition after Salter I fractures has been reported. Salter II fractures of the distal physis are more likely to result in a complete or partial growth arrest than similar injuries at other growth plates. Therefore, children who have

an injury to the distal femoral physis should be followed by clinical and radiographic examination for at least 2 years after their injury.

Salter III fractures are transverse fractures of the growth plate which have involved the bony epiphysis. No examples of this fracture have been given in this text. The Salter III fracture occurs in adolescence and is commonly seen in the distal tibia. When the physis is in the process of closing, the fracture pattern extends through the remaining open part of the physis, through the epiphysis, and into the nearby joint. Since this is an intraarticular fracture, reduction must be anatomic. This injury should be referred to an orthopaedist.

Salter IV fractures extend axially into the bony metaphysis and into the bony epiphysis. The fracture may appear to extend axially from the bony epiphysis to the bony metaphysis directly through the growth plate, or it may appear to extend axially through the bony epiphysis, transversely across part of the growth plate, then axially into the bony metaphysis. The danger of growth arrest is greatest in these fractures. Reduction must be anatomic, and close follow-up of leg-length discrepancies and angular deformities is required. The injury must be referred to an orthopaedist.

Salter V fractures are compression injuries of the growth plate. Their initial clinical characteristics are indistinguishable from those of the undisplaced Salter I fracture: no radiologic visibility, tenderness at the region of the growth plate, and eventual appearance of radiologic signs of bone healing (usually within 2 to 3 weeks). The distinction occurs much later when it becomes evident that the injured physis is either no longer growing or is growing in an asymmetric fashion. Asymmetric closure of a physis can be recognized on a roentgenogram by a bridge of sclerotic bone spanning the normal lucency of the physis. The growth arrest line may be asymmetric as well. This would be indicative of a Salter injury. Even if the injury had been recognized on the 1st day, nothing could have been done to prevent the outcome. When the undisplaced Salter I/ Salter V clinical presentation appears, parents must be warned of the poor prognosis of the Salter V fracture while the injury is treated as a Salter I fracture.

The prognosis of epiphyseal fractures differs not only among the types, but among the locations as well. Epiphyseal fractures in the upper extremity are rarely followed by growth failure, except following Salter V injuries. In the lower extremity, any epiphyseal fracture can be followed by growth failure, and the Salter III, IV, and V fractures carry a particularly guarded prognosis.

The physeal fractures presented in this text are the following: (*a*) fracture of the distal radial physis, under "Fractures of the distal third of the forearm" in Chapter 3; (*b*) slipped capital femoral epiphyses, under that heading in Chapter 6; (*c*) fracture of the distal femoral physis and fracture of the proximal tibial physis, under "Epiphyseal Fractures" in Chapter 7; (*d*) fracture of the distal tibial physis, under "Fractures of the Shafts of the Tibia and Fibula" in Chapter 8; (*e*) and axial compression injuries of the ankle in "Fractures of the Ankle" in Chapter 8.

AVULSION FRACTURES OF THE APOPHYSES

In the growing child, muscle strains about the hip may cause avulsion fractures of the apophyses about the hip. The apophyseal avulsions presented in this text are listed in Table 15.3. The mechanism, recognition, and treatment of these avulsion fractures are described under "Periarticular Myofascial Pain Syndromes" in Chapter 6.

BATTERED CHILD SYNDROME

The battered child syndrome includes nonaccidental trauma inflicted on children by parents, siblings, and other caretakers.

Table 15.3.
Apophyseal Avulsions Presented in the Text

Muscle Strained	Apophysis Avulsed
Iliopsoas	Lesser trochanter of the femur
Straight tendon of the rectus femoris	Anteroinferior iliac spine
Sartorius	Anterosuperior iliac spine
Hamstring and adductor	Ischial tuberosity

Child abuse is a term used for physical, psychological, and verbal trauma as well as sexual abuse and neglect. Physical injuries include head trauma, ruptured internal organs, and skin lesions. One-third to one-half of the children will have a bone injury. The presence of multiple bruises, certain burn and scar patterns and locations, and depression and lethargy should alert the clinician to the possibility of abuse. Vague or multiple histories that are inconsistent in themselves or inconsistent with the injury pattern support the suspicion. The clinician should not hesitate to obtain a skeletal survey in these cases; multiple fractures in various stages of healing are diagnostic. Single long bone fractures are the most common bony injury seen in abused children, however, there are several highly specific fracture patterns. Shaking of the infant, repeated blunt trauma, and pulling of the extremities result in microfractures through the primary spongiosa of the metaphyses. Radiologically, these localized bony fragments appear as transverse metaphyseal lucencies, "corner" or bucket-handle fractures, near the growth plates of the femur, proximal tibia and humerus. The corner fractures are small and triangular, while the "bucket-handle" fractures are rim-like bony fragments. Other characteristic bony injuries include complex skull fractures, posterior rib, spinal, sternal or scapula fractures. Spiral fractures indicate that a twisting force has been applied to the extremity.

Admittance of the child to the hospital is

recommended in all suspected cases. Possible occult injuries are investigated with bone scans, computed tomography scans, and magnetic resonance imaging. The health care professional is responsible for reporting the case to the appropriate agencies for investigation of the family or caretakers. Treatment of the specific injuries is important, but the protection of the child from further injury is the primary goal.

SUGGESTED READINGS

Akbarian B. The role of the orthopedist in child abuse. In: Morrisey RT, ed. Pediatric orthopedics. Philadelphia: JB Lippincott Co, 1990:365–380.

Bright RW. Physeal injuries. In: Rockwood CA Jr, Wilkins KE, King RE, eds. Fractures in children. Philadelphia: JB Lippincott Co, 1984:87–172.

Kleinman PK. Diagnostic imaging in infant abuse. AJR 1990;155:703–712.

Ogden JA. Skeletal injury in the child. 2nd ed. Philadelphia: WB Saunders Co, 1990.

CHAPTER 16

Evaluation of the Injured Patient and Basic Principles of Management

Walter J. Leclair, M.D.

Introduction

Injury is the leading cause of death in the 1- to 44-year-old age group and the fourth leading cause of death in all age groups. There are approximately 160,000 deaths per year due to injury (1). The total dollar cost to society is difficult to accurately measure. Recent estimates put the cost at approximately 25 billion dollars per year (2,3). These injuries account for 3.5 million hospital admissions yearly. While there are many subcategories of specific types of injury, motor vehicle accidents continue to be one of the leading causes. There are approximately 50,000 deaths and 4 to 5 million injuries yearly caused by motor vehicle accidents. These account for approximately 500,000 hospitalizations.

In response to this "trauma epidemic," trauma subspecialties have been developed in the fields of surgery, orthopaedics, plastic surgery, and neurosurgery. Yet often the first encounter with the trauma patient is by the primary care practitioner and not by the trauma subspecialist. It is in this first encounter when appropriate evaluation and treatment can prolong the patient's life and minimize eventual disability. In this chapter, the principles and techniques of the early management of the trauma patient will be reviewed.

The American College of Surgeons Committee on Trauma has made great strides in the establishment of standards for the care of the trauma patient. The Committee has been instrumental in the establishment of standardized care in designated trauma centers and the development of the Advanced Trauma Life Support (ATLS) Course for Physicians. The ATLS course is designed to teach physicians lifesaving skills and a standardized approach to trauma care. It is in the best interest of every physician in a position to treat trauma to become certified in ATLS, and many principles outlined in this chapter adhere to these standards.

Triage

Fifty percent of trauma deaths occur before hospitalization. Sixty-two percent of the remaining deaths occur within the first 4 hours of hospitalization (4). Delays in the recognition and transportation of the trauma patient to a facility with the appropriate level of trauma care resources can reduce survival rates.

Triage is the route by which trauma patients with severe and life-threatening injuries can be transported to facilities that have the staff and equipment immediately available to treat these patients in an aggressive and timely fashion. Patients with less severe injuries can be transported to other appropriate facilities, avoiding the expense and burden placed on the patient and the trauma center.

The use of an injury severity score (5) in some form is essential to the consistent estimation of injury. The trauma score, which has found widespread use for trauma triage,

Table 16.1.
Glasgow Coma Scale

Response	Points
Verbal	
Oriented	5
Confused	4
Inappropriate	3
Incomprehensible	2
None	1
Eye opening	
Spontaneous	4
To voice	3
To pain	2
None	1
Motor	
Obeys command	6
Localizes pain	5
Withdraws to pain	4
Flexion to pain	3
Extension to pain	2
None	1

Total Points
14–15   5
11–13   4   GCS
8–10   3   Score
5–7   2
3–4   1

Table 16.2.
Trauma Score

Parameter	Points
Respiratory rate	
≥36/min	2
25–35/min	3
10–24/min	4
0–9/min	1
None	0
Respiratory expansion	
Normal	1
Shallow	0
Retractive	0
Blood pressure (systolic)	
≥90 mm Hg	4
70–90 mm Hg	3
50–69 mm Hg	2
0–49 mm Hg	1
Pulseless	0
Capillary return	
Normal	2
Delayed	1
None	0
Glasgow Coma Scale	
14–15	5
11–13	4
8–10	3
5–7	2
3–4	1
Total	1–16

is an index composed of the Glasgow Coma Score (Table 16.1), cardiac function, and respiratory function (Table 16.2) (6). Patients with trauma scores less than 14 have been shown to benefit from expedient transport to a regional trauma center. The transport of these patients to the nearest hospital wastes precious minutes if the institution is not equipped to handle a particular patient. In a rural setting, where transport time to a trauma facility may exceed 1 hour, transport to the nearest hospital may be indicated. In this case, hospital staff should be notified as to the severity of the injuries so they may begin to mobilize their services appropriately.

In areas where an injury severity scale is not in common use, a patient should be considered a multitrauma patient if: blood pressure is less than 90 mm Hg; there is evidence of respiratory distress or airway compromise; there is penetrating injury to chest, abdomen, head or neck; and, in high-energy injuries, motor vehicle accident at 20 mph or more, fall from greater than 20 feet, etc.

Assessment and Resuscitation ABCs (Airway, Breathing, Circulation)

As in a cardiac arrest, a single physician with the most trauma training (ATLS) or experience should be in charge. An organized response is the best method to avoid missing important injuries or allowing attention to stray toward obvious but not life-threatening injuries (i.e., open fractures) (Fig. 16.1).

AIRWAY

The establishment of an adequate airway is the first priority and must be obtained as the initial step, since adequate ventilation of the patient is impossible without a clear airway. One must assume that the patient has

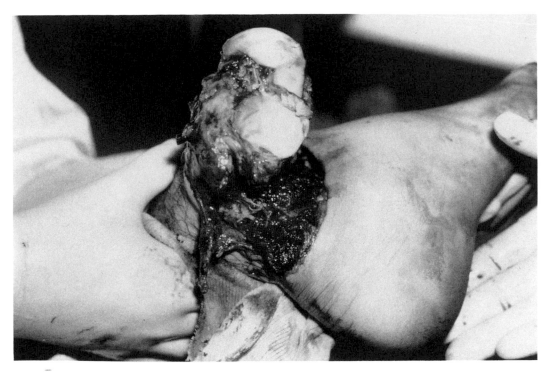

Figure 16.1.   Attention must not be drawn away from the systematic evaluation of the patient by obvious but not life-threatening injuries.

sustained a cervical spine injury until proven otherwise and must take precautions to prevent unprotected manipulation of the neck with possible spinal cord injury. The cervical spine should be secured with "in line" traction, a semirigid cervical collar, or spine board with sandbags and tape.

The oropharynx should be cleared of secretions, loose teeth, and foreign material. The airway may be maintained with the chin lift or jaw thrust maneuver, plastic oral airway, or tracheal intubation via oral or nasal route. The use of an esophageal obturator airway should be avoided when facilities are available for endotracheal intubation, as the obturator airway can result in esophageal damage, is substantially inferior in ventilatory efficiency, and does not protect the airway against nasopharynx bleeding or secretions (7). Endotracheal intubation is the preferable airway in patients needing assistance with ventilation. Intubation will even-

tually be necessary in patients who are unconscious, have maxillofacial injuries, require anesthesia, are otherwise unable to protect their own airway, or need respiratory support. In patients with proven or suspected cervical spine injuries, nasotracheal intubation rather than endotracheal intubation may be necessary.

If the patient cannot be successfully intubated in two attempts, then an airway must be established surgically. Emergency surgical access to the airway may be obtained with either a cricothyroidotomy or a tracheostomy (Fig. 16.2). Tracheostomy is not suited for the emergency situation because it can be time-consuming and is often accompanied by significant bleeding. This procedure is best left for a more controlled and elective environment.

A surgical cricothyroidotomy can be performed in the adult patient (over 12 years old) by making a midline skin incision ex-

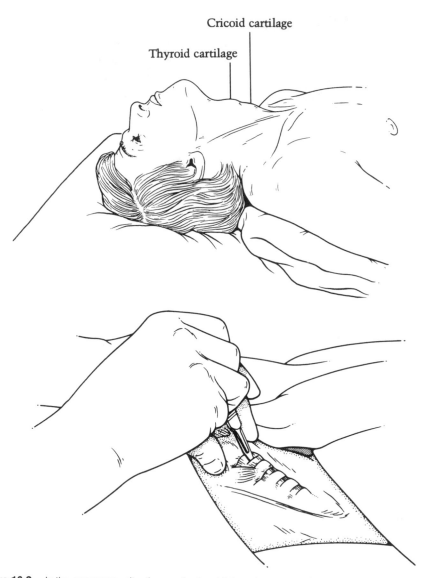

Cricoid cartilage

Thyroid cartilage

Figure 16.2.   In the emergency situation, a cricothyroidotomy has many advantages over a tracheostomy.

tending through the cricothyroid membrane into the trachea. The incision is then dilated and held open with a hemostat while a small-bore (5 to 7 mm) endotracheal tube or tracheostomy tube is inserted into the trachea and secured with tape or ties.

A needle cricothyroidotomy is preferred in patients under 12 years of age. This technique uses a 12- to 14-gauge intravenous cannula which is inserted through the cricothyroid membrane. The adaptor from a 3.5-mm pediatric endotracheal tube fits onto the hub of the cannula and allows connection to a ventilation bag.

Cricothyroidotomy and needle cricothyroidotomy are temporary emergency measures and should be replaced by a surgical tracheostomy or endotracheal intubation.

The needle cricothyroidotomy in particular can only support adequate ventilation for 45 minutes.

BREATHING

Adequate air exchange is achieved when a secure airway is obtained and 12 to 15 ml/kg oxygen-enriched air is delivered to the lungs. If this cannot be achieved, the physician must then quickly identify and correct the problem. The airway should be checked first since the most common reason for failure of ventilation is intubation of the esophagus. Three other common reasons for failure of ventilation are pneumothorax, tension pneumothorax, and flail chest.

Pneumothorax and tension pneumothorax can be managed by the insertion of a chest tube and assisted ventilation. The chest tube is inserted into the pleural space through the fifth intercostal space in the midaxillary line. The chest tube is then connected to 20 to 30 cm water seal suction. A flail chest can be managed with positive pressure, manual ventilation, or volume-cycled ventilator.

The physician should be aware that patient agitation may be a sign of hypoxia or shock. Auscultation of the chest should confirm equal movement of air within each lung.

CIRCULATION

Once satisfactory ventilation has been established, the evaluation and management of hemorrhage should then be addressed. A pulse should be palpable in the carotid or femoral arteries. If a pulse is not palpable, cardiopulmonary resuscitation should then be initiated, accompanied by volume replacement. When a pulse is palpable in the carotid or femoral arteries, the patient's systolic blood pressure is generally greater than 70 mm Hg.

Shock can be defined as inadequate perfusion of body tissues with oxygenated blood. In the setting of multiple trauma, the most likely cause of shock is hypovolemia. Unless other evidence presents itself, one should assume hypovolemia. A patient with pelvic and long bone fractures, abdominal organ injury, or injury to major vessels in the chest or abdomen can rapidly lose a large percentage of his total blood volume from the circulatory system to the third space (8). Since this does not present itself as external hemorrhage, a patient may become acutely hypovolemic without any outward signs of bleeding.

Once a pulse has been established, the physician should perform a brief examination for significant bleeding. Direct pressure should be applied to the bleeding wound. Pneumatic splints or a pneumatic antishock garment may be useful in controlling multiple areas of profuse hemorrhage. Small wounds with little bleeding should be ignored at this point; however, one must be aware that these smaller wounds can become a significant source of blood loss once volume has been replaced and blood pressure is corrected. One should not attempt to blindly ligate or clamp bleeding vessels in the depths of a wound. Bleeding from large vessels can be controlled with direct digital pressure. The use of a tourniquet for bleeding control is usually avoidable.

Two large-bore IV catheters should be started (16-gauge in the adult patient). A subclavian line or a saphenous vein cutdown may be utilized where peripheral venous access is limited. In patients who have penetrating abdominal injuries, one should avoid starting intravenous lines in the lower extremities, as an injury to the inferior vena cava would allow extravasation of infused crystalloid or blood products. At least one large-bore catheter should be started proximal to the region of injury. Once intravenous access has been established, then volume replacement should begin.

Normal circulating blood volume is approximately 7% of ideal body weight in the adult, and 8 to 9% body weight in the child.

The American College of Surgeons has divided hemorrhagic shock into four categories. *Class 1*: where up to 15% of blood volume is lost, and minimal clinical symptoms exist. *Class 2*: where 15 to 30% of blood volume is lost. Clinical symptoms present as tachycardia, tachypnea, decreased pulse pressure, CNS changes and reduced capillary refill. Blood pressure can remain unchanged (8). *Class 3*: where 30 to 40% of blood volume is lost. In addition to a worsening of previous signs, the patient with this amount of blood loss shows a deterioration in systolic blood pressure. *Class 4*: where greater than 40% of blood volume is lost.

One should assume that any trauma patient with cool extremities, flat neck veins, and tachycardia is suffering from hypovolemic shock. The hematocrit will not accurately reflect acute blood loss because this takes up to 6 hours to equilibrate. A fluid challenge should be given to the patient with signs of shock in the form of warmed lactated Ringer's solution. Warming the crystalloid solution will help avoid problems with hypothermia. An initial bolus of 2 liters in the adult or 20 ml/kg in the child should be rapidly administered. The response to the fluid challenge should be noted and a decision made as to the continued administration of crystalloid solutions and blood products. A failure to improve blood pressure, pulse rate, urine output, respiratory rate, and CNS status would be deemed an unfavorable response to the fluid challenge and indicates more severe blood loss and the need for crystalloids and blood products. In general, class 1 or class 2 shock will require crystalloid replacement, while class 3 or 4 will require both crystalloid and blood administration. In class 3 or 4 shock, where replacement cannot keep up with loss, immediate surgical intervention may be necessary to stop the source of bleeding. A continued need for volume replacement in less severe blood loss should alert the physician to an unrecognized source of bleeding. Third-

space (internal) blood loss may collect within the chest, retroperitoneal space, abdomen, or extremity fracture sites (Table 16.3). Chest, pelvic, and extremity radiographs should aid the physician in the diagnosis of these potential third-space losses.

The physician should keep in mind that myocardial infarction may proceed or follow a trauma and result in an alteration of vital signs. Spinal cord injury and head injury may also result in hypotension, yet one should not assume these to be the cause of shock. In cases where there is an immediate need for blood products, type O or type-specific blood may be used; however, these should be utilized only when there is life-threatening shock, and the physician is unable to wait for cross-matched blood products. This problem stresses the need to anticipate blood loss in the trauma setting, and to draw blood for type and cross-match on arrival. Fresh-frozen plasma and platelet transfusions are necessary to avoid coagulopathy in patients who require large amounts of blood products.

Secondary Survey

Once the initial assessment and resuscitation have been completed, a more complete secondary survey should be performed. Medical history should be obtained to include medical problems, allergies, medications, and mechanisms of injury. Much of the history must be obtained from family, witnesses, and emergency personnel on scene.

Table 16.3.
Potential Third-Space Loss of Blood from Circulating Volume with Closed Injuries

Bleeding Site	Potential Blood Loss
Chest	3000 ml/side
Abdomen	Variable
Retroperitoneum	3000 ml
Extremity fracture	1500 ml/femur if closed
	500 ml/humerus or tibia if closed

The patient must be completely examined at this stage. This should include a neurologic examination. This step is imperative, since a change in neurologic status may trigger operative intervention. It is helpful to draw sensory levels or abnormalities in ink directly on the patient as well as recording it in the medical record. The Glasgow Coma Score and trauma score should be recorded at this time.

EMERGENCY DEPARTMENT DIAGNOSTICS

On arrival in the emergency ward, the trauma patient should have diagnostic blood work drawn. This should include a hematocrit, prothrombin time, partial thromboplastin time, arterial blood gas, blood urea nitrogen, blood sugar, electrolytes, and a crossmatch specimen. An extra red top tube of blood drawn at this point and set aside may save time in the long run for later diagnostic testing.

Initial x-ray studies should include a lateral cervical spine, an anteroposterior (AP) chest film, and an AP pelvis. Additional x-ray studies should await stabilization. One must understand that a single negative cervical spine x-ray does not exclude a cervical spine injury, and cervical spine precautions must be maintained. The cervical spine series, including AP, lateral, obliques, and open-mouth odontoid films should be completed prior to discontinuation of cervical spine precautions.

A Foley catheter should be inserted. If there is suspicion of urinary tract damage (certain pelvic fractures, genital or perineal hematoma, meatal blood), a urethrogram and cystogram should be performed prior to insertion of a Foley catheter. Difficulty inserting the Foley catheter can be a sign of urethral tear, and repeated attempts at insertion may worsen the injury. A nasogastric tube should be placed if no contraindications exist. Nasogastric tubes should be avoided with patients suspected of having fractures of the cribriform plate, or penetrating trauma to their esophagus.

A systematic examination of the entire patient should be performed to include head, neck, chest, abdomen, pelvis, and extremities. All bandages and splints not applied by the examiner should be removed, the wounds inspected, and dressings reapplied. Difficult to reach areas such as the back and buttocks must not be ignored during this phase.

Head

Facial bones are palpated for evidence of instability. All wounds are palpated for evidence of open skull and facial fracture. The ear and nasal passages are examined for evidence of cerebrospinal fluid, which is often difficult to detect when mixed with blood. A drop of suspect fluid can be placed onto filter paper, and a "ring sign" will develop as the blood components remain in the center while a clear ring of cerebrospinal fluid forms around it. At this time one should repeat and record any changes in the neurologic examination and Glasgow Coma Score. An increase in intracranial pressure can cause a slowing of the respiratory rate, an elevation in blood pressure, and a change in pulse rate. If any evidence of central nervous system damage is noted, then immediate neurosurgical consultation should be obtained. Decisions for CT scan, steroids, diuretics, and operative intervention should be made by the neurosurgeon. For spinal cord injuries, high-dose steroid administration (such as methylprednisolone) is recommended by many surgeons. More detailed information on the use of steroids may be found in the chapter on spine injuries (Chapter 5).

Neck

The cervical collar should be removed with manual stabilization of the patient's cervical spine to inspect for penetrating neck wounds, subcutaneous emphysema, tracheal deviation, and hematoma, which may signal a vascular injury and endanger the airway. A penetrating neck wound will require surgical exploration. Evidence of trauma above the level of the clavicle should heighten the physician's suspicion of cervical spine injury. The cervical collar and spine precautions should not be discontinued until a full set of cervical spine x-rays are completed. All seven cervical vertebra must be visualized on x-ray. A patient with pain and cervical muscle spasm may have a ligamentous injury not apparent on the cervical spine x-rays. In this case, supervised lateral flexion and extension x-rays are needed to rule out injury, and these may be postponed until the patient is fully stabilized (Fig. 16.3).

Chest

Chest injuries that immediately threaten the airway or breathing, including flail chest, hemothorax, pneumothorax, tension pneumothorax, and cardiac tamponade, should have been treated during the primary survey. The chest should now be reassessed for these injuries. The chest x-ray should be carefully examined for widening of the mediastinum and obscuring of the aortic knob, which may signal a tear of the great vessels. An angiogram should be utilized in suspect patients when hypovolemia does not necessitate immediate surgical intervention. The ECG should be carefully monitored for cardiac arrhythmias resulting from cardiac con-

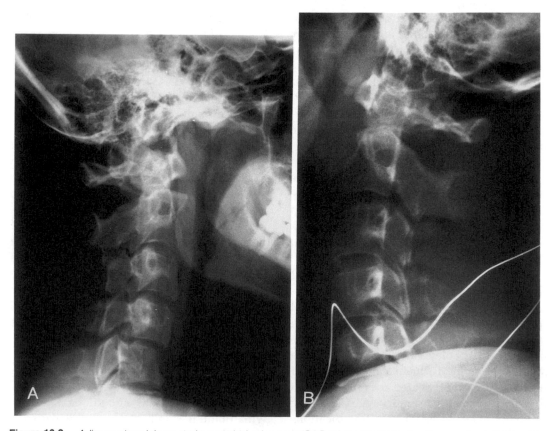

Figure 16.3.   *A,* ligamentous injury noted on cervical spine x-ray (C4-5 subluxation) following *B,* a negative initial film. Ligamentous injury must be suspected in any patient with cervical pain and spasm.

tusions. Although more than 60% of multiple trauma patients sustain some degree of cardiac contusion, only a small percentage will develop a cardiac arrhythmia or decreased cardiac output from this. Cardiac enzymes are not useful in the early evaluation and treatment phase. Pulmonary contusions are also very common. These usually cause more problems at 12 to 24 hours. Late management will include fluid restriction and intubation with volume-cycled ventilation and positive end expiratory pressure.

An elevated hemidiaphragm on chest x-ray, especially on the left, may signal a rupture of the diaphragm with herniation of abdominal organs into the chest cavity. This is a commonly missed injury, and any malposition of the chest tube (such as traversing the diaphragm) or persistent elevation of the hemidiaphragm should be investigated with an abdominal and chest CT scan.

Abdomen

The abdomen is examined for evidence of penetrating trauma. One must assume that the penetrating knife or gunshot wound has penetrated abdominal organs and, quite frequently, the diaphragm and chest organs as well. These injuries will require surgical exploration. Contusions, abrasions, and a mechanism of injury involving deceleration forces cause blunt abdominal trauma. A firm abdomen with either tenderness to palpation or rebound tenderness should be investigated. A rectal examination must be done. In the stable patient, a CT scan may be utilized for the evaluation of blunt abdominal injury; however, even under the best of circumstances a CT scan consumes a great deal of time. Peritoneal lavage may be quickly performed and is beneficial in the evaluation of intraabdominal bleeding, but it is less valuable in the detection of retroperitoneal organ injuries. Peritoneal lavage is a surgical procedure with potential iatrogenic complications and should be performed by the surgeon who will perform the laparotomy. It is difficult to diagnose significant abdominal injury in the unconscious patient or patient with spinal cord injury. Abdominal CT scan and peritoneal lavage are particularly important in these patients.

Pelvis

Tremendous force is necessary to produce pelvic ring fractures or dislocations. This force, often transmitted from the lower extremity through the pelvis and to the spine, may produce damage to the lower extremity, spine, and pelvic contents (Table 16.4). There is a high association between pelvic fractures and genitourinary injury (Fig. 16.4).

Table 16.4.
Commonly Associated Fractures with Similar Mechanism of Injury

Found	Look
Knee	Hip, spine
Wrist	Elbow
Skull	Cervical spine
Calcaneus	Knee, spine

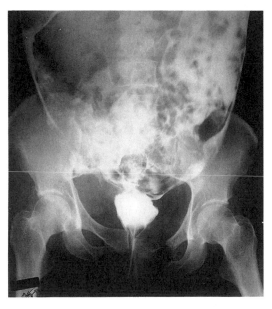

Figure 16.4. Cystogram showing extravasation of contrast into peritoneum with rupture of the bladder.

The pelvis is a well-vascularized structure, and a disruption of its architecture can produce massive hemorrhage, with third-space loss of circulating volume in the retroperitoneum and abdominal cavity. The bony pelvis itself need not fracture to produce this bleeding. A ligamentous injury to the sacroiliac joints or the symphysis pubis will produce similar results. Pelvic instability can often be diagnosed by compression and distraction of the iliac wings noting abnormal movement.

An AP pelvic x-ray will disclose injuries not apparent on examination. Pelvic ring disruptions should alert the physician to expect major blood loss, and fluid replacement should be instituted accordingly. In many cases pelvic bleeding will tamponade and stabilize. If pelvic blood loss continues and the patient manifests signs of hypovolemia, then orthopaedic stabilization of the pelvis with an external fixator is indicated in an unstable pelvic injury. Angiographic identification of the bleeding vessels and embolization or surgical ligation of those vessels may also be required. The use of a pneumatic antishock garment may be of temporary help in this situation. Open pelvic fractures represent an especially difficult problem as there is a loss of the tamponading effect of third-space hematoma. There is also a high infection and mortality rate.

Extremities

Injuries to the extremities are often quite apparent. At times these obvious injuries tend to misdirect the attention of the examiner away from the more life-threatening problems reviewed earlier. An extremity injury can be a threat to life, however, usually because of an associated vascular injury. Fortunately, even profuse bleeding from a vascular injury can usually be controlled by direct pressure. The use of a tourniquet should be avoided and used only as a life-saving measure when all other methods have failed because its use may sacrifice the limb. A closed fracture of a long bone may produce a hematoma containing 2 to 3 units of blood and contribute to hypovolemic shock.

Although limb injuries are rarely life-threatening, they are often limb-threatening. Limb-threatening injuries include dislocations of the elbow, knee, and hip, with or without immediate vascular compromise, open fractures, crush-type injuries, and fractures with circulatory compromise.

All splints and dressings should be removed, limbs inspected, and dressings reapplied. All joints and long bones should be palpated for swelling, tenderness, deformity, and crepitation. If these signs are present, range of motion examination should not be performed prior to x-ray to rule out fracture or dislocation. If these signs are absent, the joints may be placed through a range of motion looking for tenderness and crepitation. The joints are also gently stressed to detect instability.

A thorough assessment of vascular and neurologic function is performed for all four limbs. X-rays are obtained of all limbs where fracture or dislocation is suspected and these extremities must be splinted. It is important to record the neurovascular examination because the deterioration might signal the development of a compartment syndrome or subsequent vascular insufficiency. The presence of palpable pulses does not rule out all vascular injuries. Prompt orthopaedic consultation should be obtained for injuries to the extremities. Patients with open fractures should be started on broad-spectrum antibiotics and their tetanus status established. Dislocations of major joints will require immediate reduction, and open fractures will require debridement and stabilization by the orthopaedic surgeon.

Definitive Care

Following the primary and secondary survey and the evaluation and control of the emergency situation, a definitive care plan should be developed. The more urgent problems will take priority over the less urgent. The definitive care plan may include immediate surgical intervention, additional x-ray, CT scan, and angiographic evaluation or transfer to another facility where needed specialized care can be administered. This is the time for reassessment and monitoring of the patient for early changes and complications.

REFERENCES

1. Advance report of final mortality statistics, 1980. Hyattsville, MD: National Center for Health Statistics, 1983; USDHHS publication (PHS)83-1120. (Monthly vital statistics; report 32(Suppl 4):1–40.)
2. Hartunian NS, Smart CN, Thompson MS. The incidence and economic costs of cancer, motor vehicle injuries, coronary heart disease, and stroke: a comparative analysis. Am J Public Health 1980;70:1249–1260.
3. National Highway Traffic Safety Administration. The economic cost to society of motor vehicle accidents. Washington, DC: U.S. Department of Transportation, January 1983; Technical Report DOT HS-806-342.
4. American College of Surgeons Committee on Trauma. Multiple trauma outcome study, 1966.
5. Baker SP, O'Neill B, Haddon W Jr, et al. The injury severity score: a method for describing patients with multiple injuries and evaluating emergency care. J Trauma 1974;14:187–196.
6. Morris JA Jr, Auerbach PS, Marshall GA, Bluth RF, Johnson LG, Trunkey DD. The trauma score as a triage tool in the prehospital setting. JAMA 1986;256:1319–1325.
7. Blaisdell FW. Trauma myths and magic: 1984 Fitts lecture. J Trauma 1985;25:856–863.
8. O'Donnell TF Jr, Belkin SC. The pathophysiology, monitoring, and treatment of shock. Orthop Clin North Am 1978;9:589–610.

SUGGESTED READINGS

Amato JJ, Rheinlander HF, Cleveland RJ. Post-traumatic adult respiratory distress syndrome. Orthop Clin North Am 1978;9:693–713.

Baker SP, Whitfield RA, O'Neill B. Geographic variations in mortality from motor vehicle crashes. N Engl J Med 1987;317:1601–1602.

Baker SP, O'Neill B, Karpf RS. The injury fact book. Lexington, MA: Lexington Books, 1984.

Baker SP, O'Neill B, Haddon W Jr, et al. The injury severity score: a method for describing patients with multiple injuries and evaluating emergency care. J Trauma 1974;14:187–196.

Dabezies EJ, D'Ambrosia RD. Treatment of the multiply injured patient: plans for treatment and problems of major trauma. Instr Course Lect 1984;33:242–252.

Levy PS, Goldberg J, Hui S, et al. Severity measurement in multiple trauma by use of ICDA conditions. Stat Med 1982;1:145–152.

Lowe DK. Management of multiple trauma. Surg Rounds 1989;3:75–84.

Morris JA Jr, Auerbach PS, Marshall GA, et al. The trauma score as a triage tool in the prehospital setting. JAMA 1886;256:1319–1325.

Murat JE, Huten N, Mesny J. The use of standardized assessment procedures in the evaluation of patients with multiple injuries. Arch Emerg Med 1985;2:11–15.

O'Donnell TF Jr, Belkin SC. The pathophysiology, monitoring, and treatment of shock. Orthop Clin North Am 1978;9:589–610.

Index

Page numbers in italics indicate individual pp or page ranges in which figures appear.